HIV Protocols

METHODS IN MOLECULAR MEDICINE™

John M. Walker, SERIES EDITOR

METHODS IN MOLECULAR MEDICINE™

HIV Protocols

Edited by

Nelson L. Michael, MD, PhD

Walter Reed Army Institute of Research, Rockville, MD

and

Jerome H. Kim, MD

Henry M. Jackson Foundation, Rockville, MD

Humana Press ✻ Totowa, New Jersey

Cover illustration: Taken from *The Sourcebook of Medical Illustrations*, edited by Peter Cull. Copyright 1989 by the Medical College of St. Bartholomew's Hospital, London, UK. Published in the United States by The Parthenon Publishing Group, Inc., Park Ridge, NJ.

Cover design by Patricia F. Cleary.

For additional copies, pricing for bulk purchases, and/or information about other Humana titles, contact Humana at the above address or at any of the following numbers: Tel: 973-256-1699; Fax: 973-256-8341; E-mail: humana@humanapr.com or visit our website at http://www.humanapress.com

Printed in the United States of America. 10 9 8 7 6 5 4 3 2 1

Library of Congress Cataloging in Publication Data

Main entry under title:

Methods in molecular medicine™.

HIV protocols / edited by Nelson Michael and Jerome H. Kim.
       p.   cm.—(Methods in molecular medicine ; vol. 17)
    Includes index.
    ISBN 0-89603-369-4 (alk. paper)
    1. AIDS (Disease)—Laboratory manuals. 2. HIV (Viruses)—Laboratory manuals. 3. HIV infections—Laboratory manuals. I. Michael, Nelson. II. Kim Jerome H. III. Series.
    [DNLM: 1. HIV Infections—prevention & control. 2. Clinical Protocols. 3. Molecular Biology—methods. 4. Immunologic Techniques. 5. Virology—methods. WC 503.6H6765 1998]
    QR201.A37H56   1998
    616.97'92—dc21
    DNLM/DLC   98-27244
    for Library of Congress   CIP

Preface

The worldwide impact of infection with human immunodeficiency virus type 1 (HIV-1) is reflected in the cumulative number of HIV-1 infections, which is now predicted to exceed 40 million by the year 2000—equivalent to the number of humans who perished in World War II. The medical and scientific response to the HIV-1 pandemic has steadily grown since its recognition in 1981. The outlay by the United States alone for HIV research funded by the National Institutes of Health in 1997 was $1.4 billion. Laboratory-based HIV research has brought together academic clinicians, retrovirologists, molecular biologists, and immunologists in the formation of research teams attempting to dissect the viral and host factors contributing to disease pathogenesis. Increasing focus is being placed on those aspects of viral biology and host immune responses that bear on the development of vaccines to prevent HIV infection.

HIV Protocols reflects the state of HIV research in several ways. First, chapters are organized into four sections: Virology, Molecular Biology, Humoral Immunology, and Cellular Immunology. This organization is a natural consequence of the diverse scientific disciplines that have been attracted to HIV research. Second, the chapters reflect such diverse research directions as viral coreceptor usage, quantitation of viral genomes, HIV promoter function, B-cell epitope mapping, and measurements of T-cell function, each of which bears on the goal of understanding the viral and host immune responses that will be critical to the design of effective preventive vaccines. Third, *HIV Protocols* includes several chapters on the analysis of HIV-1 entry coreceptors only about two years after the first of these receptors was discovered, which is indicative of the explosion of research on these molecules.

All chapters in *HIV Protocols* open with an introduction to both a specific technique and its role in the field of HIV research. Following a thorough list of materials, a highly detailed methods section presents the technique in a clear, understandable fashion to ensure the sucessful execution of the protocol. This is followed by a Notes section that we believe many readers will perceive to be the core of these chapters. The Notes essentially go beyond the standard protocol to unlock the specifics or "tricks" inherent in the sucessful execution of the technique. A brief series of references rounds off each chapter.

Thanks are due to all of the contributing authors for the efforts each of them made in writing both highly detailed and understandable chapters. The guidance, and forbearance, of Professor John M. Walker, editor of *Methods in Molecular Medicine* series, and Mr. Thomas Lanigan, President of Humana Press, were also instrumental in bringing *HIV Protocols* to fruition.

Nelson L. Michael
Jerome H. Kim

Contents

Contributors

MAUREEN V. ABBEY • *Division of Infectious Diseases, Thomas Jefferson University, Philadelphia, PA*

MOHAMMAD AMJAD • *Division of Infectious Diseases, Thomas Jefferson University, Philadelphia, PA*

ANDREW W. ARTENSTEIN • *Division of Retrovirology, Walter Reed Army Institute of Research, Rockville, MD*

OMAR BAGASRA • *Division of Infectious Diseases, Thomas Jefferson University, Philadelphia, PA*

SANDRA C. BARRICK • *Henry M. Jackson Foundation, Rockville, MD*

DEBORAH L. BIRX • *Division of Retrovirology, Walter Reed Army Institute of Research, Rockville, MD*

PATRICK J. BLAIR • *Immune Cell Biology Program, Naval Medical Research Institute, Bethesda, MD*

LISA E. BOBROSKI • *Division of Infectious Diseases, Thomas Jefferson University, Philadelphia, PA*

D. WILLIAM CAMERON • *Department of Laboratory Medicine, Children's Hospital of Eastern Ontario, Ottawa, Ontario, Canada*

MARY CARRINGTON • *NCI-FCRDC, Frederick, MD*

RICHARD G. CARROLL • *Henry M. Jackson Foundation, Rockville, MD*

SHARON A. CASSOL • *Ottawa General Hospital Research Institute, Ottawa, Ontario, Canada*

BENJAMIN CHEN • *Aaron Diamond AIDS Research Center, New York, NY*

JOSEPHINE H. COX • *Henry M. Jackson Foundation, Rockville, MD*

FRANCISCO DIAZ-MITOMA • *Department of Microbiology and Immunology, University of Ottawa, Ottawa, Canada*

ROBERT W. DOMS • *Department of Pathology and Laboratory Medicine, University of Pennsylvania, Philadelphia, PA*

WEI DONG • *Department of Microbiology and Immunology, University of Maryland School of Medicine, Baltimore, MD*

AIMEE L. EDINGER • *Department of Pathology and Laboratory Medicine, University of Pennsylvania, Philadelphia, PA*

Bruce L. Gilliam • *Henry M. Jackson Foundation, Rockville, MD*

Paul L. Hallberg • *Henry M. Jackson Foundation, Rockville, MD*

Sook-Jin Hur • *Department of Microbiology and Immunology, Thomas Jefferson University, Philadelphia, PA*

Michelle Janes • *Ottawa General Hospital Research Institute, Ottawa, Ontario, Canada*

Robert Kaminski • *Henry M. Jackson Foundation, Rockville, MD*

Sumesh Kaushal • *Naval Medical Research Institute, Bethesda, MD*

Jerome H. Kim • *Henry M. Jackson Foundation, Rockville, MD*

Melissa Krider • *Henry M. Jackson Foundation, Rockville, MD*

Derhsing Lai • *Department of Microbiology and Immunology, Thomas Jefferson University, Philadelphia, PA*

Nathaniel R. Landau • *Aaron Diamond AIDS Research Center, New York, NY*

James R. Lane • *SRA Technologies, Inc., Rockville, MD*

Barbara Leung • *Saint Paul's Hospital, Vancouver, British Columbia, Canada*

Yen Li • *Department of Microbiology and Immunology, University of Maryland School of Medicine, Baltimore, MD*

Jen-Tsun J. Lin • *Henry M. Jackson Foundation, Rockville, MD*

Rong Liu • *Aaron Diamond AIDS Research Center, New York, NY*

Lawrence D. Loomis-Price • *Henry M. Jackson Foundation, Rockville, MD*

Mark K. Louder • *Henry M. Jackson Foundation, Rockville, MD*

David M. Margolis • *Institute of Human Virology, Medical Biotechnology Center, University of Maryland, Baltimore, MD*

Maureen P. Martin • *NCI-Frederick Cancer Research and Development Center, Frederick, MD*

John R. Mascola • *Division of Retrovirology, Walter Reed Army Institute of Research, Rockville, MD*

Gilbert McCrary • *Division of Retrovirology, Walter Reed Army Institute of Research, Rockville, MD*

Richard A. McDonald • *Division of Retrovirology, Walter Reed Army Institute of Research, Rockville, MD*

Mathew Memoli • *Division of Infectious Diseases, Thomas Jefferson University, Philadelphia, PA*

Nelson L. Michael • *Division of Retrovirology, Walter Reed Army Institute of Research, Rockville, MD*

Margaret M. Mitchell • *Henry M. Jackson Foundation, Rockville, MD*

Theresa Mo • *Saint Paul's Hospital, Vancouver, British Columbia, Canada*

Martin Nau • *Henry M. Jackson Foundation, Rockville, MD*

STEPHEN P. PERFETTO • *Henry M. Jackson Foundation, Rockville, MD*

RICHARD PILON • *Ottawa General Hospital Research Institute, Ottawa, Ontario, Canada*

SILVIA RATTO-KIM • *Henry M. Jackson Foundation, Rockville, MD*

STANLEY READ • *Department of Pediatrics, Hospital for Sick Children, Toronto, Ontario, Canada*

JAMES L. RILEY • *Walter Reed Army Institute of Research, Rockville, MD*

FABIO ROMERIO • *Institute of Human Virology, Medical Biotechnology Center, University of Maryland, Baltimore, MD*

ANINDITA ROY • *Department of Microbiology and Immunology, University of Maryland School of Medicine, Baltimore, MD*

MIKA SALMINEN • *Department of Chronic Virus Diseases, National Public Health Institute, Helsinki, Finland*

PAOLA SECCHIERO • *Institute of Human Virology, Medical Biotechnology Center, University of Maryland, Baltimore, MD*

KARL V. SITZ • *Division of Retrovirology, Walter Reed Army Institute of Research, Rockville, MD*

CHRISTOPHER A. D. SMITH • *Division of Retrovirology, Walter Reed Army Institute of Research, Rockville, MD*

LORETTA TSE • *Henry M. Jackson Foundation, Rockville, MD*

MARYANNE VAHEY • *Division of Retrovirology, Walter Reed Army Institute of Research, Rockville, MD*

JOHN L. VANCOTT • *Immunology Vaccine Center, The University of Alabama at Birmingham, Birmingham, AL*

THOMAS C. VANCOTT • *Henry M. Jackson Foundation, Rockville, MD*

FREDERIK W. VAN GINKEL • *Immunology Vaccine Center, The University of Alabama at Birmingham, Birmingham, AL*

BRUCE G. WENIGER • *Division of HIV/AIDS, Centers for Disease Control and Prevention, Atlanta, GA*

DAVIDE ZELLA • *Institute of Human Virology, Medical Biotechnology Center, University of Maryland, Baltimore, MD*

I

VIROLOGY

1

Isolation and Expansion of HIV from Cells and Body Fluids by Coculture

James R. Lane

1. Introduction

HIV can be recovered from infected patients at all stages of the disease spectrum. Typically, the quantity of biologically active virus, or viral protein, in body tissues is below the level of direct detection by either antigen capture or reverse transcriptase assays. Consequently, the virus must be expanded in culture. This may be achieved by the cocultivation of patient material with mitogen-stimulated peripheral blood mononuclear cells (PBMCs) from normal, healthy donors. These cocultures are then maintained by regularly scheduled interleukin-2 (IL-2) supplemented medium replacement, and the periodic addition of freshly stimulated normal donor PBMCs. During this cocultivation period, culture fluids are harvested at regular intervals and tested for the presence and subsequent replication of HIV. Cultures failing to demonstrate evidence of virus expression within 35 d are usually terminated.

It is well recognized that the efficiency of virus isolation is dependent on specimen type. Patient PBMCs represent a useful source of patient virus, however, isolates can be obtained from such body fluids as spinal fluid or milk. In addition, disease state also influences the isolation of virus. Isolation rates reported for patients with AIDS are consistently higher than from pre-AIDS patients. Using the Walter Reed classification system, Burke et al. *(1)* demonstrated virus isolation rate increases with CD4 cell depletion and impaired delayed hypersensitivity. Furthermore, these authors also noted that the time required for virus isolation decreased with disease progression.

To minimize genetic drift (selection) during the periods of virus isolation, it is critical that these procedures be completed as quickly as possible. This pro-

From: *Methods in Molecular Medicine, Vol. 17: HIV Protocols*
Edited by: N. L. Michael and J. H. Kim © Humana Press Inc., Totowa, NJ

cess is facilitated by utilizing target PBMCs from donors prescreened for efficient virus isolation and expansion. In the author's laboratory, PBMCs from these selected donors are routinely cryopreserved and reserved specifically for studies. This practice of standardizing assay coculture conditions not only minimizes experimental variation but also limits the opportunity for genetic drift of viruses during prolonged expansion periods and the use of PBMCs from multiple donors. The establishment and culturing procedure for isolating and expanding HIV-1 from a variety of patient specimen types is described below. Although virus isolation and expansion can also be performed using continuous cell lines, the focus of this chapter will be with the use of PBMCs.

2. Materials

2.1. Donor PBMC

Normal donor buffy coats (leukocyte-enriched whole blood, from an HIV negative donor), also known as leukopacks, may be obtained from a blood bank or donor service for processing within 12 h of collection. The donors should be screened by the standard assays currently required by the Food and Drug Administration (FDA) and the American Association of Blood Banks (AABB). To obtain the PBMCs from the leukopacks, follow the same procedure described for patient whole blood samples (**Subheading 3.1.**)

2.2. Continuous Cell Lines

There are numerous cell lines available through the AIDS Research and Reference Reagent Program (Division of AIDS, NIAID, NIH) suitable for HIV-infection and expansion of virus. In this work, H9 cells are used as an example.

2.2. Reagents

1. RPMI 1640 (Gibco [Gaithersburg, MD] or equivalent).
2. Fetal bovine serum (FBS) (Gibco or equivalent) (heat inactivated, 56°C, 30 min).
3. Pen-Strep (Gibco or equivalent): Concentration = 10,000 U Pen and 10 mg strep/mL.
4. Ficoll-Paque (Pharmacia or equivalent).
5. Trypan blue: 0.4% (Gibco or equivalent).
6. PHA (Murex cat #HA17 or equivalent, 10 mg lyophylized powder).
7. L-Glutamine (200 mM) (Gibco or equivalent).
8. IL-2 (Boehringer-Mannheim [Indianapolis, IN] cat# 663-581, or equivalent): 200 U/mL.
9. Polybrene (Sigma [St. Louis, MO] or equivalent).
10. DMSO (Sigma or equivalent).

2.3. Reagent Preparation

1. Ficoll wash medium: RPMI 1640, 2% FBS, 1% Pen-strep. Filter sterilize using a 0.2-μ filtration unit. Store at 4°C ± 2°C. Discard after 2 wk.

2. Complete medium: RPMI 1640, 15% FBS, 10% IL-2,1% Pen-strip, 2 m*M* L-Glutamine. Filter sterilize using 0.2-μ unit. Store at 4°C ± 2°C. Discard after 2 wk.
3. PHA stock solution: Reconstitute PHA (10 mg bottle) with 10 mL RPMI 1640. Filter sterilize using syringe filter. Final concentration is 1000 μg/mL. Aliquot 0.3–0.5 mL into cryovials. Store at –20°C ± 5°C. Discard after 1 yr.
4. Polybrene stock solution (0.5 mg/mL): Dissolve 100 mg of polybrene into 200 mL RPMI 1640, filter sterilize using a 0.2-μ filtration unit. Store at 4°C ± 2°C. Aliquots are stable for 1 yr.
5. Coculture medium: RPMI-1640, 15% FBS, 10% IL-2, 1% Pen-strip, 2 m*M* L-Glutamine, 2 μg/mL polybrene. Store at 4°C ± 2°C. Discard after 2 wk.
6. H9 medium: RPMI-1640, 15% FBS, 1% Pen-strip, 2 m*M* L-Glutamine, 2 μg/mL polybrene. Store at 4°C ± 2°C. Discard after 2 wk.

3. Methods
3.1. Isolation of PBMC from Whole Blood

1. In a biological safety cabinet (BSC), dilute one part of fresh whole blood sample with two parts Ficoll wash medium in a 50-mL centrifuge tube (CT) (*see* **Notes 1** and **2**). For example, 10 mL of whole blood would be added to 20 mL of wash media. Mix gently by pipeting slowly up and down three to four times.
2. Transfer no more than 30 mL of diluted blood into a 50-mL CT. Slowly layer 10 mL of Ficoll solution underneath the diluted blood mixture by placing the tip of a 10-mL pipet containing the Ficoll at the bottom of the CT (*see* **Note 3**).
3. Securely replace cap on the 50-ml CT. Centrifuge for 30–35 min at 400–440*g* with no brake at room temperature.
4. In a BSC, using a 5- or 10-mL pipet, remove the top layer (i.e., diluted plasma and most platelets) to just above the "buffy coat" and discard. Using a different 5-mL pipet each time, collect the "buffy coat" cells from each gradient tube and transfer to a 50-mL CT. "Buffy coats" from two gradients may be pooled into one 50-mL CT provided they are from the same patient or leukopack.
5. Add wash medium equaling 2–3 times the vol of the "buffy coat" layer. Centrifuge for 15–20 min at 220–240*g* at room temperature.
6. Decant supernatant, and resuspend cell pellet with 20 mL of wash medium. Remove the appropriate amount of cell suspension to perform a cell count using either a hemocytometer or an electronic counting device.
7. Take 0.1 mL of the cell suspension, and mix with 0.1 mL of 0.4% trypan blue (*see* **Note 4**). Allow dilution to incubate 3–5 min at room temperature (*see* **Note 5**).
8. Apply 0.025 mL of the trypan blue/cell mixture to a hemacytometer. This volume will ensure that the hemocytometer is not overfilled. Remove hemocytometer from the BSC and place it on the stage of a binocular microscope and focus on the cells.
9. Count the unstained (viable) and stained (nonviable) cells separately in the hemocytometer. Count to a total of 100 cells.
10. Calculate the percentage of viable cells as follows:

$$\text{viable cells } (\%) = \frac{\text{total number of viable cells counted} \times 100}{\text{total number of cells counted}}$$

11. Based on the cell count/mL obtained in **step 6**, multiply the number by the % viability. For example, if a cell count of 3×10^6/mL was obtained and the viability is 73.3%, the actual cells available equals 2.2×10^6 ($3 \times 0.733 = 2.2$).

12. Determine the amount of cells needed for the protocol of interest. For example, in the virus isolation protocol (**Subheading 3.3**), 3.3×10^6 cells are required. Divide cells needed in the particular protocol by the number of viable cells/mL to obtain the amount in mL of cell suspension required. In the example used here, this would be 3.3×10^6 cells required divided by 2.2×10^6 viable cells/mL. As a result, 1.5 mL of the cell suspension prepared above is needed in this particular example.

13. Remove volume (in the example cited it would be 1.5 mL) and place in a 15-mL conical centrifuge tube.

14. Centrifuge for 10–15 min, at room temperature, 220–$240g$. Decant supernatant. The cell pellet is now ready for use in the protocol of interest.

3.2. PHA Stimulation of Normal Donor PBMC

1. Obtain enough donor cells (prepared as described in **Subheading 3.1.**) for the appropriate protocol. As an example, assume that 60×10^6 cells will be PHA stimulated.

2. Transfer the cells into a single 15-mL CT containing 10 mL of wash media.

3. Centrifuge at 220–$240g$ for 10–15 min at room temperature. Decant the supernatant and discard.

4. Gently resuspend cell pellet in 8.0 mL complete medium, by slowly drawing cells up and down in a 10 mL pipet, transfer the cell suspension into a T-75 flask.

5. The T-75 flask now contains approx 60×10^6 cells in 8.0 mL complete medium. Add 40 µL of stock PHA to each flask.

6. Incubate at $37°C \pm 2°C$ for 15–30 min. Stand flask upright. After incubation, add 12 mL complete medium to each flask. Incubate in upright position for 18–24 h in a CO_2 incubator (5% CO_2 and 95% humidity) at $37°C \pm 2°C$.

7. After 18–24 h incubation, proceed as follows:
   a. Transfer the cell suspension from each flask into a 50-mL conical CT. Centrifuge at 220–$240g$ for 10–15 min at room temperature.
   b. Decant supernatant and discard. Resuspend each cell pellet in 10 mL of complete medium and divide equally into two new T-75 flasks (1:2 split) or one new and reuse old/original flask.
   c. Add 25 mL of fresh complete medium to each flask. Incubate in an upright position in a CO_2 incubator (5% CO_2 and 95% humidity) at $37°C \pm 2°C$ for an additional 48–72 h.

8. Cells are now ready for use in the appropriate protocol.

3.3 Virus Isolation from PBMC by Tube Coculture

1. A total of 3.3×10^6 patient PBMCs in 30 µL of coculture medium is needed for this assay. On setup day for cocultures, a total of 4×10^6 PHA-stimulated PBMCs

is needed for each patient sample tested. At d 3/4 and at d 7 intervals (i.e., d 7, 14, 21, and 28), an additional 4×10^6 PHA-stimulated PBMCs will be needed.

2. Gently resuspend the cell suspension containing 3.3×10^6 patient PBMCs with an additional 300 µL of coculture medium by pipeting slowly up and down 3–4 times using a digital pipetor and 200–1000-µL pipet tip. Total volume should now equal approx 330 µL. Add 300 µL of this patient PBMC suspension to one coculture tube labeled "A1". Add the remaining 30 µL of patient PBMC suspension to one coculture tube labeled "A2". To this latter tube ("A2"), add 270 µL of coculture medium.

3. Add 2×10^6 PHA-stimulated PBMCs in 200 µL of coculture medium to each coculture tube.

4. Incubate cocultures at 37°C ± 2°C, 5% CO_2, and 95% humidity for 30–40 min.

5. Add 2.0 mL coculture medium to each coculture tube. Gently mix cell suspension by pipeting up and down slowly 2–3 times.

6. Incubate at 37°C ± 2°C, 5% CO_2, and 95% humidity.

7. On d 3 or 4, gently remove 2.0 mL of culture supernatant without disrupting the cell pellet and discard. Add 2.0 mL of coculture medium containing 2×10^6 PHA-stimulated PBMCs to each culture tube.

8. On d 7, 14, 21, 28, and 35, remove 2.0 mL of culture supernatant without disrupting the cell pellet. Reserve 700–1000 µL of supernatant for HIV p24 assay. Discard remaining supernatant (*see* **Note 6**).

9. On d 7, 14, 21, 28, and 35, add 2×10^6 PHA-stimulated PBMCs in 2.0 mL of coculture media.

10. On d 10, 17, 24, and 31, remove 2.0 mL of culture supernatant without disrupting the cell pellet and discard. Add back 2.0 mL of coculture medium.

11. Terminate negative cocultures after obtaining p24 results of d 35 culture supernatants.

3.4. Patient Spinal Fluid (CSF) Isolation Procedures

1. Centrifuge tube containing CSF at 900*g* for 15 min.

2. Carefully remove the CSF supernatant from the tube and transfer to another tube. Do not disturb the cell pellet.

3. Resuspend the cell pellet using 200 µL of CSF supernatant removed in **step 2**. Transfer resuspension to a culture tube. Add 0.2 mL PHA stimulated normal donor PBMCs (2×10^6) and mix gently. Incubate at 37°C for 15 min, then add coculture medium for a final vol of 2.5 mL. Incubate at 37°C, feed, and sample as described in **Subheading 3.3.**

4. Save tissue culture fluids from cocultures collected at weekly intervals (d 7, 14, etc.) for subsequent p24 antigen capture ELISA. Maintain culture vol at 2.5 mL.

3.5 Patient Milk Isolation Procedures

The procedure for processing milk samples and establishing cocultures for virus (HIV) isolation involves using both the cellular and liquid portions of the milk. To increase success in isolating virus a total of six tube cultures are set up for each specimen: A1, A2, and A3 from milk suspension and C1, C2, and C3 from milk cells.

1. Culture of milk suspension
   a. Mix milk suspension gently, remove 430 μL milk to set up A1, A2, and A3 tube cultures. Save the remaining suspension for Part B. Set up cultures as follows: Transfer 300 μL milk into a culture tube labeled A1. Then transfer 100 μL milk into a culture tube (A2) + 200 μL coculture medium. Finally, transfer 30 μL milk into a culture tube (A3) + 270 μL coculture medium.
   b. To each culture tube, add 2×10^6 (200 μL) PHA-stimulated normal PBMCs, Incubate at 37°C for 30 min.
   c. After incubation, add 2.0 mL coculture medium to each tube culture and continue incubation. Feed (replace medium) and add fresh PBMCs cells as described (*see* **Subheading 3.3.**).
   e. Save tissue coculture fluids collected weekly (day 7, 14, etc.) for subsequent p24 antigen capture ELISA. Maintain culture vol at 2.5 mL.

2. Culture of milk cells:
   a. Centrifuge remaining milk at 400*g* for 15 min. Label three culture tubes C1, C2, and C3.
   b. Carefully remove milk supernatant without disturbing cell pellet.
   c. Resuspend cell pellet in 333 μL of coculture medium; then set-up cultures as follows: C1 contains a 300 μL cell suspension, C2 contains a 30 μL cell suspension + 270 μL coculture medium, and C3 contains 3 μL cell suspension + 295 μL coculture medium.
   d. To each culture, add 2×10^6 (in 200 μL) PHA-stimulated normal PBMCs, and incubate 37°C for 30 min.
   e. After incubation, add coculture medium for a final vol of 2.5 mL in each culture tube, and continue incubation. Feed (replace medium) and add PBMCs as described (*see* **Subheading 3.3**).
   f. Save tissue coculture fluids collected weekly (day 7, 14, etc.) for subsequent p24 antigen capture ELISA. Maintain culture vol at 2.5 mL.

3.6. Expansion of HIV Isolated by Tube Culture

1. Begin expansion when tube cultures demonstrate positivity.
2. Gently mix by pipeting up and down 3–4 times. Remove 1.25 mL, and place into a new coculture tube labeled "a1" or "a2" as appropriate to indicate expansion from the original A1 or A2 tube.
3. Add 2×10^6 PHA-stimulated PBMCs in 0.2 mL of coculture medium to each of the tubes. Then add 1.25 mL of coculture medium to each of tubes.
4. Incubate at 37°C ± 2°C, 5% CO_2, and 95% humidity.
5. Four days after initiating expansion, remove 2.0 mL of culture supernatant from the tubes without disrupting the cell pellet. Reserve some of the supernatant for p24 testing. Add 2.0 mL of the coculture media back into each tube. Incubate at 37°C ± 2°C, 5% CO_2, and 95% humidity.

6. Seven days after initiating expansion, remove 2.0 mL of culture supernatant from the tubes without disrupting the cell pellet. Reserve some of the supernatant for p24 testing (*see* **Note 6**). Add 2×10^6 PHA-stimulated PBMCs in 0.2 mL of coculture medium. Then add 2.0 mL of coculture medium. Incubate at 37°C ± 2°C, 5% CO_2, and 95% humidity.
7. Continue replacing media and adding cells every 3–4 d until positive cultures have been reestablished. When the culture has been determined to be positive, remove 2.0 mL of supernatant. Add 2×10^6 PHA stimulated PBMCs in 0.2 mL of coculture medium. Then add 2.0 mL of coculture medium. Incubate at 37°C ± 2°C, 5% CO_2, and 95% humidity for 3–4 more days.
8. Resuspend cell culture, and pool all tubes from a particular patient into a 15-mL centrifuge tube.
9. Centrifuge at 300–340g for 15–20 min at 4°C ± 2°C.
10. Remove supernatant and place into cryovials for storage.
11. If desired, resuspend cell pellet in complete media with 10% DMSO and aliquot into cryovials for storage.
12. Place all cryovials into a liquid nitrogen storage tank.

3.7. HIV Infection of Continuous Cells

1. H9 cells are cultured in H9 medium and incubated at 37°C ±2°C, 5% CO_2, and 95% humidity until ready for use (*see* **Note 7**).
2. Obtain 3×10^6 H9 cells and prepare as a cell pellet in a 15-mL centrifuge tube. Carefully remove the H9 medium without disturbing the cell pellet.
3. Resuspend the cells in 0.5–1 mL of virus supernatant and incubate at 37°C for 30 min. During this incubation, gently shake the centrifuge tube every 10 min to resuspend the cells.
4. Centrifuge cell suspension at 220–240g for 10–15 min at room temperature. Remove the supernatant and discard.
5. Add 2.5 mL H9 medium to the tube. Gently mix cell suspension by pipeting up and down slowly 2–3 times. Transfer cell suspension to a coculture tube.
6. Incubate at 37°C ± 2°C, 5% CO_2, and 95% humidity.
7. On d 3 or 4, gently remove 2.0 mL of culture supernatant and reserve 700–1000 μL for HIV p24 assay. Add 2.0 mL of H9 medium containing 2×10^6 H9 cells.
8. Repeat **step 7** until positive culture obtained (*see* **Note 8**).

Notes

1. All solutions and equipment coming into contact with cells must be sterile, and proper sterile technique must be used accordingly. All medium and Ficoll-Paque are to be used at room temperature. When handling patient samples or viral cultures, all work must be performed in a BSC.
2. Specimen required is a whole blood sample in anticoagulant. A minimum amount of blood that will yield 3.3×10^6 PBMCs is required. For most subjects, 7–10 mL of blood is sufficient. The blood should be processed in the laboratory within 24 h of draw. Samples showing hemolysis are not acceptable.

3. To maintain the Ficoll–blood interface, it is helpful to hold the CT at a 45° angle.

4. Trypan blue is one of several stains recommended for use in dye exclusion procedures for viable cell counting. This method is based on the principle that live (viable) cells do not take up certain dyes, whereas dead (nonviable) cells do.

5. Cells should be counted within 3–15 min of mixing with trypan blue, since longer incubation periods will lead to cell death and reduced viability counts.

6. A successful virus isolation has occurred when two consecutive cultures are positive for the presence of p24.

7. For successful infection, H9 cells should be in logarithmic growth and be highly viable.

8. If large volumes of virus are desired, transfer the cell suspension to a T-25 flask and maintain the culture at a H9 cell concentration of 2×10^6 cells/mL.

References

1. Burke, D. S, Fowler, A.K., Redfield, R.R., Dilworth, S., and Oster, C.N. (1990) Isolation of HIV-1 from the blood of seropositive adults: patient stage of illness and sample inoculum size are major determinants of a positive culture. *J. AIDS* **3(12),** 1159–1167.

2

Quantitative HIV Culture

James R. Lane

1. Introduction

This procedure is used for establishing cocultures for virus isolation by an endpoint dilution assay in a 96-well tissue culture plate. This is a cell culture assay based on the detection of HIV in patient peripheral blood mononuclear cells (PBMC) by the appearance of p24 gag protein in the culture supernatant. It can be used in a research setting as a measure of viral burden because the number of patient cells required to produce a positive culture is indicative of cellular viral load.

2. Materials
2.1. Donor PBMC

Normal donor buffy coats (leukocyte-enriched whole blood, from an anti-HIV negative donor), also known as leukopacks, may be obtained from a blood bank or donor service for processing within 12 h of collection. The donors should be screened by the standard assays currently required by the Food and Drug Administration (FDA) and the American Association of Blood Banks (AABB). To obtain the PBMC from the leukopacks, follow the same procedure described in Chapter 1 [Isolation and Expansion of HIV from Cells and Body Fluids by Co-Culture], Section 3.1.

2.2. Reagents

1. RPMI 1640 (Gibco [Gaithersburg, MD] or equivalent).
2. Fetal bovine serum (FBS) (Gibco or equivalent) (heat-inactivated, 56°C, 30 min).
3. Pen-Strep (Gibco or equivalent) Concentration = 10,000 U Pen and 10 mg strep/mL.
4. Ficoll-Paque (Pharmacia or equivalent).
5. 0.4% Trypan blue (Gibco or equivalent).

From: *Methods in Molecular Medicine, Vol. 17: HIV Protocols*
Edited by: N. L. Michael and J. H. Kim © Humana Press Inc., Totowa, NJ

6. PHA (Murex cat #HA17 or equivalent, 10 mg lyophylized powder).
7. 200 m*M* L-Glutamine (Gibco or equivalent).
8. 200 U/mL Interleukin-2 (IL-2) (Boehringer-Mannheim cat# 663-581, or equivalent).
9. Polybrene (Sigma [St. Louis, MO] or equivalent).

2.3. Reagent Preparation

1. Ficoll wash medium: RPMI 1640, 2% FBS, 1% Pen-Strep. Filter sterilize using a 0.2 μ filtration unit. Store at 4°C ± 2°C. Discard after 2 wk.
2. Complete medium: RPMI 1640, 15% FBS, 10% IL-2,1% Pen-Strep, 2 m*M* L-Glutamine. Filter sterilize using 0.2 μ filtration unit. Store at 4°C ± 2°C. Discard after 2 wk.
3. PHA stock solution: Reconstitute PHA (10 mg bottle) with 10 mL RPMI 1640. Filter sterilize using syringe filter. Final concentration is 1000 μg/mL. Aliquot 0.3–0.5 mL into cryovials. Store at –20°C ± 5°C. Discard after 1 yr.
4. Polybrene stock solution (0.5 mg/mL): Dissolve 100 mg of polybrene into 200 mL RPMI 1640, filter sterilize using a 0.2 μ filtration unit. Store at 4°C ± 2°C. Aliquots are stable for 1 yr.
5. Coculture medium: RPMI-1640, 15% FBS, 10% IL-2, 1% Pen-strep, 2 m*M* L-Glutamine, 2 μg/mL polybrene. Store at 4°C ± 2°C. Discard after 2 wk.

3. Methods

1. Label four sterile cluster "A", "B", "C", and "D".
2. Resuspend a cell pellet containing 2.2×10^6 patient cells processed as described in Chapter 1 [Isolation and Expansion of HIV from Cells and Body Fluids by Coculture], Section 3.1., in 350 μL of coculture medium Gently mix suspension 2–3 times using a 200–1000-μL pipet tip.
3. Transfer all of the resuspended cell pellet from step 2 into Tube A.
4. Gently mix and transfer 120 μL of cell suspension from Tube A into tube B containing 260 μL of coculture medium.
5. Gently mix and transfer 120 μL of cell suspension from Tube B into Tube C containing 260 μL of coculture medium.
6. Gently mix and transfer 120 μL of cell suspension from Tube C into Tube D containing 260 μL of coculture medium.
7. Dispense four replicates of each cell dilution into a 96-well microtiter plate according to the format in **Table 1**.
   a. 50 μL of Tube A cell suspension into wells 3C–3F.
   b. 50 μL of Tube B cell suspension into wells 4C–4F.
   c. 50 μL of Tube C cell suspension into wells 5C–5F.
   d. 50 μL of Tube D cell suspension to wells 6C–6F.
8. Obtain 4.0×10^6 PHA stimulated, viable, PBMC prepared as described in Chapter 1 [Isolation and Expansion of HIV from Cells and Body Fluids by Coculture], Section 3.).
9. Centrifuge at 220–240*g* for 10–15 min at room temperature. Decant supernatant.
10. Resuspend pellet in 2.0 mL of coculture medium.

Table 1
Suggested Plate Format: Cells/Coculture (Log$_{10}$)

	1	2	3	4	5	6	7	8	9	10	11	12
A	PBS	PBS	PBS	PBS	PBS	PBS	PBS	PBS	PBS	PBS	PBS	PBS
B	PBS							PBS				PBS
C	PBS		$10^{5.5}$	10^5	$10^{4.5}$	10^4		PBS				PBS
D	PBS		$10^{5.5}$	10^5	$10^{4.5}$	10^4		PBS				PBS
E	PBS		$10^{5.5}$	10^5	$10^{4.5}$	10^4		PBS				PBS
F	PBS		$10^{5.5}$	10^5	$10^{4.5}$	10^4		PBS				PBS
G	PBS							PBS				PBS
H	PBS	PBS	PBS	PBS	PBS	PBS	PBS	PBS	PBS	PBS	PBS	PBS

PBS = 200 μL phosphate-buffered saline or RPMI-1640 to minimize medium evaporation loss from inner wells.

Numbers reflect amount of patient cells in Log$_{10}$

11. Add 100 μL of this cell suspension to each of the appropriate wells (3C–3F, 4C–4F, 5C–5F, and 6C–6F) shown above.
12. Incubate at $37°C \pm 2°C$, 5% CO_2 and 95% humidity for 30–40 min.
13. Add 100 μL coculture medium to each well containing the mix of patient and PHA-stimulated donor cells. Add 200 μL of sterile PBS or RPMI-1640 to each of the outer wells designated "PBS" as shown in the plate format to minimize evaporation loss. The outer wells may be filled earlier if convenient.
14. Incubate at $37°C \pm 2°C$, 5% CO_2 and 95% humidity.
15. Remove 175 μL of supernatant at d 3–4, 7, 10, 14, 17, 24, and 28. Be careful not to disrupt the cells at bottom of wells. On d 21 "split" culture by pipeting up and down three times to resuspend cells and remove only 150 μL. On d 7, 10, 24, and 28, transfer the 175 μL to an identically labeled 96-well U-bottom microtiter plate. Cover supernatant plate with plate sealer. On d 7 and 28, measure p24 present in the supernatants. On d 3–4, 14, 17, and 21, supernatant is discarded.
    a. On d 3–4, 7, 14, and 21, add back 175 μL of fresh coculture medium containing 2×10^5 PHA-treated PBMC.
    b. On d 10, 17, and 24, add back 175 μL of fresh coculture medium without PHA stimulated cells.
16. Terminate cultures after 28 d of incubation. If desired, save original plate by sealing with a plate sealer and storing at $-70°C \pm 10°C$.
17. Calculations of TCID$_{50}$:
    a. TCID$_{50}$ values are calculated by the method of Spearman and Karber. For those patient viruses that are "slow-growing," more useful information may be obtained from the d 28 values compared to d 7.
    Spearman-Karber Formula:

$$M = xk + d[0.5 - (1/n) \times (\text{sum of } r)]$$

where M = TCID$_{50}$ expressed as Log$_{10}$, xk = dose of highest dilution (1.5 in this case), r = the number of negative wells, d = spacing between dilutions (0.5 in this case), and n = wells/dilution (4 in this case).

Table 2
Conversion Table

# Negative wells	No. of cells for 50% infection ($TCID_{50}$)
16	≥ 564286
15	421333
14	316000
13	237594
12	177528
11	133333
10	100000
9	74882
8	56228
7	42133
6	31600
5	23688
4	17773
3	13327
2	10000
1	7493
0	≤ 5620

Used		d
3.16×10^5		10^0 "Undiluted"
1.0×10^5		$10^{0.5}$
3.16×10^4	4 replicates each	10^1
1.0×10^4		$10^{1.5}$

b. The following is an example for calculating the result using the Spearman-Karber equation. A well is considered positive if the p24 value as determined by ELISA is 15.625 pg/mL or greater.

Example: No. of negative wells = 9

$$M = 1.5 + 0.5 \, [0.5 - (1/4) * 9]$$
$$= 1.5 + 0.5 \, [-1.75]$$
$$= 1.5 - 0.875$$
$$= 0.625$$

The antilog of M ($10^{0.625} = 4.22$) is the relative dilution of starting cells resulting in a 50% infection rate. To calculate the $TCID_{50}$, the original input of patient cells (316,000) is divided by M. Therefore, 316,000/4.22 = 74882 = number of cells needed to infect 50% of cultures. Alternatively, using the conversion table **(Table 2)**, one can calculate the $TCID_{50}$ manually if necessary.

References

1. Dimitrov, D. H., Melnick, J. L., and Hollinger, F. B. (1990) Microculture assay for the isolation of human immunodeficiency virus type 1 and for titration of infected peripheral blood mononuclear cells. *J. Clin. Microbiol.* **28,** 734–737.
2. ACTG Virology Manual for HIV Laboratories. (1993) (Hollinger, F.B., ed.) Version 2.0, MIC-1 to MIC-4.

3

Quantitation of Cell-Free HIV
by Reverse Transcriptase Activity

James R. Lane

1. Introduction

This assay measures the activity of reverse transcriptase (RNA-dependent-DNA polymerase), an enzyme that synthesizes DNA using RNA as the template. The detection of reverse transcriptase activity (RT) indicates the presence of HIV-1 in in vitro cultures of human peripheral blood mononuclear cells (PBMCs). Because active HIV-1 infection results in lysis of lymphocytes and release of free virions, the associated enzyme activity can be found in cell culture supernatants. Virus is concentrated from the supernatant and separated from soluble cellular contaminants by pelleting in polyethylene glycol and resuspended in a minimal volume of suspension buffer prior to assay.

A portion of this suspension is added to a reaction solution containing a detergent which disrupts the virus and frees the polymerase enzyme, a synthetic RNA template (poly rA), a short DNA primer (oligo dT), and a radiolabelled nucleotide ^{3}H-thymidine triphosphate (^{3}H-TTP). The reaction solution also contains Tris buffer (at optimal pH), metal salts (to provide needed ionic strength and required Mg), and dithiothreitol (to stabilize the enzyme-free sulfhydryl groups). Presence of RT causes the extension of the RNA–DNA primer complex by incorporation of the ^{3}H-TTP into a newly-synthesized DNA strand complementary to the exiting RNA strand. The RNA–^{3}H-DNA hybrid produced is precipitated with TCA, isolated by filtration, and quantitated by measuring the radioactivity. The level of radioactivity is generally proportional to the amount of active RT enzyme present.

An estimate of cellular DNA-polymerase activity, which has a low-level, nonspecific RT activity is made by adding a portion of the test specimen to reaction solution containing a synthetic, primed DNA template (dAdT) instead of an RNA template.

From: *Methods in Molecular Medicine, Vol. 17: HIV Protocols*
Edited by: N. L. Michael and J. H. Kim © Humana Press Inc., Totowa, NJ

In the presence of ^{3}H-dTT, production of relatively little ^{3}H-radiolabeled DNA–DNA hybrid indicates little contamination by cellular or nonspecific polymerases.

2. Materials

2.1. Reagents and Special Preparations

1. Polyethylene glycol (30% solution). Polyethylene glycol (PEG MW 6000), 30.0 g is dissolved in phosphate-buffered saline (PBS) (without CaCl$_2$), brought to a volume of 100 mL with PBS, and filter sterilized. Store at 4°C. Make fresh every month.
2. Sample suspension buffer (SB)

Stock	Add	Final concentration in SB
5 M NaCl	10.0 mL	0.1 mL
1 M Tris base (DNase free)	25.0 mL	50 mM
0.1 M NaEDTA (DNase free)	5.0 mL	1 mm

   Fill a 500-mL graduated cylinder to the 350 mL mark with dH$_2$O. Add the above ingredients, and stir with a magnetic stirring bar. Adjust the pH to 7.6 using 1 M HCl, and bring the total volume to 500 mL. Filter sterilize into two 250-mL plastic bottles. Store at 4°C.
3. Polymerase reaction mixtures (*see* **Table 1**).
4. Polymerase stop solution (3X)

Stock	Volume added
Sodium pyrophosphate	500.0 mg
5 M NaCl	1.5 mL
Bovine serum albumin (BSA)	50.0 mg

   Fill a 100-mL graduated cylinder to the 60 mL mark with dH$_2$O. Add the above ingredients in order, and dissolve completely with a magnetic stirring bar. The BSA must be added slowly to avoid clumping and foaming. Bring the total volume to 100 mL. Do not adjust the pH. Filter sterilize into a plastic bottle. Store at 4°C. Dilute 1:3 using sterile dH$_2$0 at time of assay.
5. Trichloroacetic acid (TCA) solution (store at 4°C):

100% (1 g/mL):	454 TCA + 182 mL dH$_2$0
60%:	60 mL (100% TCA) + 40 mL dH$_2$0
6%:	100 mL (60% TCA) +
	10 mL (10% sodium pyrophosphate) + 890 mL dH$_2$0

6. Preparation of standard RT enzyme solutions: Immediately before use, dilute commercial RT enzyme to make three standard solutions as follows:

Dilution	Method	# U enzyme in 10 μL
1:10	To original 10 μL, add 90 μL SB	20 U
1:25	Take 30 μL of 1:10 dilution, add 45 μL SB	8 U
1:100	Take 20 μL of 1:25 dilution, add 60 μL SB	2 U

Table 1
Polymerase Reaction Mixtures

Stock	Polymerase reaction mix			Final concentration in polymerase reaction
	A	B	C	
DH_2O	11.52 mL	10.88 mL	10.88 mL	
0.05 *M* Tris-HCl, pH 8.3	2.00 mL	2.00 mL	2.00 mL	0.0625 *M*
5 *M* NaCl	0.40 mL	0.40 mL	0.40 mL	0.1250 *M*
1 *M* MgCl$_2$	0.12 mL	0.12 mL	0.12 mL	0.0075 *M*
0.5 *M* DTT	0.40 mL	0.40 mL	0.40 mL	0.0125 *M*
Oligo dT[a] (1 mg/mL)	0.08 mL	0.00 mL	0.00 mL	0.005 mg/mL
Poly rA[b] (10 mg/mL)	0.08 mL	0.00 mL	0.00 mL	0.050 mg/dL
rAdT[a] (1.4 mg/mL)	0.00 mL	0.80 mL	0.00 mL	0.070 mg/mL
dAdt[b] (1.4 mg/mL)	0.00 mL	0.00 mL	0.80 mL	0.070 mg/mL
10% NP-40	0.40 mL	0.40 mL	0.40 mL	0.25%
3H-TTP (1.9 µ*M*)	1.00 mL	1.00 mL	1.00 mL	0.1562 mCi/mL
Total volume	16.00 mL	16.00 mL	16.00 mL	

[a]*See* **Note 1**.
[b]Reconstitute the lyophilized solid using dH$_2$O.

7. Preparation of controls:
   a. Negative control (H9 cell line): Cell line supernatant is decanted into 50-mL tubes and centrifuged at 1500 rpm for 10 min. The supernatant is decanted into a second 50-mL tube, swirled, and aliquoted into 1.5-mL centrifuge tubes. It is then spun at 10,000 rpm for 5 min. Add 1.0 mL of supernatant to 1.5-mL centrifuge with 0.5 mL cold PEG. The vials are vortexed and kept on ice overnight in the refrigerator. The following day, the vials are spun at 10,000 rpm for 10 min. After the pellet is blotted dry, it is resuspended in 100 µL SB and vortexed for 2 h. The vials are then frozen in the –85°C freezer and thawed individually for the RT assay. Just prior to assay, a vial is thawed at room temperature and vortexed gently. It is assayed (10 µL in each of three wells) as described.
   b. Positive control (HIV-infected H9 cell line): The same procedure as used for the negative control. Just prior to assay, a vial is thawed at room temperature and vortexed gently. It is assayed (10 µL in each of three wells) as described.

3. Methods

3.1. Specimen Preparation

1. This procedure is performed on cell-free, culture supernatant samples, obtained from routine lymphocyte cocultures.
2. For RT testing, pipet 1.5 mL of the sample into a microcentrifuge tube, and centrifuge at 10,000 rpm for 5 min in a Beckman microfuge-12 or equivalent.
3. Remove 1.0 mL of the supernatant, and add to a 1.5-mL microfuge tube containing 0.5 mL of 30% cold PEG.
4. Vortex each sample thoroughly, and place on ice at 4°C for no less than 90 min (may be left overnight). This will precipitate the virus.
5. Pellet the precipitate by centrifugation for 10 min at 10,000 rpm.
6. Decant the supernatant into a conical tube, and discard.
7. Invert each tube on absorbent material, and blot dry. Carefully dry the pellet and tube further by using a cotton-tipped applicator (*see* **Note 2**). Do not touch the pellet with the applicator.
8. Resuspend each pellet in 100 μL of suspension buffer. This usually requires 2–4 h on a shaker. Pellets may be left overnight with suspension buffer to soften and dissolve. Agitate occasionally. Samples can be stored frozen at –85°C until assayed. However, freeze-thaw cycles and long standing reduce RT activity.

3.2. Assay Procedure (see Note 3)

1. The assay is performed in a 96-well, round-bottom microtiter plate. Each test run includes the following types of samples: a blank (i.e., suspension buffer), positive controls, negative control, a standard, and unknowns. For each type of sample, assign a series of 3 microtiter wells. Dispense 30 μL of polymerase reaction mix A into each of the first two wells, and then 30 μL of polymerase reaction mix C into the third well (do not allow to dry).
2. Add 10 μL of each sample (or control) to the appropriate wells and swirl to mix. Samples should be added directly into the reaction mix. Change tip for each well. Freeze remaining samples.
3. Incubate for 2 h at 37°C in a humid atmosphere.
4. After incubation, add 130 μL of ice-cold polymerase stop solution (lX) and swirl. A multichannel pipet may be used for this purpose.
5. Precipitate the reaction by adding 30 μL of ice-cold 60% TCA to each well, and keep the plate at 4°C on ice for at least 30 min.
6. Collection of the precipitate using a Skatron Harvester:
   a. Flush water from lines using 6% TCA. Close the valve leading to the dH_2O carboy. Open the valve to the 6% TCA container. Turn on the vacuum. Make sure that vacuum is set for 15–17 in. Hg. Adjust each of the three wash settings to read "9". Align a glass filtermat on the Skatron Harvester. Place the harvest manifold into an empty 96-well plate and press "prewet". When indicated, press "wet". Repeat twice more to flush all water from the inlet lines.

    b. Harvest samples: Remove this filter and replace with another. "Prewet" again using the empty plate. The unit is now ready to harvest the first 12 samples. Place the harvest manifold into the first row of samples to be filtered. Press "wet" to start. Once the wash cycle has been completed, move the filter to the next setting. "Prewet" again using the blank plate.

    c. Flush 6% TCA from lines using dH_2O: After all the samples have been harvested, remove the filtermat, clamp the TCA supply valve, and open the H_2O valve. Using an empty plate and filtermat, flush the unit with H_2O at least five times. Turn the vacuum off when this has been completed. Brush the rubber O-rings and screens to remove residual glass fibers. Dry the filtermats completely under a heat lamp before punching out the filter discs and adding to scintillation vials. Fill vials with 3 mL of scintillation fluid and count to determine the amount of label incorporation. Express the data in disintegrations per minute (DPM).

7. To verify total DPM added in each reaction, add 30 μL of Mix A (in duplicate) and Mix B (in duplicate) directly to scintillation vials, add 3 mL scintillation fluid as above, and determine DPM. Also, measure radioactive DPM in swabs of hood area and Skatron bench.

3.3. Calculations

If desired, a curve of DPM vs activity units can be plotted from the three dilutions of commercial standard RT enzyme. Then the RT activity of the unknown patient coculture specimens can be expressed in activity units by comparisons of the DPM obtained with the DPM from the standard curve.

3.4. Results and Interpretation

A specimen is considered positive for the presence of RT activity if the following criteria are met: Using the RNA template (polymerase reaction mix A or B), the DPM of the specimen (S) must be at least 10,000; specimens must exhibit at least five times the DPM of the PBMC negative control (i.e., S/C ratio [ratio of DPM of specimen to DPM of uninoculated donor cells] > 5) when the RNA template is used (i.e., polymerase reaction mix A or B); and the S/C ratio using the RNA template (i.e., polymerase reaction mix A or B) must be at least twice the S/C ratio using the DNA template (i.e., polymerase reaction mix C).

3.5. Quality Control

A negative control is included in each assay tray. A set of two dilutions of positive controls is included in each assay. These specimens come from the same master lot and are frozen in small aliquots so that the RT activity should be constant to test for interassay variability. Therefore, the activity of these specimens should be comparable between runs. Specimens are run in duplicate, and a third tube is included to check for nonspecific reverse transcriptase activity.

Notes

1. This material is sold as a lyophilized solid in quantities measured in A_{260} units. Check the certificate of analysis included with the shipment of this product to determine the exact weight (mg) of material per A_{260} unit. Reconstitute using sterilized dH20
2. This is important since PEG has been shown to inhibit the activity of RT enzyme.
3. The assay described is a modification of the procedure reported by David Waters (Frederick Cancer Research Institute) in a personal communicatiuon to Arnold K. Fowler (SRA Technologies, Inc.).

References

1. Hoffman, A. D., Banapour, B., and Levy, J. (1985) Characterization of the AIDS-associated retrovirus reverse transcriptase and optimal conditions for its detection in virions. *Virology* **147,** 326–335.
2. Lee, M. H., Sano, J., Morales, F. E., and Imagawa, D. T. (1987) Sensitive reverse transcriptase assday to detect and quantitate human immunodeficiency virus. *J. Clin. Microbiol.* **25,** 1717–1721.

4

Determination of Syncytium-Inducing Phenotype of Primary HIV-1 Isolates Using MT-2 cells

Mark K. Louder and John R. Mascola

1. Introduction

HIV-1 is routinely isolated by cocultivation of patient PBMC with mitogen-stimulated HIV-uninfected donor PBMC (*see* Chapter 1). In this culture system, HIV-1 primarily replicates in CD4$^+$ T-lymphocytes, and such viruses are termed clinical or primary isolates. As early as 1986, the in vitro replicative capacity and cell tropism of primary HIV-1 isolates were shown to be important in the pathophysiology of HIV-1 infection *(1)*. High replication capacity in PBMC and virus growth and syncytium formation in neoplastic T-cell lines were found to correlate with severity of HIV-1-disease *(2–5)*. Compared to syncytium-inducing (SI) isolates, nonsyncytium-inducing (NSI) strains did not replicate in neoplastic T-cell lines and showed preferential replication in cells of the monocyte-macrophage lineage *(6,7)*. Thus, NSI viruses have often been termed macrophage tropic, whereas SI strains are termed T-cell line tropic.

In 1989, Koot et al. showed that cocultivation of patient PBMC with a human T-cell leukemia virus type I-transformed lymphoblastoid cell line (MT-2) could readily detect SI isolates *(8)*. Using similar methods of MT-2 phenotyping for identification of SI viruses, several studies confirmed that the SI phenotype was an independent marker for progression to AIDS *(9–11)*. The predominance of NSI viruses isolated during primary or early stage HIV-1 infection suggested that NSI viruses were preferentially transmitted *(12,13)*, and longitudinal studies showed that emergence of SI variants was generally associated with progression of disease *(7,12,14)*. Thus, the association of viral phenotype with HIV-1 transmission and disease progression has made determination of this biologic characteristic of HIV-1 an important laboratory methodology.

From: *Methods in Molecular Medicine, Vol. 17: HIV Protocols*
Edited by: N. L. Michael and J. H. Kim © Humana Press Inc., Totowa, NJ

The recent discovery that cellular entry of HIV-1 requires binding to both CD4 and a chemokine coreceptor has helped clarify the virology of HIV-1 cell tropism *(15–21)*. Primary NSI strains enter cells almost exclusively via CD4 and the chemokine receptor CCR5, whereas SI isolates preferentially utilize the CXCR-4 coreceptor. MT-2 cells and most neoplastic T-cell lines (e.g., H9, CEM, Sup-T1) express CXCR-4, but lack CCR5, explaining the tropism of SI strains for these cell lines *(22)*. The physiologic importance of the chemokine coreceptors and their relationship to viral SI phenotype, in vivo, have recently been demonstrated by studies of HIV-1-infected individuals heterozygous for a deletion in the gene coding the CCR5 coreceptor. In several HIV-1 seropositive cohort studies, the heterozygous (CCR5/Δccr5) genotype was associated with a significant decrease in progression to AIDS *(23–25)*. However, consistent with our understanding of the virus-cell tropism, this protective effect on disease progression was lost when the infecting virus used CXCR-4 as a coreceptor *(25)*. Although the biologic mechanisms associating HIV-1 SI phenotype, in vivo coreceptor utilization, and HIV-1 disease progression are not fully understood, the determination of viral SI phenotype will continue to be important in studies of HIV-1 pathogenesis. The method described below is a microtiter plate assay for determination of SI-phenotype based on visual inspection for syncytia after HIV-1 infection of MT-2 cells. This method is adapted from the standardized microtiter assay described by Japour et al. *(26)* for the United States AIDS Clinical Trials Group of the National Institute of Allergy and Infectious Diseases.

2. Materials

1. Culture Media (cRPMI)—RPMI 1640, without L-Glutamine (Quality Biological, Inc., Gaithersburg, MD), supplemented with 15% heat-inactivated fetal bovine serum (PAA Laboratories, Inc., Newport Beach, CA), 2 mM L-glutamine, 100 U/mL Penicillin, 100 µg/mL streptomycin (all from Quality Biological, Inc.).
2. MT-2 cells (NIH AIDS Research and Reference Reagent Program, Rockville, MD; *see* **Note 1**).
3. Control SI (IIIB) and NSI (JR-CSF) viruses (NIH AIDS Research and Reference Reagent Program, Rockville, MD).
4. Ninety-six-well flat-bottom microtiter plates (Costar, Cambridge, MA).
5. Inverted transmitted-light microscope (Telaval-31, Carl Zeiss Inc., Thornwood, NY).

3. Methods

1. MT-2 cells are cultured in cRPMI and split every 3–4 d to maintain a cell density of ~1 × 10^6 cells/mL. The assay is performed with cells in exponential growth phase (i.e., 1–2 d after split).
2. Virus stocks are pre-titered on donor PBMC to determine $TCID_{50}$/mL (*see* **Note 2**).

3. On the day of the assay, MT-2 cells are counted and resuspended at 1×10^6 cells/ mL, 5×10^4 cells (50 µL) are aliquoted into a 96-well flat-bottom microtiter plate (duplicate wells per virus).
4. Control and test viruses are thawed in a 37°C water bath and diluted to 200 $TCID_{50}/50$ µL in cRPMI.
5. Fifty microliters of each diluted viral stock are added to duplicate wells of MT-2 cells; cRPMI is added to duplicate control wells. Virus and cells are incubated for 2 h at 37°C and 100 µL of cRPMI are added to each well for a total volume of 200 µL/well.
6. The cells are visually examined for syncytium formation using an inverted microscope at X100 magnification (low-power field). Test wells are scored positive (SI) if three or more syncytial cells are observed per low-power field (*see* **Note 3**). Discordance between duplicate wells is considered uninterpretable, and the assay is repeated.
7. The cells are split every 3–4 d by removing 125 µL of cell suspension/well and adding back an equal amount of fresh cRPMI.
8. The assay is continued for 21 d. Viruses not producing MT-2 syncytium formation at termination day are scored NSI (*see* **Note 4**).

4. Notes

1. MT-2 cells are a human T-cell leukemia virus type I-transformed lymphoblastoid cell line.
2. Virus titration is performed as described in Chapter 33, Subheading 3.4. Normalization of infectious titer assures that an adequate amount of infectious virus is added to MT-2 cells. This prevents false-negative NSI readings owing to low or noninfectious virus inoculum.
3. MT-2 cells are generally examined every 1–2 d. Noting the day that syncytia are first observed is helpful as a semiquantitative measure of virus SI phenotype. Typically, prototype T-cell line-adapted SI strains, such as HIV-IIIB and MN, produce syncytia by d 2–3. Once a virus produces syncytia, the infection generally spreads throughout the well; results are rarely equivocal.
4. Some investigators terminate the assay at 14 d. In our experience, approx 1 in 10 SI viruses will first demonstrate syncytia between days 14 and 21.

References

1. Asjo, B., Morfeldt-Manson, L., Albert, J., Biberfeld, G., Karlsson, A., Lidman, K., and Fenyo, E. M. (1986) Replicative capacity of human immunodeficiency virus from patients with varying severity of HIV infection. *Lancet* **2,** 660–662.
2. Tersmette, M., Lange, J. M. A., de Goede, R. E. Y., de Wolf, F., Eeftink-Schattenkerk, J. K. M., Schellekens, P. T. A., Coutinho, R. A., Huisman, J. G., Goudsmit, J., and Miedema, F. (1989) Association between biological properties of human immunodeficiency virus variants and risk for AIDS and AIDS mortality. *Lancet* **1,** 983–985.
3. Cheng-Mayer, C., Seto, D., Tateno, M., and Levy, J. (1988) Biologic features of HIV-1 that correlate with virulence in the host. *Science* **240,** 80–82.

 4. Fenyo, E. M., Morfeldt-Manson, L., Chiodi, F., Lind, B., von Gegerfelt, A., Albert, J., Olausson, E., and Asjo, B. (1988) Distinct replication and cytopathic characteristics of human immunodeficiency virus isolates. *J. Virol.* **62,** 4414–4419.
 5. Tersmette, M., Gruters, R. A., de Wolf, F., de Goede, R. E. Y., Lange, J. M. A., Schellekens, P. T. A., Goudsmit, J., Huisman, H. G., and Miedema, F. (1989) Evidence for a role of virulent human immunodeficiency virus (HIV) variants in the pathogenesis of acquired immunodeficiency syndrome: Studies on sequential HIV isolates. *J. Virol.* **63,** 2118–2125.
 6. Fenyo, E. M., Albert, J., and Asjo, B. (1989)Replicative capacity, cytopathic effect and cell tropism of HIV. *AIDS* **3 Suppl. 1,** S5–S12.
 7. Schuitemaker, H., Kootstra, N. A., de Goede, R. E. Y., de Wolf, F., Miedema, F., and Tersmette, M. (1991) Monocytotropic human immunodeficiency virus type 1 (HIV-1) variants detectable in all stages of HIV-1 infection lack T-cell line tropism and syncytium-inducing ability in primary T-cell culture. *J. Virol.* **65,** 356–363.
 8. Koot, M., Vos, A. H. V,, Keet, R. P. M., de Goede, R. E. Y., Dercksen, M. W., Terpstra, F. G., Coutinho, R. A., Miedema, F., and Tersmette, M. (1992) HIV-1 biological phenotype in long-term infected individuals evaluated with an MT-2 cocultivation assay. *AIDS* **6,** 49–54.
 9. Koot, M., Keet, I. P. M., Vos, A. H. V., de Goede, R. E. Y., Roos, M. T. L., Coutinho, R. A., Miedema, F., Schellekens, P. T. A., and Tersmette, M. (1993) Prognostic value of HIV-1 syncytium-inducing phenotype for rate of CD4$^+$ cell depletion and progression to AIDS. *Ann. Intern. Med.* **118,** 681–688.
10. Bozzette, S. A., McCutchan, J. A., Spector, S. A., Wright, B., and Richman, D. D. (1993) A cross-sectional comparison of persons with syncytium- and non-syncytium-inducing human immunodeficiency virus. *J. Infect. Dis.* **168,** 1374–1379.
11. Karlsson, A., Parsmyr, K., Sandström, E., Fenyö, E. M., and Albert, J. (1994) MT-2 cell tropism as prognostic marker for disease progression in human immunodeficiency virus type 1 infection. *J. Clin. Microbiol.* **32,** 364–370.
12. Roos, M. T. L., Lange, J. M. A., de Goede, R. E. Y., Coutinho, R. A., Schellekens, P. T. A., Miedema, F., and Tersmette, M. (1992) Viral phenotype and immune response in primary human immunodeficiency virus type 1 infection. *J. Infect. Dis.* **165,** 427–432.
13. Zhu, T., Mo, H., Wang, N., Nam, D. S., Cao, Y., Koup, R. A., and Ho, D. D. (1993) Genotypic and phenotypic characterization of HIV-1 in patients with primary infection. *Science* **261,** 1179–1181.
14. Connor, R. I. and Ho, D. D. (1994) Human immunodeficiency virus type 1 variants with increased replicative capacity develop during the asymptomatic stage before disease progression. *J. Virol.* **68,** 4400–4408.
15. Feng, Y., Broder, C. C., Kennedy, P. E., Berger, E. A. (1996) HIV-1 entry cofactor: Functional cDNA cloning of a seven-transmembrane, Gprotein-coupled receptor. *Science* **272,** 872–877.
16. Choe, H., Farzan, M., Sun, Y., Sullivan, N., Rollins, B., Ponath, P. D., et al. (1996) The b-chemokine receptors CCR3 and CCR5 facilitate infection by primary HIV-1 isolates. *Cell* **85,** 1135–1148.

17. Alkhatib, G., Combadiere, C., Broder, C. C., Feng, Y., Kennedy, P. E., Murphy, P. M., and Berger, E. A. (1996) CC CKR5: A RANTES, MIP-1a, MIP-1b receptor as a fusion cofactor for macrophage-tropic HIV-1. *Science* **272**, 1955–1958.

18. Deng, H. K., Liu, R., Ellmeier, W., Choe, S., Unutmaz, D., Burkhart, M., et al. Identification of a major co-receptor for primary isolates of HIV-1. Nature. 1996;381:661-666.

19. Dragic, T., Litwin, V., Allaway, G. P., Martin, S. R., Huang, Y. X., Nagashima, K. A., et al. (1996) HIV-1 entry into CD4$^+$ cells is mediated by the chemokine receptor CC-CKR-5. *Nature* **381**, 667–673.

20. Trkola, A., Dragic, T., Arthos, J., Binley, J. M., Olson, W. C., Allaway, G. P., et al. (1996) CD4-dependent, antibody-sensitive interactions between HIV-1 and its co-receptor CCR-5. *Nature* **384**, 184–187.

21. Wu, L. J., Gerard, N. P., Wyatt, R., Choe, H., Parolin, C., Ruffing, N., et al. (1996) CD4-induced interaction of primary HIV-1 gp120 glycoproteins with the chemokine receptor CCR-5. *Nature* **384**, 179–183.

22. Wu, L. J., Paxton, W. A., Kassam, N., Ruffing, N., Rottman, J. B., Sullivan, N., et al. (1995) CCR5 levels and expression pattern correlate with infectability by macrophage-tropic HIV-1, in vitro. *J. Exp. Med.* **185**, 1681–1691.

23. Dean, M., Carrington, M., Winkler, C., Huttley, G. A., Smith, M. W., Allikmets, R., et al. (1996) Genetic restriction of HIV-1 infection and progression to AIDS by a deletion allele of the CKR5 structural gene. *Science* **273**, 1856–1862.

24. Huang, Y. X., Paxton, W. A., Wolinsky, S. M., Neumann, A. U., Zhang, L. Q., He T, et al. (1996) The role of a mutant CCR5 allele in HIV-1 transmission and disease progression. *Nature Med.* **2**, 1240–1243.

25. Michael, N. L., Chang, G., Louie, L. G., Mascola, J. R., Dondero, D., Birx, D. L., et al. (1997) The role of viral phenotype and CCR-5 gene defects in HIV-1 transmission and disease progression. *Nature Med.* **3**, 338–340.

26. Japour, A. J., Fiscus, S. A., Arduino, J.-M., Mayers, D. L., Reichelderfer, P. S., and Kuritzkes, D. R. (1994) Standardized microtiter assay for determination of syncytium-inducing phenotypes of clinical human immunodeficiency virus type 1 isolates. *J. Clin. Microbiol.* **32**, 2291–2294.

5

Determination of HIV-1 Chemokine Coreceptor Tropism Using Transduced Human Osteosarcoma (HOS) Cells

Mark K. Louder and John R. Mascola

1. Introduction

CD4 was identified in 1984 as the receptor for HIV-1 *(1,2)*. However, it was soon apparent that a second receptor was necessary for HIV-1 infection of CD4$^+$ cells. This coreceptor was first identified by Berger and colleagues who showed that fusion and entry of T-cell line-adapted strains of HIV-1 into CD4$^+$ cells were mediated by a member of the seven transmembrane chemokine receptor family *(3)*. This protein was initially termed "fusin" and later found to be the α-chemokine receptor CXCR4. Subsequent reports by several laboratories rapidly identified a β-chemokine receptor, CCR5, that mediated entry of macrophage tropic HIV-1 isolates into CD4$^+$ cells *(4–8)*. Since these initial reports, our understanding of HIV-1 cell entry has continued to evolve. It now seems clear that primary HIV-1 strains with a nonsyncytium-inducing phenotype (in MT2 cells) utilize the CCR5 coreceptor and are designated "R5," whereas syncytium-inducing viruses preferentially utilize CXCR4, but may be dual tropic and are designated either "X4" or X4R5, respectively *(9,10)*. Some viruses also appear to be able to utilize chemokine receptors CCR2B and CCR3 *(7–10)*. In addition, the role of chemokine coreceptors in the pathophysiology of HIV-1 infection and disease progression is just beginning to be understood. Individuals who are homozygous for a 32-bp deletion in the CCR5 gene are only rarely found to be HIV-1-infected, and the heterozygous CCR5/Δccr5 genotype has been associated with a survival advantage against HIV-1 disease progression *(11–14)*. The protective effect of the CCR5/Δccr5 genotype is lost when the infecting virus uses the CXCR-4 coreceptor *(14)*.

From: *Methods in Molecular Medicine, Vol. 17: HIV Protocols*
Edited by: N. L. Michael and J. H. Kim © Humana Press Inc., Totowa, NJ

   In order to determine the coreceptor phenotype of HIV-1 isolates, the assay described below utilizes $CD4^+$ human osteosarcoma (HOS) cells that have been transduced to express a chemokine coreceptor. The cells were transduced using the retroviral expression vector pBABE-puro and provided to the United States NIH AIDS Research and Reference Reagent Program by Landau and colleagues (5,15,16). Thus, replication of HIV-1 in control cells (HOS-CD4.pBABE) can be compared to HOS-CD4 cell lines that express CXCR4 (HOS-CD4.fusin) or CCR5 (HOS-CD4.CCR5). HOS-CD4 cell lines that express CCR1, CCR2B, CCR3, and CCR4 are also available from the AIDS Research and Reference Reagent Program. This method is a microtiter plate assay that determines virus replication in HOS-CD4 cell lines by measuring expression of HIV-1 p24-antigen in culture supernatants.

2. Materials

1. Culture medium (cDMEM)—DMEM, without L-glutamine, with 4.5 g glucose per liter (Quality Biological, Inc., Gaithersburg, MD), supplemented with 10% heat-inactivated fetal bovine serum (PAA Laboratories, Inc., Newport Beach, CA), 2 mM L-glutamine, 100 U/mL penicillin, 100 µg/mL streptomycin (each from Quality Biological, Inc.), and 1 µg/mL puromycin (Sigma Chemical Co., St. Louis, MO).
2. Trypsin–EDTA solution—Trypsin (0.05%)–EDTA (0.1%), without calcium and magnesium (Quality Biological, Inc.) (see Note 1).
3. HOS-CD4 cell lines—HOS-CD4.pBABE-puro, HOS-CD4.CCR5, HOS-CD4.fusin(CXCR4) (NIH AIDS Research and Reference Reagent Program, Rockville, MD).
4. Control laboratory-adapted (e.g., HIV-MN, IIIB) and macrophage tropic (e.g., BAL, JRCSF) virus stocks (NIH AIDS Research and Reference Reagent Program).
5. T-75 vented tissue culture flasks (Costar, Cambridge, MA).
6. Ninety-six-well flat-bottom microtiter plates (Costar).
7. Twelve-Channel manual ELISA aspirator (Corning ELISA Plate Washer, #26305-72, Corning, NY).
8. HIV-1 p24 antigen-capture ELISA kit (Coulter Corp., Miami, FL).
9. V_{max} ELISA plate reader (Molecular Devices Corp., Sunnyvale, CA).

3. Methods
3.1. Maintenance of HOS-CD4 Cell Lines

   HOS-CD4 are adherent cell lines and require trypsinization for culture maintenance and for preparation of the phenotyping assay. Trypsinized cells are handled under cold conditions (4°C) in order to avoid cell loss due to adherence to tubes, pipets, and so forth.

1. Ongoing cultures are maintained in 30 mL cDMEM in a T-75 vented tissue culture flask and laid flat in a 5% CO_2 incubator kept at 37°C. Cultures are examined frequently and are split on reaching ~ 90% confluence (see Note 2).

2. Trypsin-EDTA solution is quickly thawed in a 37°C water bath, and 1 mL is diluted 1:1 with cold PBS for an initial rinse of the culture flask.

3. Working quickly and with one culture at a time, culture medium is removed and discarded. Two milliliters of diluted trypsin solution are added, and the culture flask is rinsed by gently rocking from side to side, so that the entire surface area is covered. This rinse is discarded.

4. Five milliliters of undiluted trypsin solution (37°C) are added to the flask, being sure to cover the entire surface area, and the flask is incubated for 2 min at 37°C (*see* **Note 3**).

5. Cells are dislodged from the flask by firmly tapping the sides. The cell suspension is then transferred to a 50-mL conical tube containing 10 mL cold, heat-inactivated fetal bovine serum, and pelleted by centrifugation at 1000 rpm (~210g) at 4°C. Cells are resuspended in cold cDMEM and counted, 2.5×10^4 cells are placed back into the T-75 flask, and cDMEM is added to a final volume of 30 mL.

3.2. Coreceptor Phenotyping Assay

1. On the day prior to infection, HOS-CD4 cells are counted, resuspended at 1.25×10^4 cells/mL, 2.5×10^3 cells (200 µL) aliquoted into a 96-well flat-bottom microtiter plate (triplicate wells per cell line per test virus), and allowed to adhere overnight at 37°C.

2. On the day of HOS-CD4 cell infection, control and test viruses are quickly thawed in a 37°C water bath and diluted to ~500 $TCID_{50}$/100 µL in cDMEM (*see* **Note 4**).

3. Culture medium is slowly aspirated from the seeded plate using a 12-channel manual ELISA plate aspirator, taking care not to remove all media (*see* **Note 5**).

4. One hundred microliters of each diluted viral stock are added to triplicate wells of each cell line to be infected. One hundred microliters of cDMEM is added to triplicate control wells for each cell line. Virus and cells are incubated for 2 h at 37°C and 100 µL of cDMEM are added for a final volume of 200 µL/well.

5. After overnight incubation, cells are washed four times with cDMEM to remove initial viral stock p24 antigen. Culture supernatant is carefully aspirated, and for each wash, 250 µL of cDMEM is added to each well. After the last wash, 230 µL of cDMEM are added to each well, and the plate is incubated at 37°C for 3–4 d.

3.3. HIV-1 p24 Antigen Quantitation and Primary Receptor Determination

p24 antigen expression by infected HOS-CD4 cell lines reaches detectable levels at varying rates, depending on the virus stock and HOS-CD4 cell line. Culture supernatant is generally collected beginning 3 d postinfection and every 2 d thereafter. The assay may be terminated when the p24 data permit discernment of cell line coreceptor use (*see* **Note 6**).

1. One hundred microliters of culture supernatant are removed from each well and transferred to a corresponding microtiter plate containing 80 µL of PBS and 20 µL of Coulter lysis buffer/well (i.e., final dilution of 1:2). The harvest plate is then

frozen at –20°C until p24 determination. Fresh cDMEM is added back to the experiment plate if the culture is to be continued.

2. On the day of p24-antigen determination, plates are thawed and brought to 37°C. The Coulter p24-antigen ELISA is performed according to the manufacturer's instructions.

3. For each virus, the p24 antigen level produced by each cell line is compared to determine coreceptor use. P24 antigen produced by infection of the HOS-CD4.pBABE-puro line is considered background growth and should be subtracted from results of corresponding infections before making a final determination (*see* **Note 7**).

4. Notes

1. Trypsin solutions are subject to self-digestion. The stock solution should be divided into smaller aliquots, frozen at –20°C, and thawed just prior to use.

2. Maintenance of HOS-CD4 cell lines in a T-75 tissue culture flask yields approx $20–25 \times 10^6$ cells at ~90% confluence. The size of cultures may be scaled up or down, according to the needs of the user.

3. Occasionally, this 2 min incubation may not be adequate to dislodge all adherent cells. The flask should be visually inspected and if adherent cells remain, the incubation period may be extended 1–2 min further.

4. Viral stocks are pre-titered on HIV-negative donor PBMC to determine $TCID_{50}/$ mL. The titration is performed as described in Chapter 33, Subheading 3.4. Although $TCID_{50}$ measured on mitogen stimulated PBMC may not correlate with infectious titer on HOS cells, normalization of the infectious titer helps to ensure consistent infection of the HOS cell lines. If there is no detectable infection of any HOS cell line, the assay may be repeated with a higher viral inoculum.

5. Medium is aspirated to a residual volume of approx 25–50 µL. Removal of all media may result in cell loss or dehydration. It is recommended that this aspiration technique be practiced and evaluated by visual inspection of individual wells before actual performance of the assay.

6. Definitive results are obtained for most high titer viruses between day 4 and 7. After this time, the HOS-CD4 cells have outgrown their environment and trypsinization is required to continue the assay. Whereas this will occasionally yield high enough p24-antigen levels to determine coreceptor utilization, in our experience it is preferable to repeat the assay with a higher virus inoculum.

7. HOS-CD4 cells appear to constitutively express some CXCR4 and highly tropic CXCR4 using viruses (e.g., HIV-MN and IIIB) will infect the control HOS-CD4.pBABE-puro cells. However, the p24-antigen expression by the HOS-CD4.fusin cells is generally two- to threefold higher than the control cells. Prototypic macrophage tropic viruses that use CCR5 do not infect control HOS-CD4.pBABE-puro cells.

Reference

1. Dalgleish, A. G., Beverley, P. C., Clapham, P. R., Crawford, D. H., Greaves, M. F., and Weiss, R. A. (1984) The CD4 (T4) antigen is an essential component of the receptor for the AIDS retrovirus. *Nature* **312,** 763–767.

2. Klatzmann, D., Champagne, E., Chamaret, S., Gruest, J., Guetard, D., Hercend, T., et al. (1984) T-lymphocyte T4 molecule behaves as the receptor for human retrovirus LAV. *Nature* **312,** 767–768.

3. Feng, Y., Broder, C. C., Kennedy, P. E., and Berger, E. A. (1996) HIV-1 entry cofactor: Functional cDNA cloning of a seven-transmembrane, Gprotein-coupled receptor. *Science* **272,** 872–877.

4. Alkhatib, G., Combadiere, C., Broder, C. C., Feng, Y., Kennedy, P. E, Murphy, P. M., et al. (1996) CC CKRS: A RANTES, MIP-1a, MIP-1b receptor as a fusion cofactor for macrophage-tropic HIV-1. *Science* **272,** 1955–1958.

5. Deng, H. K., Liu, R., Ellmeier, W., Choe, S., Unutmaz, D., Burkhart, M., et al. (1996) Identification of a major co-receptor for primary isolates of HIV-1. *Nature* **381,** 661–666.

6. Dragic, T., Litwin, V., Allaway, G. P., Martin, S. R., Huang, Y. X., Nagashima, K. A., et al. (1996) HIV-1 entry into CD4$^+$ cells is mediated by the chemokine receptor CC-CKR-5. *Nature* **381,** 667–673.

7. Choe, H., Farzan, M., Sun, Y., Sullivan, N., Rollins, B., Ponath, P. D., et al. (1996) The b-chemokine receptors CCR3 and CCR5 facilitate infection by primary HIV-1 isolates. *Cell* **85,** 1135–1148.

8. Doranz, B. J., Rucker, J., Yi, Y. J., Smyth, R. J., Samson, M., Peiper, S. C., et al. (1996) A dual-tropic primary HIV-1 isolate that uses fusin and the b-chemokine receptors CKR-5, CKR-3, and CKR-2b as fusion cofactors. *Cell* **85,** 1149–1158.

9. Dittmar, M. T., McKnight, A., Simmons, G., Clapham, P. R., Weiss, R. A., and Simmonds, P. (1997) HIV-1 tropism and co-receptor use. *Nature* **385,** 495,496.

10. Rana, S., Besson, G., Cook, D. G., Rucker, J., Smyth, R. J., Yi, Y. J., et al. (1997) Role of CCR5 in infection of primary macrophages and lymphocytes by macrophage-tropic strains of human immunodeficiency virus: Resistance to patient-derived and proto-type isolates resulting from the Deltaccr5 mutation. *J. Virol.* **71,** 3219–3227.

11. Dean, M., Carrington, M., Winkler, C., Huttley, G. A., Smith, M. W., Allikmets, R., et al. (1996) Genetic restriction of HIV-1 infection and progression to AIDS by a deletion allele of the CKR5 structural gene. *Science* **273,** 1856–1862.

12. Huang, Y. X., Paxton, W. A., Wolinsky, S. M., Neumann, A. U., Zhang, L. Q., He T, et al. (1996) The role of a mutant CCR5 allele in HIV-1 transmission and dis-ease progression. *Nature Med.* **2,** 1240–1243.

13. Samson, M., Libert, F., Doranz, B. J., Rucker, J., Liesnard, C., Farber, C. M., et al. (1996) Resistance to HIV-1 infection in Caucasian individuals bearing mutant alleles of the CCR-5 chemokine receptor gene. *Nature* **382,** 722–725.

14. Michael, N. L., Chang, G., Louie, L. G., Mascola, J. R., Dondero, D., Birx, D. L., and Sheppard, H. W. (1997) The role of viral phenotype and *CCR-5* gene defects in HIV-1 transmission and disease progression. *Nature Med.* **3,** 338–340.

15. Landau, N. R. and Littman, D. R. (1992) Packaging system for rapid production of murine leukemia virus vectors with variable tropism. *J. Virol.* **66,** 5110–5113.

16. He, J. and Landau, N. R. (1995) Use of a novel human immunodeficiency virus type 1 reporter virus expressing human placental alkaline phosphatase to detect an alternative viral receptor. *J. Virol.* **69,** 4587–4592.

6

Use of Luciferase Reporter Viruses for Studying HIV Entry

Rong Liu, Benjamin Chen, and Nathaniel R. Landau

1. Introduction

HIV replication is classically measured by quantitating virus present in the supernatant of infected cells over time. Typically, cells are infected at low multiplicity of infection (MOI) and washed extensively to remove input virus. Samples of culture supernatant are then removed over approximately a two week period and frozen. Virus in the supernatants is then quantitated by reverse transcriptase assay or by ELISA for p24^{gag} antigen. Using live virus for studying virus replication is appropriate for many applications but has several drawbacks. Generating growth curves is relatively labor-intensive, requiring frequent sampling and passaging of the infected cultures. Input virus may be carried over and mistaken for virus production at early points in the growth curve. In addition, there is the biohazard associated with working with live virus.

Single-cycle reporter virus offers a useful alternative for several applications, particularly those concerning virus entry. Using reporter viruses generally provides rapid and accurate results, necessitating only a single time point assay (typically three to five days post-infection). In addition, the problem of carry-over of input virus is substantially decreased since reporter gene activity is not present in the virus stock but requires active production in the target cells. In the case of luciferase, the assay is very sensitive (<0.001 pg of enzyme), rapid, and accurate. In addition, because the viruses are competent only for a single round of replication, conclusions can be drawn concerning virus entry. Reporter viruses present reduced biohazard to the researcher, since they are typically replication-defective and therefore do not mediate a spreading infection. They cannot be considered completely harmless, however, since

From: *Methods in Molecular Medicine, Vol. 17: HIV Protocols*
Edited by: N. L. Michael and J. H. Kim © Humana Press Inc., Totowa, NJ

stocks may contain low levels of replication-competent virus resulting from recombination during transfection.

There are at least three different classes of reporter viruses. Perhaps the most commonly used encode an easily assayed enzyme such as chloramphenicol acetyl transferase *(1)* or luciferase *(2,3)*. These viruses allow for rapid determination of the relative infection frequency in a culture. However, because quantitating these enzymes involves lysing the cells, these viruses cannot be used for experiments in which it is necessary to count single infected cells; the data generated reflect relative amounts of reporter gene product in the entire culture. In two infected cultures, one might have a large fraction of infected cells each expressing a small amount of enzyme, whereas the other culture might contain a small number of infected cells each producing a large quantity of the reporter enzyme. The cultures could show similar amounts of reporter gene activity. A second class of reporter virus contains marker genes such as heat stable antigen (CD24) *(4)*, Thy-1 *(5)*, alkaline phosphatase *(6)*, or green fluorescent protein *(7)*, that can be measured by flow cytometery or by microscopic counting of infected cells. These allow quantitation of the number of infected cells in a culture and the amount of reporter gene activity per cell. A third class of reporter virus includes those containing a selectable marker gene, for example, *gpt (8)*. These viruses allow counting of colonies arising from single infected cells and also allow isolation of individual infected cell clones for further analysis.

Replication-defective reporter viruses containing a mutation in *env* are particularly useful for studying virus entry, since they undergo only a single cycle of replication. Expression of the reporter gene requires only the early steps of the virus replication cycle (entry, reverse transcription, integration, and provirus transcription). Thus, later steps in virus replication (virus assembly and budding) are not measured. Furthermore, the viruses can be produced as pseudotypes bearing heterologous Env glycoproteins. This can allow for definitive studies on virus entry. Pseudotyping with amphotropic murine leukemia virus Env (A-MLV) *(9)* or with VSV-G *(10)* produces virus that enters cells independent of CD4 or chemokine receptors. These serve as controls for ruling out postentry effects on reverse transcription, integration, or provirus transcription. For example, the target of a drug that inhibits HIV replication can be rapidly determined using reporter viruses. If the drug inhibits reporter virus infection, it must target the first half of the virus life cycle. If A-MLV pseudotypes are also inhibited, the drug probably affects a postentry step somewhere between fusion and assembly. If M-tropic or T-tropic HIV-1 pseudotypes are inhibited, whereas A-MLV pseudotypes are not, then it is likely that inhibition is at entry implicating the entry coreceptors CCR5 or CXCR4, respectively, as the likely targets.

Luciferase reporter viruses have been particularly useful for detecting HIV coreceptor activity when used in combination with cultured cell lines stably expressing CD4 and various transfected coreceptor expression vectors *(11)*. HOS.CD4 and U87.CD4 cells expressing different CC-chemokine receptors or CXCR4 are available through the National Institutes of Health AIDS Research and Reference Reagent Program. HOS.CD4 cells have the advantage of rapid growth, but the disadvantage of expressing trace amounts of endogenous CXCR4 detectable by RT-PCR, but not by FACS (unpublished observations). Endogenous coreceptor expression can result in increased experimental background owing to a small amount of virus entry in the absence of transfected coreceptor. U87.CD4 cells, although being somewhat more difficult to culture, do not have detectable endogenous CXCR4 mRNA.

2. Materials

2.1. Plasmids

pNL-Luc-R⁻Env⁻ and pNL-Luc-R⁺-Env⁻ are based on the HIV-1 proviral clone pNL4-3 *(2,3)*. Both plasmids contain the firefly luciferase gene in the *nef* position, and are *env⁻* owing to a frameshift near its 5'-end. pNL-Luc-R⁻Env⁻ has a frameshift in *vpr*, such that the infected cells do not become arrested in G_2. The plasmids are prepared from *Escherichia coli* grown with ampicillin selection. M-tropic (JR.FL, ADA, BAL *[2]*, T-tropic (HXB2 *[8]*), and A-MLV *(9)* Env genes are cloned into the simian virus-40-based expression vector pSV7d.

2.2. Cell Lines

HOS and U87 cells are cultured in DMEM/10% FBS/1% penicillin/streptomycin. Suspension cells are cultured in RPMI/10% FBS/1% penicillin/streptomycin. To maintain long-term expression of chemokine receptors transduced by the retroviral vector pBABE-puro *(12)*, puromycin (1 μg/mL) is added to the medium.

2.3. Reagents for Ca_2PO_4 Transfection

1. 2X HBS: 1.0 g HEPES, 1.6 g NaCl, 0.074 g KCl, 0.025 g Na_2HPO_4 (for 7·H_2O use 0.047 g). Adjust pH to 7.05–7.15. Add dH_2O to 100 mL. Accurate pH and the amount of phosphate are crucial. Filter sterilize and store at 4°C.
2. 2.0 *M* $CaCl_2$: 29.40 g $CaCl_2$. H_2O. Add dH_2O to 100 mL. Filter sterilize.
3. Sterile dH_2O.

2.4. Reagents for Infection and Luciferase Assay

1. Polybrene (Sigma). Prepare an 8 mg/mL solution in PBS. Store at –20°C.
2. Luciferase assay substrate (Promega). Store at –20°C.
3. Lysis buffer (Promega). Store at –20°C.

3. Methods

3.1. Preparation of Reporter Virus Stocks

1. The day before transfection, seed 10-cm tissue culture dishes with 2×10^6 293 or 293T cells in 10 mL DMEM/10% FBS.
2. Cotransfect cells with a mixture of 10 µg luciferase reporter virus DNA, pNL-Luc-R$^-$ Env$^-$ and 10 µg Env expression vector DNA. EtOH precipitate the DNA and resuspend in 450 µL dH$_2$O. Add 70 µL 2 M CaCl$_2$. To the DNA CaCl$_2$ mixture, add 500 µL 2X HBS, dropwise. Incubate on ice for 30 min. Add the precipitate dropwise to a dish of cells.
3. Change medium 24 h posttransfection.
4. Harvest the supernatant 48 h posttransfection and remove cell debris by filtering through a 0.45-µm syringe filter.
5. Freeze the supernatant at –80°C in 1-µL aliquots. Quantitate virus by p24 ELISA or reverse transcriptase assay.

3.2. Infection of HOS.CD4 or U87.CD4 Transfectants with Luciferase Reporter Viruses

1. One day before infection, plate 5×10^3 HOS-CD4 or U87.CD4 cells expressing transduced chemokine receptors in 24-well plates in 1 mL DMEM/10% FBS (without puromycin).
2. Replace the medium with luciferase reporter virus (10 ng p24) in 0.5 mL DMEM/10% FBS. Polybrene can be added to the culture (8 µg/mL) to increase infectivity if desired.
3. Replace medium 5–18 h later.
4. Three days postinfection, harvest the culture. Wash the cells with 1 mL PBS, remove supernatant and resuspend in 200 µL commercial (Promega) lysis buffer. Incubate 2 min at room temperature and freeze at –80°C for subsequent assay.
5. Thaw cell lysate at 37°C; clarify lysate by centrifuging at 14,000 rpm for 2 min at 4°C. Take 20 µL of the supernatant for luciferase assay. Add 80 µL of luciferase substrate and measure in a luminometer or scintillation counter.

3.3. Infection of CEM Cells

1. CEM cells (3×10^4) are mixed with 10 ng p24 pseudotyped luciferase reporter viruses in 300 µL RPMI/10% FBS in 24-well plates. If desired, polybrene (8 µg/mL) can be added to increase infectivity.
2. After incubating 3–5 h at 37°C, add 0.5 mL RPMI/10% FBS.
3. Three days postinfection, transfer cells into 1.5-mL Eppendorf tubes and pellet cells at 1,200 rpm for 5 min.
4. Wash pellet once with PBS, lyse in 200 µL commercial lysis buffer and freeze in aliquots at –80°C.
5. Follow **step 5** above.

4. Notes

1. The viruses can be used to infect most any cell-line or primary cells such as peripheral blood mononuclear cells or monocytes. Primary cells generally should be assayed at later time points (d 5–10 postinfection).

2. High-efficiency transfection is important for getting reporter virus in usable amounts. If p24^{gag} levels are low (e.g., <50–100 ng/mL) there may be a problem. Transfection efficiencies can be improved by changing reagents or thawing new batches of 293 cells. 293 cells are delicate. If they are split from overly confluent dishes they are generally not in good shape for transfection the next day. We have not found that there is much difference between 293 and 293T with respect to virus production. We have not tried using cholorquine in transfections; however this might boost virus production significantly.

3. Promega luciferase substrate produces light efficiently but briefly with a half life of about 5 min. Luc-Lite reagents from Packard produce light with a longer half-life (in our hands, approx 1 h) which offers practical advantages.

4. Controlling for day to day consistency of the luciferase assay is recommended. This can be done using a highly dilute solution of pure luciferase enzyme (Sigma), and measuring a fixed amount of it for each independent experiment.

5. Reporter virus aliquots can be re-used with a loss of approx 50% activity on each freeze-thaw.

6. Some Envs work much better than others. The A-MLV and VSV-G will yield the most active viruses; BAL and HXB2 seem to be the weakest. We routinely use 5 ng instead of 10 ng p24^{gag} for A-MLV pseudotypes.

References

1. Helseth, E., Kowalski, M., Gabuzda, D., Olshevsky, U., Haseltine, W., and Sodroski, J. (1990) Rapid complementation assays measuring replicative potential of human immunodeficiency virus type 1 envelope glycoprotein mutants. *J. Virol.* **64,** 16–20.

2. Chen, B. K., Saksela, K., Andino, R., and Baltimore, D. (1994) Distinct modes of human immunodeficiency virus type 1 proviral latency revealed by superinfection of nonproductively infected cell lines with recombinant luciferase-encoding viruses. *J. Virol.* **68,** 654–660.

3. Connor, R. I., Chen, B. K., Choe, S., and Landau, N. R. (1995) Vpr is required for efficient replication of human immunodeficiency virus type-1 in mononuclear phagocytes. *Virology* **206,** 936–944.

4. He, J. Choe, S., Walker, R., Di Marzio, P., Morgan, D. O., and Landau, N. R. (1995) Human Immunodeficiency Virus Type-1 Viral Protein R (Vpr) arrests cells in the G2 phase of the cell cycle by inhibiting p34cdc2. *J. Virol.* **69,** 6705–6711.

5. Jowett, J. B., Planelles, V., Poon, B., Shah, N. P., Chen, M. L., and Chen, I. S. (1995) The human immunodeficiency virus type 1 vpr gene arrests infected T cells in the G2 + M phase of the cell cycle. *J. Virol.* **69,** 6304–6313.

6. He, J. and Landau, N. R. (1995) Use of a novel Human Immunodeficiency virus Type 1 reporter virus expressing human placental alkaline phosphatase to detect an alternative viral receptor. *J. Virol.* **69,** 4587–4592.

7. Page, K. A., Liegler, T., and Feinberg, M. B. (1997) Use of a green fluorescent protein as a marker for human immunodeficiency virus type 1 infection. *AIDS Res. Hum. Retroviruses.* **13,** 1077–1081.

8. Page, K. A., Landau, N. R., and Littman, D. R. (1990) Construction and use of a human immunodeficiency virus vector for analysis of virus infectivity. *J. Virol.* **64,** 5270–5276.

9. Landau, N. R., Page, K. A., and Littman, D. R. (1991) Pseudotyping with human T-cell leukemia virus type I broadens the human Immunodeficiency virus host range. *J. Virol.* **65,** 162–169.

10. Yee, J. K., Friedmann, T., and Burns, J. C. (1994) Generation of high-titer pseudotyped retroviral vectors with very broad host range. *Meth. Cell. Biol.* **43,** 99–112.

11. Deng, D., Liu, R., Ellmeier, W., Choe, S., Unutmaz, D., Burkhart, M., et al. (1996) Identification of a major co-receptor for primary isolates of HIV-1. *Nature* **381,** 661–666.

12. Morgenstern, J. P. and Land, H. (1990) Advanced mammalian gene transfer: high titre retroviral vectors with multiple drug selection markers and a complementary helper-free packaging cell line. *Nucleic Acids Res.* **18,** 3587–3596.

7

A Cell–Cell Fusion Assay to Monitor HIV-1 Env Interactions with Chemokine Receptors

Aimee L. Edinger and Robert W. Doms

1. Introduction

Biological membrane fusion is an important part of many cellular processes and is a critical step in the entry of enveloped viruses, such as HIV-1, into cells. For HIV-1 to infect cells, the virus must bind to the cell surface, after which the viral Env protein must be triggered to undergo a conformational change that mediates membrane fusion. Cell-surface binding has long been known to occur via a high-affinity interaction between Env and CD4. However, the cell-surface molecules responsible for triggering the fusion-inducing conformational change in the Env protein have been only recently identified, permitting the study of HIV-1 Env-mediated membrane fusion in much greater detail (for review, *see 1*). These molecules, termed coreceptors, have been shown to be members of the nine-transmembrane domain receptor family. The most important HIV-1 coreceptors are the chemokine receptors CCR5 and CXCR4 *(2–7)*, although at least nine other chemokine receptors or orphan receptors have been shown to support cellular entry for subsets of HIV-1 or SIV strains *(3,5,8–11)*. The ability of a given virus strain to utilize particular chemokine receptors is a major determinant of cellular tropism. Thus, it is desirable to identify the receptors used by virus strains in a rapid, quantitative, and reproducible manner.

To identify the repertoire of coreceptors that can be used by HIV-1, HIV-2, and SIV strains, to identify novel receptors, and to analyze Env-coreceptor interactions, we have refined the cell-cell fusion assay first described by Nussbaum *(12)*. In this assay, effector cells expressing the viral Env protein and T7 RNA polymerase are mixed with target cells expressing CD4, the desired coreceptor, and luciferase under the control of the T7 promoter *(5)*. T7

From: *Methods in Molecular Medicine, Vol. 17: HIV Protocols*
Edited by: N. L. Michael and J. H. Kim © Humana Press Inc., Totowa, NJ

polymerase is expressed via recombinant vaccinia virus, but all other constructs are expressed by transfection. If cell-cell fusion occurs, cytoplasmic mixing results in luciferase production and is readily quantifiable with high sensitivity (signal-to-noise ratios of 50–1000 to one can be routinely obtained) using a luminometer or scintillation counter with luminescence capabilities. Such a cell–cell fusion assay is ideally suited for screening envelope proteins cloned from primary isolates, for the study of mutant and chimeric receptors and envelopes, and for blocking studies with antibodies, chemokines, and inhibitory compounds. Advantages of the cell–cell fusion assay include:

1. The biosafety concerns associated with live HIV work are mitigated by studying the envelope in isolation from an infectious genome.
2. A large number of envelopes and coreceptors can be tested more quickly and easily than in intact virus systems.
3. Signals in this assay are often more robust than in infection assays, allowing the study of chimeras and mutants, which may give only weak signals by infection.
4. Blocking studies are performed with short incubation periods making the replenishment of expensive or scarce blocking reagents unnecessary.

It is important to remember, however, that there are occasional discrepancies between cell–cell fusion and infection assays. Once a result has been obtained in a cell–cell fusion system, it must be verified by infection studies, for instance, with luciferase reporter viruses and by infection of relevant primary cells when possible. Nonetheless, the fusion assay has proven to be a valuable technique in the study of HIV and SIV coreceptor utilization. For an in-depth discussion of the cell–cell fusion assay and its variations, the interested reader should refer to Rucker et al. *(13)*.

2. Materials
2.1. Cells and Media

1. The requirements for target cells are that they lack a functional coreceptor prior to transfection and that they are readily transfectable. We routinely use quail QT6 fibrosarcoma cells (ATCC # CRL-1708), since they give a low background signal and can be transfected with very high efficiency (up to 100%). These cells grow quite well in Dulbecco's modified Eagle's medium (DMEM) supplemented with 10% fetal calf serum (DMEM-10) and 2-mM penicillin-streptomycin if desired. This medium is used exclusively in our lab with no obvious ill-effects, although the recommended media is Medium 199 (M199, Gibco BRL,Gaithersburg, MD) supplemented with 1% chicken serum, 5% fetal calf serum, 2 mM glutamine, 2 mM penicillin-streptomycin, and 10% tryptose phosphate broth (29.5 g/L, Gibco BRL). Quail cells should not generally be split at ratios >1:10, since they grow best at higher cell densities; 1:2 or 1:4 splits are recommended.

2. The requirements for effector cells are that they show minimal cytopathic effect (CPE) with vaccinia infection and that they are readily transfectable. The envelope must also be correctly glycosylated and cleaved to gp120 + gp41 in the cells selected. Effector cells of several types have been used successfully in our lab. QT6 or human 293T cells are two suitable cell lines. 293T cells also grow well in DMEM-10.

3. Virus trypsin (bovine pancreatic trypsin, Sigma, St. Louis, MO) is prepared at 0.25 mg/mL and is stored in 1- to 5-mL aliquots at –20°C.

4. Rifampicin (Sigma) is used because it inhibits vaccinia virus assembly thereby minimizing CPE and background *(14)*. Rifampicin is prepared as a 1000X stock solution (100 mg/mL) in sterile DMSO and stored in aliquots at –20°C.

5. Cytosine arabinoside (AraC, Sigma) is also used to decrease background. AraC inhibits vaccinia virus DNA replication and transcription from the vaccinia late promoter. T7 RNA polymerase is under the control of the late promoter in the recombinant vaccinia vTF1.1 whereas vTF7.3 carries T7 RNA polymerase under the control of the synthetic early–late (SEL) promoter. For this reason, only vTF1.1 *(14)* should be used in this assay. AraC is prepared as a 100X stock solution (10 μM) in sterile water, and stored in aliquots at –20°C.

6. Other standard tissue culture supplies, such as 24-well plates, T25 flasks, cell trypsin/EDTA, sterile PBS, sterile 50- or 15-mL screw-cap tubes, sterile Eppendorfs, sterile pipets, and sterile pipet tips (filter tips should be used when working with vaccinia), will also be required. It is also necessary to maintain an incubator at 32°C for the overnight incubation of effector cells between days 1 and 2.

2.2. Expression Vectors

1. T7 polymerase is expressed in effector cells by the use of a recombinant vaccinia virus, vTF1.1 *(14)*. This recombinant vaccinia virus can be obtained from Bernard Moss (NIH, Bethesda, MD).

2. Envelopes can be expressed either by a recombinant vaccinia virus (*see* **Notes 1** and **2**) if one is available (making a recombinant vaccinia requires roughly 3 wk) or by transfection. This protocol describes the use of envelope expressed by transfection. Envelope constructs should be in a eukaryotic expression vector under the control of the CMV promoter (pcDNA3, Invitrogen, has been used with success by our lab).

3. Receptors and coreceptors must also be in eukaryotic expression vectors under the control of a constitutive promoter, such as the CMV promoter. Our lab generally uses receptors cloned into pcDNA3. It may be useful to prepare all receptors in the same vector to help standardize expression levels. It is always important to consider relative expression levels when comparing signals obtained with different receptors and chimeras (*see* **Note 3**).

2.3. Transfection Solutions

1. The DNA used for transfection should be pure, that is, prepared by cesium chloride gradient purification, PEG precipitation, or with a Qiagen kit (Chatsworth,

CA; in our hands, other kits have not given satisfactory results). Transfections are more variable and often fail with low quality DNA.

2. We use the calcium phosphate precipitation protocol for transfection. Other transfection protocols may be substituted, but this technique is relatively reliable and inexpensive. The transfection solutions used in our lab are:
   a. 0.5 M HEPES, pH 7.1 (pH is critical).
   b. 2.0 M NaCl.
   c. 1 M Na$_2$HPO$_4$, pH 7.0 (use phosphoric acid to adjust pH).
   d. 2.0 M CaCl$_2$.
   e. 10X NTE: 8.77 g NaCl; 10 mL 1 M Tris, pH 7.4, 4 mL 0.25 M EDTA, pH 8.0; bring up to 100 mL in sterile water.

   All solutions should be sterile-filtered before use and tested for efficacy before a large experiment is attempted owing to variable transfection efficiencies with different batches of transfection solutions.

2.4. Luminescence Reagents

1. When using the luciferase reporter gene, a luminometer or scintillation counter with luminescence capabilities is required. We use a Wallac (Turku, Finland) 1450 Microbeta Plus liquid scintillation counter.
2. Luciferase substrate may be purchased from Promega (Madison, WI).

3. Methods
3.1. Plating Cells for the Experiment

Cells are plated the day before the experiment, such that they are roughly 80% confluent on the following morning. For QT6 cells, this means plating at 50% confluence, and for 293T cells, at about 40% confluence. Target cells are prepared in 24-well plates, and effectors can be prepared in six wells, T25 flasks, or 10-cm dishes, depending on the number of effector cells needed. A T25 should easily provide cells for 8–10 different coreceptor wells.

3.2. Day 1: Preparing the Effector and Target Cells

1. Confluence of the effector cells is estimated, and cells are infected at an MOI of 10 with the vTF1.1 vaccinia encoding the T7 RNA polymerase (*see* **Note 4**). Enough virus for all effectors is trypsinized with an equal volume of virus trypsin for 30 min at 37°C with vortexing every 10 min. After 30 min, DMEM supplemented with 2.5% fetal calf serum is added to quench the trypsin and dilute the virus. The medium is aspirated from the effector cells and replaced with the medium containing virus. Infection volumes should be small, but cover the cells; 3 mL for a 10-cm dish and 1 ml for a T25 or six-well work well. Infection is allowed to proceed for 1 h at 37°C.
2. DNA mixes can be prepared during trypsinization. The chart below shows our standard protocols for transfection in various flasks and plates:

	DNA, µg	10X NTE, µL	2 *M* CaCl$_2$, µL	Total volume, µL
24 Well	2	2.5	3.1	25
6 Well	6	15	18.8	150
T25	15	25	31	250
10 cm dish	30	50	62.5	500

Sterile water is used to make up the mix to the total volume. DNA should be added last to avoid contamination and because it is the most precious reagent. Both envelope and target cell transfections must be prepared. Transfectant should be prepared in a batch for all wells with the same receptor/coreceptor combination. Plan for one extra well so that the last well transfected does not receive less transfectant than the others.

3. Just before transfection, the DNA mix is combined with an equal volume of freshly prepared 2X transfection buffer made with the following recipe: 1 mL 0.5 *M* HEPES, pH 7.1, 8.1 mL sterile water, 0.9 mL 2 *M* NaCl, 20 µL 1 *M* Na$_2$HPO$_4$, pH 7.0. The DNA and 2X transfection buffer are mixed by adding the DNA solution to the buffer **dropwise**, while vortexing at **low speed** (3 out of 10) just to aerate the mixture without actually forming a vortex. The solution should become cloudy following mixing. If the precipitate is chunky, it is likely that it was vortexed too hard during mixing, and it should be prepared again and mixed at a slower speed. Clear snap-cap tubes allow for evaluation of the quality of the precipitate formed, but microfuge tubes have also been used for mixing with success. Allowing the precipitate to stand at room temperature for 10–15 min may increase precipitate formation, but is not absolutely required. The amount of precipitant added should not exceed 10% of the volume of medium in the well to avoid dramatic pH changes.

4. Mixed transfection solution is added dropwise to the target cells, 50 µL/24-well. The plate is gently shaken front to back and side to side, and placed in a 37°C incubator for 4 h. At 4 h, media on the target cells should be replaced with 0.5–1 mL fresh DMEM-10. QT6 cells are very sensitive to calcium phosphate transfection and it is important to change the medium by 6 h posttransfection, or cell viability will be reduced.

5. One hour after the effectors were infected with vTF1.1, the medium is changed to DMEM-10, and the cells transfected using transfection mixes prepared as above. Transfectant is added dropwise, and the effectors are incubated at 37°C for 4 h when the medium is changed to DMEM-10 plus rifampicin. Rifampicin affects the subcellular localization of a vaccinia virus structural protein, thereby preventing the formation of new virus particles. This helps prevent introduction of nascent vTF1.1 into the target cells following cell mixing, which would result in nonspecific luciferase production. Rifampicin also reduces CPE in some cell types. Effectors are incubated overnight at 32°C to reduce vaccinia CPE further (*see* **Note 5**).

3.3. Day 2: Cell Mixing

1. Effector cells can generally be lifted from the plate simply by banging the flask, but cells will be easier to count (fewer clumps) if they are washed once very gently with PBS and then lifted with 0.5 mM EDTA in PBS (0.5 mL per T25 works well).

2. After 2–3 min, the EDTA is quenched by adding 5 mL DMEM-10 per T25. Effectors are transferred to 15 mL screw-cap tubes, and cells pelleted at 1000 rpm for 5–10 min at 4° in a tabletop centrifuge.

3. While preparing the effectors, the medium on the target cells should be replaced with 0.5 mL/24-well of DMEM-10 with rifampicin and AraC. Enough of this medium should be prepared to change the medium on the targets and to resuspend the effectors (about 1.5 mL per T25 of effectors).

4. Effector cells are washed with 5 mL cold (4°C) PBS and pelleted as above.

5. Effectors are resuspended in 5 mL cold PBS and counted with a hemocytometer. Remember that these cells contain vaccinia, and therefore, should be handled with care when manipulating them outside of the hood. Effector cells should be kept cold while counting to minimize background from vaccinia production.

6. Cells are pelleted as above and resuspended at $2–4 \times 10^6$ cells/mL in DMEM-10 with rifampicin and AraC.

7. Prepared effectors are added to the target cells, 50 μL/well, and incubated at 37°C for 7–8 h to allow cell-cell fusion.

8. To quantify fusion, cells are lysed by adding 150 μL of 0.5% NP-40 or TX-100 in PBS. Before lysing cells, it is often helpful to look for syncytia by eye to help localize problems when troubleshooting. Not all cell/envelope combinations form readily visible syncytia without staining; the presence of syncytia is meaningful, whereas its absence is difficult to interpret (*see* **Notes 6** and **7**).

9. We use a Wallac 1450 Microbeta Plus for luminescence counting (*see* **Note 8**). Solid white luminescence plates (Wallac) are loaded with 20 μL of cell lysate from the 24-well plates. When the entire plate is loaded, 50 μL of luciferase substrate is added rapidly with a multichannel pipeter, and the plate counted immediately, since luciferase has a short half-life. It is good practice to add luciferase under dim light, since it is light-sensitive (*see* **Note 9**).

10. Lysates may be frozen at −20 or −70°C, and thawed and recounted later, but signals will degrade 10–50% depending on how long the lysate is stored and should not be left more than several days without counting. Samples should be at room temperature when counted to obtain the maximum signal.

4. Notes

1. Vaccinia virus should be handled with Biosafety Level 2 procedures. Hoods should be sprayed down with 70% ethanol following virus use, and materials that have contacted virus should be bleached before disposal. *Current Protocols in Molecular Biology* contains a comprehensive chapter on the recombinant vaccinia system *(15)*. Protocols for vaccinia use at your institution should be investigated, and vaccination options discussed with Environmental Health and Safety personnel.

2. Recombinant vaccinia viruses can also be used to express the viral envelope in the effector cells. The signals with vaccinia-encoded envelopes are often higher, presumably owing to higher expression levels, and the experiments tend to show less day-to-day variability. Many vaccinia constructs encoding HIV envelope genes can be obtained from the National Institutes of Health AIDS Research and

Reference Reagent Program (NIH, Bethesda, MD) or the American Type Culture Collection (ATCC, Rockville, MD). HeLa cells are usually used as effectors, since they show minimal vaccinia CPE. Effectors are coinfected with the envelope vaccinia and vTF1.1 and the infection allowed to proceed for 2 h at 37°C. To prepare effectors for overnight incubation, they are:
   a. Washed with PBS.
   b. Trypsinized with trypsin/EDTA (GIBCO-BRL).
   c. Resuspended in 10 mL (10-cm dish) or 5 mL (T25 or 6-well) of DMEM-10.
   d. Spun at 1000 rpm in 50 mL screw-cap tubes in a tabletop centrifuge to pellet cells.
   e. Washed once with 10 or 5 mL of PBS.
   f. Resuspended in 10 or 5 mL of DMEM-10 with rifampicin and incubated overnight in a 32°C incubator in a rack tilted at about 30°C from horizontal (e.g., one side propped with a 96-well plate) to increase surface area for gas exchange. The following morning, cells are spun down and the protocol is the same starting at **Subheading 3.3.3.**

3. The fusion assay is a complicated procedure that can make troubleshooting difficult, and the intelligent use of positive and negative controls is essential. Positive controls should include (where possible): (a) Control envelopes that use the coreceptors of interest and (b) coreceptors that the envelope being studied is known to use. Negative controls should include: (a) CD4 without coreceptor and (b) CD4 with a nonfunctional receptor. Including envelopes that do not use a certain receptor (e.g., HIV-1 IIIB on CD4/CCR5) is very helpful in identifying contamination problems.

4. Preliminary work using a plasmid-encoded T7 RNA polymerase rather than vTF1.1 to eliminate vaccinia from this assay did not give acceptable signals when the envelope and T7 polymerase plasmid were cotransfected. This may relate to the fact that vaccinia replicates in the cytoplasm, whereas transfected DNA must be imported into the nucleus before translation. With further investigation, a plasmid-encoded T7 RNA polymerase might be successfully used in this assay.

5. Blocking studies have been successfully performed by shortening the time allowed for fusion to 5 h (if the experiment is allowed to proceed longer, blocking compounds are harder to evaluate owing to the robust fusion seen in this assay) and by preincubating target cells with the putative inhibitor for 30 min before the addition of effectors. Blocking protocols can be adapted to suit the individual experiment.

6. The problem most commonly encountered is no or low signal. If the protocol is re-examined and no obvious sources of error are uncovered and the envelope and coreceptors being evaluated are known to be functional and expressed on the cell surface, the most likely problem is transfection efficiency. One should begin by making new transfection solutions, and it may be worthwhile to check transfection efficiency using a reporter construct under the control of a constitutive promoter (e.g., ß-galactosidase under the CMV promoter). Duplicates using independently prepared transfection solutions may also be useful. Thawing new cells may also be beneficial, particularly if the cells have been passaged for long periods. Vaccinia is a hardy virus and is rarely the problem, but the vTF1.1 can

be retitered if problems persist. Plasmids should be checked for degradation by agarose-gel electrophoresis, and concentration verified from these gels. Mycoplasma infection should also be considered.

7. Another possible scenario is high background. Two potential sources of background are (a) the presence of a molecule on the surface of the target cells which can function as a viral receptor (e.g., a quail homolog of the receptor of interest) or (b) inadequate rifampicin, AraC, or washing resulting in residual or nascent vaccinia virus present during mixing. These problems should be distinguishable by visual examination prior to lysis; if there are syncytia in the negative control well (usually CD4 alone), then the problem is likely a receptor homolog. As mentioned above, QT6 cells are used as target cells owing to their extremely high transfection efficiency and their avian origin, which lessens the likelihood that they contain a functional HIV/SIV coreceptor. Other cells may be substituted as long as they are transfectable and endogenous coreceptors are considered. Another possible source of syncytia in the negative controls is contamination of a plasmid or vaccinia stock.

8. The detector system should be carefully evaluated. Detectors have detection limits above which they are no longer linear, and this can distort results. We use a Wallac 1450 Microbeta Plus for luminescence counting and have found that the linear range varies with the model. Pure luciferase is available from Promega and can be used to evaluate the linear range of your counter. Red luminescence foil (Wallac) is used to bring the signal into the linear range and to prevent crosstalk between wells. Clear filters can be used for lower signals. Ideally, the coincidence circuit should be turned off; alternatively, a linear relationship between luciferase concentration and cpm can be obtained by calculating the square root of sample cpm minus background cpm. Background cpm can be obtained by reading lysate from a nontransfected well. In addition, the amount of lysate and substrate suggested in this protocol have been determined to be appropriate under the experimental conditions described above. If changes are made in the protocol, it may be necessary to re-evaluate the amount of substrate required.

9. Both luciferase substrate and luminometers are expensive. This assay can be used with other, less-expensive reporter systems, although we have found the luciferase-based system to be the most sensitive. If ß-galactosidase is used as the reporter gene, care must be taken that the recombinant vaccinias employed do not also encode ß-galactosidase, which is sometimes used as a selection marker when making recombinant vaccinia viruses.

Reference

1. Doms, R. W. and Peiper, S. C. (1997) Unwelcome guests with master keys: How HIV uses chemokine receptors for cellular entry. *Virology* **235,** 179–190.
2. Alkhatib, G., Combadiere, C., Broder, C. C., Feng, Y., Kennedy, P. E., Murphy, P. M., and Berger, E. A. (1996) CC CKR5: A RANTES, MIP-1α, MIP-1ß receptor as a fusion cofactor for macrophage-tropic HIV-1. *Science* **272,** 1955–1958.
3. Choe, H., Farzan, M., Sun, Y., Sullivan, N., Rollins, B., Ponath, P. D., et al. (1996) The ß-chemokine receptors CCR3 and CCR5 facilitate infection by primary HIV-1 isolates. *Cell* **85,** 1135–1148.

4. Deng, H., Liu, R., Ellmeier, W., Choe, S., Unutmaz, D., Burkhart, M., et al. (1996) Identification of a major co-receptor for primary isolates of HIV-1. *Nature* **381,** 661–666.
5. Doranz, B. J., Rucker, J., Yi, Y., Smyth, R. J., Samson, M., Peiper, S. C., et al. (1996) A dual-tropic primary HIV-1 isolate that uses fusin and the ß-chemokine receptors CKR-5, CKR-3, and CKR-2b as fusion cofactors. *Cell* **85,** 1149–1158.
6. Dragic, T., Litwin, V., Allaway, G. P., Martin, S. R., Huang, Y., Nagashima, K. A., et al. (1996) HIV-1 entry into CD4+ cells is mediated by the chemokine receptor CC-CKR-5. *Nature* **381,** 667–673.
7. Feng, Y., Broder, C. C., Kennedy, P. E., and Berger, E. A. (1996) HIV-1 entry cofactor: functional cDNA cloning of a seven-transmembrane domain, G-protein coupled receptor. *Science* **272,** 872–877.
8. Deng, H., Unutmaz, D., Kewalramani, V. N., and Littman, D. R. (1997) Expression cloning of new receptors used by simian and human immunodeficiency viruses. *Nature* **388,** 296–300.
9. Farzan, M., Choe, H., Martin, K., Marcon, L., Hofmann, W., Karlsson, G., et al. 1997. Two orphan seven-transmembrane segment receptors which are expressed in CD4-positive cells support simian immunodeficiency virus infection. *J. Exp. Med.* **186,** 405–411.
10. Liao, F., Alkhatib, G., Peden, K. W. C., Sharma, G., Berger, E. A., and Farber, J. M. (1997) STRL33, a novel chemokine receptor-like protein, functions as a fusion cofactor for both macrophage-tropic and T cell line-tropic HIV-1. *J. Exp. Med.* **185,** 2015–2023.
11. Rucker, J., Edinger, A. L., Sharron, M., Samson, M., Lee, B., Berson, J. F., et al. (1997) Utilization of chemokine receptors, orphan receptors, and herpesvirus encoded receptors by diverse human and simian immunodeficiency viruses. *J. Virol.* **71,** 8999–9007.
12. Nussbaum, O., Broder, C. C., and Berger E. A. (1994) Fusogenic mechanisms of enveloped-virus glycoproteins analyzed by a novel recombinant vaccinia virus-based assay quantitating cell fusion-dependent reporter gene activation. *J. Virol.* **68,** 5411–5422.
13. Rucker, J., Doranz, B. J., Edinger, A. E., Long, D., Berson, J. F., and Doms, R. W. (1997) Use of a cell-cell fusion assay to study the role of chemokine receptors in human immunodeficiency virys type 1 (HIV-1) entry. *Meth. Enzymol.* **288,** 118–133.
14. Moss, B., Rosenblum, E. N., Katz, E., and Grimley, P. M. (1969) Rifampicin: a specific inhibitor of vaccinia virus assembly. *Nature* **224,** 1280–1284.
15. Earl, P. and Moss, B. (1991) Expression of proteins in mammalian cells using vaccinia viral vectors, in *Current Protocols in Molecular Biology* (Ausubel, F. M., Brent, R., Kingston, R. E., Moore, D. D., Seidman, J. G., Smith, J. A., et al., eds.), Wiley-Interscience, New York, pp. 16.15.1–16.18.10.

8

Methods of Culturing HIV-1 from Semen

Bruce L. Gilliam

1. Introduction

The predominant mode of transmission of HIV-1 worldwide is sexual intercourse. Therefore, there has been growing interest in studying HIV-1 in genital secretions. Given the urgency to develop a vaccine to protect against HIV-1, techniques have been developed to isolate and quantitate HIV-1 from genital secretions.

Semen is a major vehicle in the transmission of HIV-1. In order to be able to develop effective vaccines and decrease transmission of HIV-1, the qualities of HIV-1 in semen must be carefully characterized. Recovery of the virus from semen is integral to this goal. This may be done in a qualitative, semiquantitative, or quantitative manner. However, even in experienced laboratories, the yield of HIV-1 seminal cell cocultures is 9–50% *(1,2,4–10,13–16)*. The yield of seminal plasma cocultures is worse, usually <15% *(1,2,5–9,15,16)*. Because of this fact, it is very important to optimize collection and processing of specimens.

The protocol presented here describes the qualitative culture of seminal cells and plasma for HIV-1 as previously described by Vernazza et al. *(1)*. It can be easily adapted to be semiquantitative or quantitative (*see* **Note 16**).

2. Materials
2.1. Specimen Collection

1. Viral transport medium (VTM) or alternative medium (i.e., HBSS, PBS, RPMI): This can be easily prepared using the following formula and stored at 4°C for 6 mo. The final concentrations of the components are 200 U/mL of nystatin, 1000 U/mL of penicillin, and 1000 µg/mL of streptomycin (*see* **Note 1**).

From: *Methods in Molecular Medicine, Vol. 17: HIV Protocols*
Edited by: N. L. Michael and J. H. Kim © Humana Press Inc., Totowa, NJ

   a. 1 mL penicillin/streptomycin (100,000 U/mL each).
   b. 2 mL nystatin suspension (10,000 U/mL).
   c. RPMI 1640 to bring to 100 mL.
2. Sterile specimen container.

2.2. Ficoll-Hypaque Isolation of PBMC

See protocol as described in Chapter 38.

2.3. Qualitative Seminal Cell
and Seminal Plasma Culture Procedure

1. Fresh semen (*see* **Note 17**).
2. Hank's buffered saline solution (HBSS) or phosphate-buffered saline (PBS).
3. Culture medium (*see* **Note 2.**): RPMI 1640 medium, 2 mM glutamine, 20% heat-inactivated fetal bovine serum (FBS), 5% human interleukin-2 (IL-2), 100 U/mL penicillin, 100 µg/mL streptomycin.
4. PBMC suspension.
5. Hemocytometer.
6. Trypan blue, 0.4%.
7. Incubator with temperature, CO_2, and humidity controls.
8. Low-speed centrifuge (Model GPR-5, Beckman Instruments, or equivalent).
9. p24 antigen assay (Coulter, Hialeah, FL).

3. Methods

3.1. Specimen Collection

1. The subject is asked to refrain from any form of sexual activity for 48 h prior to semen donation (*see* **Note 4**).
2. The subject cleans the head of the penis with a Rantex or similar medicated towel to remove dead skin and loose bacteria (*see* **Note 5.**)
3. The subject masturbates without the use of lubricants and avoids touching the area of the penis near the urethral meatus (*see* **Note 6**).
4. The subject ejaculates into a sterile specimen container being careful not to touch the inside of the container with his hands or penis (*see* **Note 7**).
5. VTM or alternative medium is added to semen as soon as possible following ejaculation (*see* **Notes 1** and **11**). If specimen is produced near lab facility, the semen should be diluted 1:1 with medium as soon as possible. If specimen produced away from a lab facility, a standard amount of VTM (usually 2.5–3.0 mL) should be added by the patient immediately following ejaculation (*see* **Note 8**).
6. Transport specimen to laboratory and begin processing within 4 h of ejaculation (*see* **Note 9**).

3.2. Ficoll-Hypaque Isolation of PBMC

See protocol in Chapter 38. Note that in this protocol, the target concentration of the PBMC is 2×10^6 PBMC/mL (*see* **Note 10**).

3.3. Qualitative Seminal Cell Culture Procedure

1. Semen volume is measured, and semen is diluted 1:1 with VTM or alternative medium (*see* **Notes 1** and **11**).
2. Diluted, well-mixed semen is placed in a 15-mL conical tube and centrifuged at 600g (approx 1800 rpm) for 15 min (*see* **Note 12**).
3. Seminal plasma is carefully pipeted off and seminal cells are resuspended with 10 mL of HBSS (*see* **Note 13**).
4. Resuspended cells are centrifuged at 600g for 10 min.
5. Supernatant is carefully pipeted off or discarded by single-motion pouring while being careful not to disturb the cell pellet.
6. The supernatant is discarded, and the seminal cells are resuspended in 10 mL of HBSS. The cell suspension is then centrifuged at 600g for 10 min (*see* **Note 14**).
7. The seminal cells are resuspended in 3 mL of culture medium. Half of the cells (1.5 mL) are placed in a 25 mL culture flask containing 3.5 mL of culture medium. To this flask, 5 mL of 2×10^6 PBMC/mL with 100 µL of nystatin suspension (10,000 U/mL) and 40 µL of penicillin/streptomycin are added (*see* **Notes 10, 15,** and **16**).
8. The culture flask is then placed in a 37°C, 5% CO_2, 95% humidity incubator with the cap loosened.
9. The remaining seminal cells should be mixed 1:1 with freezing medium and frozen in approx 1-mL aliquots at –70°C for 24 h. The aliquots should then be moved to liquid nitrogen for storage (*see* **Note 17**).
10. Half of the culture medium is removed twice weekly (without disturbing the cells at the bottom of the flask) and is alternately replaced with 2×10^6 PBMC/mL and culture medium alone.
11. The supernatant is removed and tested for either p24 antigen (according to the manufacturer's instructions) on d 14 and 21. The culture is considered positive if the supernatant contains more than 30 pg/mL of p24 antigen.
12. If the culture is positive, the isolate may be harvested by removing the supernatant, centrifuging it at 600g for 10 min, and freezing the resulting supernatant at –70°C. It may also be frozen as a mixture of cells and supernatant.

3.4. Qualitative Seminal Plasma Culture Procedure

1. Follow **steps 1–3** of **Subheading 3.3.**
2. Pass approx 1–1.5 mL of seminal plasma through a 0.45 µm filter, and place 0.5 mL of filtered seminal plasma in a small, snap-cap tube (*see* **Notes 18** and **19**).
3. Add 1 mL of PBMC suspension (2×10^6 PBMC/mL) made with HBSS or RPMI to the seminal plasma (*see* **Notes 2** and **10**).
4. Incubate the seminal plasma and PBMC at 37°C and 5% CO_2 for 1.5–4 h (*see* **Note 20**).
5. After the incubation, wash the cells with 2 mL of HBSS and centrifuge at 600g for 5 min (*see* **Note 20**).
6. Decant the supernatant, resuspend the cells in 2 mL of HBSS, and centrifuge at 600g for 5 min.

7. Decant the supernatant, resuspend the cells in 1 mL of culture medium (*see* **Notes 2** and **10**), and transfer to a well of a 24-well plate (*see* **Notes 21** and **22**).

8. Maintain and test cultures as described in **steps 10–12** of the seminal cell culture procedure.

4. Notes

1. Viral transport medium is not essential, but it may decrease bacterial and fungal contamination. In addition, tlhe use of VTM may, by suppressing bacterial and fungal growth, enhance viral recovery. As listed, alternative media which may be used to dilute the semen include HBSS, PBS, or RPMI.

2. Contamination of the culture may be reduced by the use of antimicrobials in the medium, Antimicrobials are not toxic to the cells and do not affect culture results *(1)*. In feeding cultures, it may be beneficial to use a total of 5X penicillin/strep-tomycin and 1X nystatin. This is described in **Note 10**. It is important to note that the use of antimicrobials in semen culture has not been documented to improve culture recovery and good, careful technique may obviate the need for them.

3. PBMC can be counted with either trypan blue or Turk's solution. The only advantage to trypan blue is the ability to determine cell viability. If one is unfamiliar with the cell viability of PMBC in the lab, it would be wise to use trypan blue.

4. It is important that the subject refrain from sexual activity for at least 48 h. The number of white blood cells (WBC) in semen decreases with frequent ejaculation. Therefore, a recent ejaculation prior to donation by the patient may decrease the number of WBC in the semen and thus the culture yield.

5. Rantex towels contain 50% witch hazel and 7% alcohol and serve to remove dead skin cells and loose bacteria. They are generally used by patients to clean around the urethra for a clean-catch urine collection. Any similar product may be used.

6. It is also important that care be taken by the patient not to use saliva or other lubricants to masturbate with, since this may increase risk of contamination and inhibit viral recovery. Interrupted sexual intercourse (anal, vaginal, or oral) is unacceptable for the above reasons.

7. It is a good idea to record time of ejaculation, time of initial processing, and the time culture is completed.

8. The use of a standard amount of VTM in a snap-cap tube for the patient to add, although not as exact as a 1:1 dilution, may be advantageous when patients are reluctant or unable to ejaculate in the lab, clinic, or hospital setting. It is recommended to keep the VTM refrigerated until use.

9. It is important to remove the seminal plasma from the cells quickly because the seminal plasma is toxic to the cells. Vernazza et al. have shown that culture yield decreases the longer cells are exposed to seminal plasma *(1)*. The semen should be allowed to liquify prior to processing. This usually occurs in 20–30 min.

10. If the decision is made to use antimicrobials, the following concentrations are recommended. For initial culture, additional antibiotics are added to the PBMC in order to obtain overall concentration of 5X penicillin/streptomycin and 1X nystatin in the culture. Therefore, it is necessary to add 8X penicillin/streptomy-

cin (i.e., 8 μL of penicillin/streptomycin/mL of PBMC suspension) and 2X nystatin (i.e., 20 μL of nystatin/mL of PBMC suspension). Remember that the culture medium already has 1X penicillin/streptomycin. For feeding cultures, 4X penicillin/streptomycin (i.e., 4 μL of penicillin/streptomycin/mL of PBMC or culture medium) and 1X nystatin (i.e., 10 μL of nystatin/mL of PBMC of culture medium) are added to the culture medium (*see* **Note 2**).

11. It is a good idea to record semen volume prior to dilution, or if already diluted with a standard volume of VTM, to record this volume.

12. It is important to mix the semen and medium well, but gently, in order to avoid lysing the seminal cells.

13. Semen can be very viscous at times, especially in late-stage AIDS patients. It can be difficult at times to remove the seminal plasma without disturbing the cell pellet. Techniques that sometimes work are centrifuging again, using a small pipet (i.e., 1–2 mL pipet) and aspirating carefully as far from the pellet as possible, and leaving some seminal plasma behind and washing with HBSS. At times, with extremely viscous specimens, a large portion of the seminal plasma may need to be left to maintain the integrity of the cell pellet. This seminal plasma is removed by washing with HBSS. In andrology labs, incompletely liquefied viscous semen has been passed through a 19-gauge needle to decrease viscosity. However, introducing needles into a retrovirology lab presents risks to the lab personnel and using this method could shear DNA that is present. An alternative is to try passing the semen through a micropipet tip which removes the risk of hollow needle exposure.

14. It is not important to separate the WBC from the spermatozoa, since the spermatozoa do not interfere with HIV-1 recovery in culture. In addition, Ficoll-Hypaque separation does lead to loss of some WBC in the separation process.

15. If the cell pellet is small, or one does not wish to freeze cells, the whole cell pellet can be used in culture.

16. Quantitative seminal cell culture can be done by using a protocol adapted from the ACTG PBMC microculture assay *(4)*. If one wishes to do quantitative seminal cell culture, at **step 7** half of the cells (1.5 mL) would be taken and added to a small snap-cap tube with 1.5 mL of culture medium (Tube A). Add 2.4 mL of culture medium to 5 more small snap-cap tubes making sure to label them (Tubes B-F). Then remove 600 μL from tube A after careful mixing, and place in tube B. Continue to make fivefold dilutions by adding 600 μL of each dilution to the next tube. Make sure to change pipet tips with each transfer to a new tube. A 24-well plate is used for the culture, and the culture is done in duplicate wells. One milliliter of each dilution is placed in the appropriate two wells for that dilution, with each well already containing 1 mL of PBMC with extra antibiotics. Like the qualitative culture, the culture is monitored by p24 antigen on d 14 and 21. The number and pattern of wells positive by p24 antigen are used to obtain quantitative results. This is done by reference to an algorithm published by Myers *(11)*. The results can be expressed as infectious units/ejaculate. If one wishes to be more quantitative, the protocol by Anderson to count the WBC in semen may be followed *(12)*. The results may then be expressed as infectious units /WBC.

17. Frozen cells may be snap-thawed and cultured. When done quantitatively, this results in approx a one dilution drop in recovery of HIV-1 from the culture plate.
18. Filtering the seminal plasma may improve culture recovery by removal of potential contaminants.
19. This culture can be performed with more than 0.5 mL of seminal plasma if more sample is available. The volumes of reagents have to be adjusted for larger amounts of seminal plasma. Although it would seem that this would increase the culture recovery rate, there is no data to support or refute this at the present time.
20. The incubation should be carried out in media without FBS, since it has been shown to enhance the toxicity of the seminal plasma on cells *(1)*. The standard incubation period is 1.5 h; however, it may enhance HIV-1 recovery to extend the incubation to 4 h. There is no evidence documenting this at the present, but Vernazza et al. *(1)* have shown that increasing the incubation time to 4 h does not significantly increase toxicity in the absence FBS. An incubation period <1.5 h would not be recommended, since it might not allow adequate time for the virus to infect the cells.
21. Given the poor culture recovery of seminal plasma culture, there is little to no experience with quantitative seminal plasma culture. It could, however, be done in a method similar to quantitative seminal cell culture.
22. It is not necessary to use a 24-well plate to perform this culture. It has been convenient in some experiments, but any culture flask or plate may be used that can contains the appropriate volume.

References

1. Vernazza, P. L., Eron, J. J., and Fiscus, S.A. (1996) Sensitive method for the detection of infectious HIV in semen of seropositive individuals. *J. Virol. Methods* **56,** 33–40.
2. Van Voorhis, B., Martinez, A., Mayer, K., and Anderson, D. J. (1991) Detection of human immunodeficiency virus type 1 in semen from seropositive men using culture and polymerase chain reaction deoxyribonucleic acid amplification techniques. *Fertil. Steril.* **55,** 588–594.
3. Mermin, J. H., Holodniy, M., Katzenstein, D. A., and Merigan, T. C. (1991) Detection of human immunodeficiency virus DNA and RNA in semen by the polymerase chain reaction. *JID* **164,** 769–772.
4. Dyer, J., Gilliam, B. L., Eron, J. J. Jr., Grosso, L., Cohen, M. S., and Fiscus, S. (1996) Quantitation of human immunodeficiency virus type 1 RNA in cell-free seminal plasma: comparison of NASBA and amplicor reverse transcription PCR amplification. *J. Virol. Methods* **60,** 161–170.
5. Vernazza, P. L., Eron, J. J. Jr., Cohen, M. S., van der Horst, C. M., Troiani, L., and Fiscus, S. A. (1994) Detection and biologic characterization of infectious HIV-1 in semen of seropositive men. *AIDS* **8,** 1325–1329.
6. Krieger, J. N., Coombs, R. W., Collier, A. C., Koehler, J. K., Ross, S. O., Chaloupka, K., et al. (1991) Fertility parameters in men infected with human immunodeficiency virus. *JID* **164,** 464–469.

7. Krieger, J. N., Coombs, R. W., Collier, A. C., Ross, S. O., Speck, C., Corey, L. (1995) Seminal shedding of human immunodeficiency virus type 1 and human cytomegalovirus: evidence for different immunologic controls. *JID* **171**, 1018–1022.
8. Krieger, J. N., Coombs, R. W., Colllier, A. C., Ross, S. O., Zeh, J. E., et al. (1995) Intermittent shedding of human immunodeficiency virus in semen: implications for sexual transmission. *J. Urol.* **154**, 1035–1040.
9. Anderson, D. J., O'Brien, T. R., Politch, J. A., Martinez, A., Seage, G. R. III, Padian N., et al. (1992) Effects of disease stage and zidovudine therapy on the detection of human immunodeficiency virus type 1 in semen. *JAMA* **267**, 2769–2774.
10. Gilliam, B. L., Dyer, J., Fiscus, S. A., Marcus, C., Zhou, S., Wathen, L., Freimuth, W. W., Cohen, M. S., Eron, J. J. Jr. (1997) Effects of reverse transcriptase inhibitor therapy on HIV-1 viral burden in semen. *J. Acquir. Immun. Defic. Syndr. Hum. Retrovirol.* **15**, 54–60.
11. Myers, L. E., McQuay, L. J., and Hollinger, F. B. (1994) Dilution assay statistics. *J. Clin. Microbiol.* **32**, 732–739.
12. Wolff, H., and Anderson, D. J., (1988) Immunohistologic characterization and quantitation of leukocyte subpopulations in human semen. *Fertil. Steril.* **49**, 497–504.
13. Vernazza, P. L., Gilliam, B. L., Dyer, J., Fiscus, S. A., Eron, J. J., Frank, A. C., and Cohen, M. S. (1997) Quantitation of HIV in semen: Correlation with antiviral treatment and immune status. *AIDS* **11**, 987–993.
14. Vernazza, P. L., Gilliam, B. L., Flepp, M., Dyer, J. R., Frank, A. C., Fiscus, S. A., et al. (1997) Effect of antiviral treatment on shedding of HIV-1 in semen. *AIDS* **11**, 1249–1254.
15. Krieger, J. N., Coombs, R. W., Collier, A. C., Ross, S. O., Chaloupka, K., Cummings, D. K., et al. (1991) Recovery of human immunodeficiency virus type 1 from semen: minimal impact of stage of infection and current antiviral chemotherapy. *JID* **163**, 386–388.
16. Cooms, R. W., Speck, C. E., Hughes, J. P., Lee, W., Sampoleo, R., Ross, S. O., et al. (1998) Association between culturable human immunodeficiency virus type 1 (HIV-1) in semen and HIV-1 RNA levels in semen and blood: evidence for compartmentalization of HIV-1 between semen and blood. *JID* **177**, 320–330.

II

MOLECULAR BIOLOGY

Select vaccine reflects this quasi-species state

9

Detection of HIV-1 Nucleic Acids by Southern Blotting

Richard A. McDonald

1. Introduction

Replication of the human immunodeficiency virus type 1 (HIV-1) is associated with a high degree of viral sequence variation *(1)* that has been shown to correlate with disease state *(2–8)*. The genetic diversity of the viral swarm within an HIV-1 infected individual is so extensive that this entity has been termed as quasi-species. Geographic distributions of HIV-1 reveal sequence clustering into a major group M and a minor (outlier) group O. Group M HIV-1s are further divided into a growing number of subtypes (A through H at this writing). Although DNA sequence analysis is the gold standard technique for HIV-1 genetic subtyping, molecular hybridization of untyped viral sequences with subtype-specific probes is frequently used as a subtyping screen.

This chapter will discuss HIV-1 specific molecular hybridization using the general DNA transfer/hybridization technique pioneered by E. M. Southern *(9)* universally known as "Southern blotting." Southern blotting is a method that transfers DNA fragments from an agarose gel onto nitrocellulose or nylon membranes. The membrane is then probed with a labeled double-stranded DNA (dsDNA), oligonucleotide, or complementary RNA probe specific to a DNA sequence of interest.

Although there are many techniques available for Southern blotting, this chapter will describe a method for genomic DNA isolation from cells and tissue, two DNA transfer (blotting) techniques, and two methods of generating nonradioactive hybridization probes. For the purposes of this chapter, dsDNA will be used as the probe for genomic DNA while oligonucleotides will be used as the probe for PCR products.

From: *Methods in Molecular Medicine, Vol. 17: HIV Protocols*
Edited by: N. L. Michael and J. H. Kim © Humana Press Inc., Totowa, NJ

2. Materials
2.1. Solutions and Buffers for Genomic DNA Isolation

1. 1X Phosphate-buffered saline (PBS): PBS (magnesium and calcium-free). PBS may be conveniently obtained commercially in sterile bottles. If desired, it may be made using the following recipe and sterile filtered:
   a. 1.15 g anhydrous Na_2HPO_4.
   b. 0.23 g anhydrous NaH_2PO_4.
   c. 9.00 g NaCl.
   d. Distilled H_2O to 950 mL; adjust pH to between 7.2 and 7.4 with either 1 M HCl or 1 M NaOH; add distilled H_2O to 1000 mL.
   e. Filter sterilize by passage through a 0.45-μM pore size filter unit.
2. Mammalian cell lysis buffer: 10 mM Tris-HCl, pH 7.4 (autoclaved), 20 mM ethylenediamine tetra-acetic acid (EDTA), 200 mM NaCl, 0.5% sodium dodecyl sulfate (SDS) and 100 µg/mL freshly prepared proteinase K.
3. Extraction buffer: Phenol/chloroform/isoamyl alcohol (25:24:1). The phenol is buffer-equilibrated and treated with 8-hydroxyquinoline.
4. Precipitation solution: Ammonium acetate (final concentration of 3 M) and 200-proof ethanol.
5. TE buffer: 10 mM Tris-HCl, pH 8.0 (autoclaved) and 1 mM EDTA.
6. RNA degradation dolutions:
   a. DNA (A): DNase-free RNase A.
   b. DNA (B): 0.5% SDS and 100 µg/mL proteinase K (final concentration).

2.2 Solutions, Buffers and Materials for Blotting and Hybridization

1. Gel running buffer for genomic DNA (1X TBE Buffer): 90 mM Tris-borate and 1 mM EDTA.
2. Gel running buffer for PCR products (1X TAE Buffer): 40 mM Tris-acetate, pH 8.0, and 1 mM EDTA.
3. Agarose: A high quality agarose.
4. Membrane filter: Nitrocellulose or nylon.
5. Blotting paper or paper towels.
6. Whatman 3MM paper.
7. Gel denaturation solution for genomic DNA (A): 0.5 N NaOH and 1.5 M NaCl.
8. Gel neutralization solution for genomic DNA (B): 0.5 M Tris-HCl (pH 7.4) and 1.5 M NaCl.
9. Gel depurination solution for PCR products: 0.25 N HCl.
10. Gel denaturation solution for PCR products (C): 0.4 N NaOH
11. Gel neutralization solution for PCR products: (D) 0.25 M Tris-acetate, pH 8.0, and 0.1 M NaCl. (E) 0.025 M Tris-acetate, pH 8.0, and 0.01 M NaCl.
12. Reagents supplied by Amersham's enhanced chemiluminesence (ECL™) system: Hybridization component, blocking agent, blocking buffer, fluorescein-11-dUTP, antifluorescein-horseradish peroxidase (HRP)-conjugate nucleotide mix,

primers, DNA polymerase (Klenow fragment), cacodylate buffer, terminal transferase, and detection reagents 1 and 2.

13. 20X SSC: 3 M NaCl and 0.3 M Na$_3$citrate.
14. Hybridization buffer (dsDNA probing genomic DNA): 0.5X SSC, 0.1 % SDS, 0.5% blocking agent, 5% dextran sulfate and 100 µg/mL boiled, sheared, heterologous, herring sperm DNA.
15. Hybridization buffer (oligonucleotide probing for PCR products): 5X SSC, 0.02% SDS, 0.1% of hybridization component and 1X liquid block.
16. Labeling dsDNA (random prime labeling, for dsDNA >2,500 bp): 200 ng dsDNA (50 ng/µL) (*see* **Note 1**), 10 µL fluorescein-11-dUTP, 10 µL nucleotide mix, 5 µL primers, 1 µL Klenow (4 U) and distilled water to 50 µL. Incubate for 1 h at 37°C and terminate with 20 mM EDTA and store at –20°C (*see* **Note 2**). Assume 100% labeling efficiency (*see* **Note 3**).
17. Labeling of probe (3'-end) for PCR products: 100 pmoles oligonucleotide, 10 mL fluorescein-11-dUTP, 16 µL cacodylate buffer, 112.9 to 144 µL water and 16 µL terminal transferase. Incubate at 37°C for 60–90 min and store at –20°C (*see* **Note 2**). Assume 100% labeling efficiency (*see* **Note 3**).
18. Wash buffer for genomic DNA:
    a. (A) 1X SSC and 0.1%SDS.
    b. (B) 0.5X SSC and 0.1% SDS.
19. Wash buffer for PCR products: (C) 5X SSC and 1% SDS. (D) 1X SSC and 1% SDS.
20. Antibody wash buffer: 100 mM Tris-HCl, pH 7.5, and 150 mM NaCl.
21. Buffer 1: 0.15 M NaCl and 0.1 M Tris-HCl, pH 7.5.
22. Buffer 2: 0.4 M NaCl and 0.1 M Tris-HCl, pH 7.5.
23. BSA-fraction V.

3. Methods

Prior to starting, one must first observe the biosafety handling of HIV infected material.

3.1. Genomic DNA Isolation from Primary Human Monocyte/Macrophages, T Lymphocyte, or Neoplastic Cell Lines

1. For the nonadherent cells, pellet cells by centrifugation at 300g for 10 min at 4°C.
2. Lyse the cell pellet with 1 mL of the mammalian cell lysis buffer. For the monocyte/macrophages wash in 1X PBS in flask; and then lyse with 1–5 mL of the mammalian cell lysis buffer (*see* **Note 4**).
3. Transfer the viscous solution to an appropriate size tube (*see* **Note 5**) and incubate at 37°C overnight on a mechanical rocker at gentle speed.
4. Extract with equal volume of the extraction buffer twice with chloroform/isoamyl alcohol. Centrifuge at 208g for 10 min.
5. Precipitate DNA with the precipitation solution (*see* **Note 6**). Centrifuge at 208g for 10 min.
6. Wash genomic DNA sequentially with 70, 95, and 100% ethanol (*see* **Note 7**).

7. Resuspend DNA in 5–10 mL of TE, and incubate overnight at 37°C on a mechanical rocker at gentle speed (*see* **Note 8**).
8. Add 50 μg/μL the RNA degradation Solution A, and incubate for 1 h at 37°C on a mechanical rocker at gentle speed.
9. Add the RNA degradation solution B.
10. Repeat **steps 3–6**, and resuspend DNA in 2–5 mL TE (*see* **Note 8**).
11. Incubate overnight at 37°C on a mechanical rocker at gentle speed.
12. Check for the quality and for the integrity of the DNA by OD (*see* **Note 9**) and on a 0.7% agarose gel.

3.2. Tissue Genomic DNA Isolation

1. The tissue is first minced in 1X PBS then homogenized with a Dounce homogenizer in 1X PBS.
2. After homogenizing the tissue, the protocol is as for the cells in **Subheading 3.1.**

3.3. Southern Blotting

Genomic DNA can be digested (partial or complete) with one or more restriction endonucleases for either localizing a gene or for cloning purposes. The DNA is separated according to size by electrophoresis (as with the PCR products) through an agarose gel. In general, at least 10 μg of digested genomic DNA is needed for a good genomic analysis.

1. Load genomic DNA (*see* **Note 10**) and PCR product with appropriate molecular weight markers in the appropriate percent agarose gels (*see* **Note 12**) and run in the appropriate gel running buffer (*see* **Note 8**). Voltage also varies with genomic DNA as well as with PCR products (*see* **Note 13**).
2. After electrophoresis, soak the gel for 20 min at room temperature in running buffer adjusted to 0.5 μg/mL ethidium bromide. Visualize the gel with UV transillumination and photograph. Cut the loading wells off the gel and a corner for orientation of the gel during transfer.
3. For genomic DNA, soak the gel in the denaturation solution A (*see* **Note 14**) for 1 h at ambient temperature with agitation, briefly rinse the gel in distilled water, and soak the gel in neutralization solution B for 1 h at ambient temperature with agitation, then rinse in distilled water.
4. For PCR products, soak the gel first in the depurination solution for PCR products for 15 min at ambient temperature with agitation, then rinse in distilled water, and soak twice in denaturation solution C for 15 min at ambient temperature with agitation with distilled water rinses between soaks. Following this, soak the gel in the neutralization solution D for 15 min at ambient temperature with agitation, rinse in distilled water, then soak in neutralization solution E for 15 min at ambient temperature with agitation and then rinse with distilled water.
5. For the gel containing genomic DNA, soak for 10 min in 10X transfer buffer, and for the gel containing the PCR products soak in 1X transfer buffer.

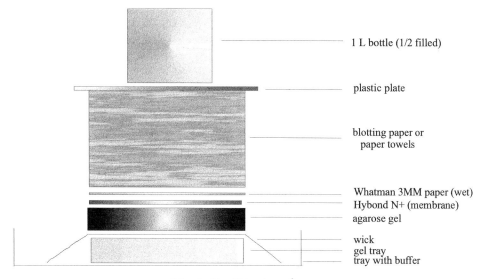

Fig. 1. Capillary transfer.

1 L bottle (1/2 filled)

plastic plate

blotting paper or
paper towels

Whatman 3MM paper (wet)
Hybond N+ (membrane)
agarose gel

wick
gel tray
tray with buffer

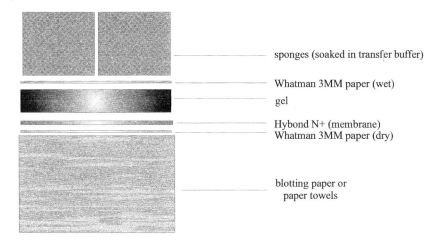

Fig. 2. Gravitational transfer.

sponges (soaked in transfer buffer)

Whatman 3MM paper (wet)
gel

Hybond N+ (membrane)
Whatman 3MM paper (dry)

blotting paper or
paper towels

6. Set up gel capillary transfer system. For the gel containing genomic DNA use the system set-up in **Fig. 1** (*see* **Note 15**), and for the gel containing PCR products use system setup in **Fig. 2** (*see* **Note 15**).
7. Transfer gel for appropriate times (*see* **Note 16**).
8. After transfer, crosslink membrane using an UV crosslinker (*see* **Note 17**).
9. Prehybridize the membrane containing genomic DNA in a sealable bag containing the prehybridization buffer for genomic DNA (*see* **Note 18**) for 1 h at the

appropriate temperature (*see* **Note 19**). Prehybridize the membrane containing the PCR products in the prehybridization buffer for PCR products in a sealable bag (*see* **Note 18**) for 15–30 min at the appropriate temperature (*see* **Note 20**).

10. Following prehybridization (*see* **Note 21**), add the appropriate amount of probe (*see* **Note 22**) and hybridize 18–20 h for the membrane containing the genomic DNA and at least 1 h to overnight for the gel containing the PCR products at the prehybridization temperatures.

11. For the dsDNA-probed genomic DNA-containing membrane (*see* **Notes 21** and **23**), incubate with gentle agitation, in excess prehybridization fluid, at the same hybridization temperature used in **steps 9** and **10**, once with prewarm wash buffer A for 15 min, then a wash with prewarm wash buffer B for 15 min.

12. Rinse with antibody wash buffer, and add 0.5 mL/cm^2 blocking agent (0.5%). Incubate, with gentle agitation, for 60 min at ambient temperature.

13. Rinse with antibody wash buffer, and incubate with gentle agitation and at ambient temperature, with 0.25 mL/cm^2 antibody wash buffer containing 0.5% BSA with 1000-fold HRP.

14. Rinse several times with antibody wash buffer.

15. Incubate with gentle agitation at ambient temperature twice in an excess of antibody wash buffer for 10 min.

16. Wash twice in an excess of antibody wash buffer containing 0.1% Tween-20.

17. In the dark room (red light on), transfer the membrane to a dry flat-bottom plastic box (*see* **Note 24**), add equal volumes of reagents 1 and 2 (0.125 mL/cm^2) and incubate with swirling for 1 min.

18. Drain off excess solution and wrap the membrane with plastic wrap.

19. Expose the membrane to film at ambient temperature (*see* **Note 25**).

20. For the oligonucleotide probed PCR product-containing membrane (*see* **Notes 21** and **23**), incubate, with gentle agitation, in excess, at the same hybridization temperature used in **steps 9** and **10**, twice with prewarm buffer C for 30 min and twice with prewarm wash buffer D.

21. Rinse with excess buffer 1 and incubate for 30 min, with gentle agitation and at ambient temperature, with the liquid blocking buffer (0.5 mL/cm^2).

22. Follow this incubation with another incubation, with gentle agitation and at ambient temperature, with buffer 2 (0.25 mL/cm^2), supplemented with 1X (1000-fold dilution) HRP-conjugate and 0.5% BSA fraction, for 30 min at ambient temperature.

22. In the dark room (red light on), transfer the membrane to a dry flat-bottom plastic box (*see* **Note 24**), add equal volumes of reagents 1 and 2 (0.125 mL/cm^2) and incubate with swirling for 1 min.

23. Drain off excess solution and wrap the membrane with plastic wrap.

24. Expose the membrane to film at ambient temperature (*see* **Note 25**).

4. Notes

1. Prior to labeling, the dsDNA must first be heated in a boiling water bath for 5 min and snap-cooled on wet ice. An 8.8-kb dsDNA has been successfully labeled in this manner to probe 1.4-kb HIV fragments.

2. Although manufacturer's probe life stability is 6 mo, probes that have been stored at −20°C in aluminum foil for over 2 yr have been used successfully.
3. Assuming 100% labeling efficiency and using 1–10 µL of probe, without any dilutions, saves time and works well.
4. The amount of lysis buffer required is cell number dependent (<1 × 10⁶ use 1 mL, 1 × 10⁶ to 5 × 10⁶ use 3 mL, >5 × 10⁶ use 5 mL). If 5 mL of the lysis buffer is not sufficient to lyse all the cells more can be added. Lysis of the cells is verified by light microscopy.
5. There should be enough room in the tube to see the mixture roll from end to end.
6. During the precipitation procedure, the DNA appears as a white cottony mass.
7. No centrifugation is necessary when washing genomic DNA with ethanol.
8. Resuspending the DNA in TE will greatly depend on the DNA going into solution.
9. An OD 260/280 ratio ≥1.8 is an indicator of the relative paucity of protein and enrichment for DNA. A >1.8 ratio indicates RNA contamination and a <1.8 ratio indicates protein contamination.
10. The DNA should be heated at 56°C for 2–3 min and snap-cooled prior to loading on the gel.
11. While both genomic DNA and PCR products can be loaded on the same kind of agarose, the percentages differ. For genomic DNA, 0.7% agarose gel is used, while for PCR products a range of 0.7–2.5% agarose gel is used (the larger the fragment the smaller the percent agarose). Likewise, if two similar size bands are present, a lower percentage gel is recommended.
12. For genomic DNA, the gel running buffer for genomic DNA is used during electrophoresis, while the gel running buffer for PCR products is used during electrophoresis PCR products (*see* **Note 8**). 1X TBE (or even 0.5X TBE) instead of TAE during electrophoresis because TBE results in a tighter banding pattern on the agarose gel, essential for identifying fragments of genomic DNA.
13. 1–2 V/cm for 8–16 h is used to separate digested genomic DNA. For PCR products, voltage varies on size and on separating two fragment size products. For small PCR products (50–300 bp) 6–8 V/cm can be applied to the gel, while 4–6 V/cm can be applied to the gel for larger fragments.
14. Depurination of the DNA for 10 min with 0.2 *N* HCl solution at ambient temperature will improve transfer for DNA fragments larger than 15 kb as the subsequent base treatment will cause strand scission at the apurinic sites.
15. Ensure that the wick, membrane, blotting paper, and paper towels are the same size as the gel.
16. For gels containing genomic DNA, complete DNA transfer occurs at 14–16 h. For the gel containing PCR products, complete transfer occurs within 30–60 min for fragments <3,000 bp and overnight (at least 12 h) for larger fragments.
17. After crosslinking the membrane, it can be stored at +4°C. If desired, the agarose gel can be restained with ethidium bromide the estimate the transfer efficiency.
18. Prehybridize and hybridize the membrane in the minimal amount of buffer necessary to cover the gel (2–5 mL/cm² is recommended, 5 mL/cm² is normally used). More than one filter can be hybridized in one bag at a time, but more buffer should be added (about 1.5 mL/cm² per additional filter).

19. The prehybridization and hybridization temperature of 56°C for HIV dsDNA probe works well (an initial range of 55–65°C is generally tested first). Mild agitation of the membrane while incubating is only necessary when there is more than one membrane in the sealed bag.
20. For an oligonucleotide probe against HIV PCR products, 56°C also works well, though, 37°C has been used with no background. Shaking is not necessary when only probing one membrane.
21. After prehybridization or hybridization, the sealable bag containing the buffer and membrane may be stored at –20°C.
22. For genomic DNA, the amount of probe is 5–10 μL. The dsDNA probe must first be heated in a boiling water bath, boiled for 5 min, then snap-cooled on wet ice. For PCR products the amount of probe used is 1–5 μL. Both for the dsDNA and oligonucleotide probes, the amount is dependent on the number of filters used.
23. The solution containing the probe has been successfully reused (stored at –20°C).
24. The dry, plastic box can be a pipet tip box, as long as the membrane will fit into it.
25. The exposure time depends on the intensity of the band (from 5 s to 1 min is a good starting point). In some cases, a band not visible by ethidium bromide staining is detected after an extended (8 min) exposure to film.

References

1. Ho, D.D., Neumann, A.U., Perselson, A..S, Chen, W., Leonard, J.M., and Markowitz, M. (1995) Rapid turnover of plasma virions and CD4 lymphocytes in HIV-1 infection. *Nature* **373,** 123–126.
2. Hahn, B. H., Shaw, G. M., Taylor, M. E., Redfield, R. R., Markham, P. D., Salahuddin, S. Z., et al. (1986) Genetic variation in HTLV-111/LAV over time in patients with AIDS or at risk for AIDS. *Science* **232,** 1548–1553.
3. Meyerhans, A., Cheynier, R., Albert, J., Seth, M., Kwok, S., Sninsky, J., et al. (1989) Temporal fluctuations in HIV quasispecies in vivo are not reflected by sequential HIV isolations. *Cell* **58,** 901–910.
4. Holmes, E. C., Zhang, L. Q., Simmonds, P., Ludlam, C. A., and Leigh-Brown, A. J. (1992) Convergent and divergent sequence evolution in the surface envelope glycoprotein of human immunodeficiency virus type 1 infection: low viral RNA copy numbers in serum and maintenance of high HIV-1 p24-specific, but not V3-specific antibody levels. *J. Infect. Dis.* **171,** 811–821.
5. Zhu, T., Mo, H., Wang, N., Nam, D. S., Cao, Y., Koup, R. A. et al. (1993) Genotypic and phenotypic characterization of HIV-1 in patients with primary infection. *Science* **261,** 1179–1181.
6. Wolinsky, S. M., Wike, C.M., Korber, B.T., Hutto, C., Parks, W. P., Rosenblum, L. L., et al. (1992) Selective transmission of human immunodeficiencv virus type-1 variants from mothers to infants. *Science* **255,** 1134–1137.
7. Lamers, S. L., Sleasman, J. W., She, J. X., Barrie, K. A., Pomeroy, S. M. , Barrett, D. J., et al. (1994) Persistence of multiple maternal genotypes of human immunodeficiency virus type I in infants infected by vertical transmission. *J. Clin. Invest.* **93,** 380–390.

8. McDonald, R. A., Mayers, D. L., Chung, R. C. Y., Wagner K. F., Ratto-Kim, S., Birx, D.L., et al. (1997) Evolution of human immunodeficiency virus type 1 env sequence variation in patients with diverse rates of disease progression and T-cell function. *J. Virol.* **71,** 1871–1879.
9. Southern, E. M. (1975) Detection of specific sequences among DNA fragments separated by gel electrophoresis. *J. Mol. Biol.* **98,** 503.

10

Detection of HIV-1 Nucleic Acids by Northern Blotting

Richard A. McDonald and Christopher A. D. Smith

1. Introduction

Northern blotting *(1)* is one of many tools used in understanding the human immunodeficiency virus type 1 (HIV-1). In the process of Northern blotting, RNA is first separated by size through a denaturing agarose gel and transferred onto a membrane. With this transfer or blotting, and subsequent hybridization with a DNA or RNA probe, quantitation, expression levels of the RNA, size of the RNA, and mapping of the 5'- and 3'-terminal end of the RNA can be determined from primary and cultured cells, blood, and tissue. For HIV research, Northern blotting has been utilized for determining the expression levels and splicing patterns of HIV RNA regulatory genes *(2–4)*, HIV RNA protease gene *(5)*, cytokine effects on the levels of spliced and genomic HIV RNA *(6,7)*, steady-state transcriptional levels and splicing patterns of HIV RNA as a result of antiviral constructs *(8)*, and receptor studies *(9,10)*. In addition, Northern blotting has be utilized to answer questions on the effect on the HIV RNA level of expression of the envelope protein on calmodulin *(11)* and carbohydrate binding proteins *(12)*.

A large number of extraction methods are available in the literature that isolate the different RNA subtypes with varying efficiencies. Also, there are several commercial RNA isolation kits available that provide a convenient way to obtain good-quality RNA from tissues and cell lines. Here is described a hot phenol/guanidinium isothiocyanate method, which can be used for large-scale and small-scale isolation of total RNA from most source material.

From: *Methods in Molecular Medicine, Vol. 17: HIV Protocols*
Edited by: N. L. Michael and J. H. Kim © Humana Press Inc., Totowa, NJ

2. Reagents

2.1. Isolation of RNA from Cells and Tissues

1. 1X PBS: Phosphate-buffered saline (magnesium- and calcium-free): 1.15 g anhydrous Na_2HPO_4, 0.23 g anhydrous NaH_2PO_4, 9.00 g NaCl, distilled H_2O to 950 mL; adjust pH to between 7.2 and 7.4 with either 1 M HCl or 1 M NaOH; add distilled H_2O to 1000 mL. Filter-sterilize by passage through a 0.45-micron pore size filter unit.
2. 1 M Tris-HCl (pH 7.2).
3. 500 mM EDTA (pH 8.0).
4. 200 mM sodium acetate (pH 5.2).
5. GT buffer: 4 M guanidinium isothiocyanate, 10 mM EDTA, 1% ß-mercaptoethanol, 2% (w/v) sodium lauryl sulfate, and 50 mM Tris-HCl (pH 7.6).
6. Ultra-pure phenol equilibrated with 100 mM Tris-HCl (pH 8.0)
7. TAE buffer: 40 mM Tris-acetate, pH 8.0, 1 mM EDTA.
8 CI buffer: Chloroform and isoamyl alcohol solution (24:1).
9. 95% Ethanol and 70% ethanol.
10. TE buffer: 10 mM Tris (pH 8.0) and 1 mM EDTA.
11. Ficoll-hypaque.
12. NP-40 lysis buffer: 0.65% NP-40, 0.15 M NaCl, 0.01 M Tris-HCl (pH 7.8), and 1.5 mM $MgCl_2$.
13. Monocyte media: RPMI 1640 supplemented with penicillin (100 U/mL), streptomycin (100 μg/mL), 2 mM L-glutamine, and 20% heat-inactivated fetal bovine serum, supplemented with 10% normal human serum.
14. T lymphocyte media: RPMI 1640 supplemented with penicillin (100 U/mL), streptomycin (100 μg/mL), 2 mM L-glutamine, and 20% heat-inactivated fetal bovine serum, supplemented with 10% interleukin-2 (20 U/mL).

2.2. Electrophoresis and Blotting

1. 10X gel running buffer (10X GRB): formaldehyde gels—200 mM sodium 3-(N-morpholino)propanesulfonic acid (MOPS), 50 mM sodium acetate, and 10 mM EDTA (adjust to pH 7.0 with acetic acid). Glyoxal gels—100 mM Na_2HPO4/NaH_2PO_4 (pH 6.5).
2. 10X tracking dye: 0.1% (w/v) bromophenol blue and 0.1% (w/v) xylene cyanol in 50% (v/v) glycerol.
3. 37% Formaldehyde (reagent grade).
4. Formamide (deionized).
5. 6 M Glyoxal (40% solution).
6. Dimethyl sulfoxide.
7. Sample buffer: formaldehyde gels: 500 μL formamide, 175 μL 37% formaldehyde, 200 μL 10X GRB. Glyoxal gels: 500 μL DMSO, 175 μL 6 M glyoxal, and 200 μL 10X GRB.
8. Agarose: ultra-pure, low-conductivity molecular biology grade.
9. Hybond N+ membrane (Amersham Corp., Inc.)—cut to size of gel.

10. Filter paper strips or paper towels cut to RNA gel size.
11. Whatman 3MM paper or equivalent to act as a wick.
12. Transfer buffer: 25 mM Na$_2$HPO4/NaH$_2$PO$_4$ (pH 6.5).
13. 20X SSC: 3 M sodium citrate and 1.5 M sodium chloride.

2.3. Hybridization

1. 10% (w/v) sodium lauryl sulphate (SLS).
2. 20X SSC: 3 M sodium citrate, and 1.5 M sodium chloride.
3. Formamide (deionized).
4. Reagents supplied by Amersham's enhanced chemiluminesence (ECL™) system: hybridization component, blocking agent, blocking buffer, fluorescein-11-dUTP, anti-fluorescein-horse radish peroxidase (HRP) conjugate nucleotide mix, primers, Klenow, cacodylate buffer, terminal transferase, and detection reagents 1 and 2.
5. Prehybridization solution (*see* **Note 1**): 50% formamide, 5X SSC, 1% SLS, 1.25% (w/v) blocking agent, and 100 µg/mL sonicated salmon sperm or calf thymus DNA.
6. Hybridization solution (*see* **Note 1**): 50% formamide, 3X SSC, 1% SLS, 0.5% (w/v) blocking agent, 100 µg/mL sonicated salmon sperm or calf thymus DNA.
7. Appropriate HIV specific probe: DNA or RNA probe (*see* **Note 2**).
8. Labeling dsDNA (*see* **Note 3**) (random prime labeling, for dsDNA >2,500 bp): 200 ng dsDNA (50 ng/mL) (*see* **Note 4**), 10 µL fluorescein-11-dUTP, 10 µL nucleotide mix, 5 µL primers, 1 µL Klenow (4U) and distilled water to 50 µL. Incubate for 1 h at 37°C and terminate with 20 mM EDTA and store at –20°C (*see* **Note 5**). Assume 100% labeling efficiency (*see* **Note 6**).
9. Labeling oligonucleotide (3'-end): 100 pmoles oligonucleotide, 10 µL fluorescein-11-dUTP, 16 µL cacodylate buffer, 112.9 to 144 µL water and 16 µL terminal transferase. Incubate at 37°C for 60–90 min and store at –20°C (*see* **Note 5**). Assume 100% labeling efficiency (*see* **Note 6**).
10. Wash solution 1: 2X SSC, 1% SLS.
11. Wash solution 2: 1X SSC, 0.1% SLS.
12. Wash solution 3: 0.1X SSC, 0.1 % SLS.
13. Antibody wash buffer: 100 mM Tris-HCl (pH 7.5) and 150 mM NaCl.
14. Buffer 1: 0.15 M NaCl and 0.1 M Tris-HCl (pH 7.5).
15. Buffer 2: 0.4 M NaCl and 0.1 M Tris-HCl (pH 7.5).
16. BSA-fraction V.

3. Experimental Procedures

All biosafety protocols for handling and disposal of HIV-infected material should be carried out throughout these procedures.

3.1. Precautions To Be Taken for RNA Isolation

It is important for the isolation of good RNA preparations, from any source material, to eliminate endogenous and exogenous RNAse activity. This can be achieved successfully by taking the following steps.

1. Work as much as possible in a clean, dust-free laboratory, and wear disposable gloves at all times.
2. The inclusion of RNase inhibitors, such as RNasin, vanadyl ribonucleotide complex, and placental RNase inhibitor, in cell lysis buffers is recommended.
3. The employment of methods that simultaneously lyse cells and denature RNases (guanidine hydrochloride and guanidinium isothiocyanate) is advisable for the isolation of intact RNA.
4. The use of dedicated laboratory glassware and plasticware, agarose electrophoresis equipment, and chemicals to minimize RNase contamination from other experimental sources is important. Disposable, sterile plasticware, tips, tubes, and pipets is preferable to glassware. If glassware must be used, thoroughly clean and rinse with distilled water followed by ethanol, and subsequently bake at 180°C overnight.
5. Make up solutions using diethylpyrocarbonate-(DEPC) treated, distilled water. DEPC-treated water is prepared by adjusting to a 0.1% (v/v) with DEPC, standing for 2 h at 37°C, and autoclaving. Aqueous buffers (except GT buffer) should be autoclaved following preparation.

3.2. Total RNA Extraction from Cells

1. Collect cells (HIV-infected) in a screw-capped polypropylene tube. Wash twice with ice-cold PBS (centrifugation of 208g for 10 min at 4°C.).
2. Heat the GT buffer, phenol, and TAE buffer to 60°C in a water bath.
3. Resuspend and lyse the cell pellet in 5–10 vol (original volume) of hot GT buffer. When the cell suspension is clear, pass the solution six times through a plastic syringe with a 19- to 25-gauge needle attached to shear DNA.
4. Add an equal volume of hot phenol, and pass through syringe and needle six times.
5. Add a half original volume of TAE buffer, and mix vigorously at 60°C.
6. Add an original volume of CI buffer, mix vigorously, and incubate at 60°C for 10 min, followed by 5 min on ice.
7. Centrifuge the tubes at 2000–2,500g for 10 min at 10°C.
8. After centrifugation, three phases should be visible in the tubes (phase separation) (*see* **Note 7**): An upper aqueous layer containing the RNA, a lower organic phase containing hydrophobic cell components, and a central interface (white) containing protein and DNA.
9. Carefully transfer the upper aqueous phase to a fresh tube (do not take any of the interface), and incubate at 60°C for 5 min. Then re-extract with the original volume of phenol and CI buffer as before.
10. Repeat **steps 7–9** two more times or until the interface area between the aqueous and organic phases is clear (all protein and DNA are removed).
11. Extract the aqueous phase with an equal volume of CI buffer, centrifuge as in **step 7**, and carefully remove the final RNA solution to an appropriate size ultracentrifuge tube, add 2 vol of ice-cold 95% ethanol, mix, and precipitate the RNA overnight at –20°C.

12. Recover the RNA by centrifugation at 15,000g for 20 min at 4°C, carefully wash the pellet with 70% ethanol (ice-cold), and air-dry or lyophilize.
13. Dissolve the pellet in a minimal volume of ice-cold TE or sterile distilled water, and check the amount and quality of the RNA spectrophotometrically by OD_{260} measurements and the OD_{260}/OD_{280} ratio of a small amount of the solution. An OD_{260} of 1 represents a 40 µg/mL solution of RNA, and a 260/280 ratio approaching 2.0 represents an RNA preparation essentially free of protein and DNA. Dilute the RNA to 2.5–5.0 µg/mL (*see* **Note 8**).
14. Store the RNA (*see* **Note 9**) in 20-µL aliquots at –20°C or colder.

3.3. RNA Extraction from Tissues

1. Cut the tissue (HIV-infected) into small fragments, and then homogenize in a small volume of ice-cold 1X PBS in a Dounce homogenizer.
2. Centrifuge cells in a screw-capped polypropylene tube at 208g for 10 min at 4°C.
3. After centrifugation proceed to **Subheading 3.2., step 2**.

3.4. Extraction of Nuclear and Cytoplasmic RNA

1. Centrifuge cells (HIV-infected) in a screw-capped polypropylene tube at 208g for 10 min at 4°C.
2. Wash twice with ice-cold PBS (centrifugation of 208g for 10 min at 4°C).
3. Resuspend cells in 2 vol of ice-cold NP-40 lysis buffer.
4. Let cells stand on ice for 5 min.
5. Centrifuge cells at 208g for 10 min at 4°C. The supernatant is the cytoplasmic fraction, and the pellet is the nuclear fraction.
6. Transfer the supernatant (cytoplasmic fraction) to a clean screw-capped polypropylene tube and proceed to **Subheading 3.2., step 2**.
7. Resuspend the nuclear fraction in 5 vol of NP-40 lysis buffer and centrifuge at 208g for 10 min at 4°C.
8. Discard the nuclear supernatant from **step 7** and proceed to **Subheading 3.2., step 2**.

3.5. RNA Extraction of Peripheral Blood Mononuclear Cells

1. Dilute the heparinized HIV-infected blood or sodium citrate-treated blood one to two volumes of PBS to a final volume of 30 mL in a 50-mL conical centrifuge tube.
2. Underlay the diluted blood with 12 mL of Ficoll-hypaque solution.
3. Centrifuge for 45 min at 407g at ambient temperature.
4. The mononuclear cells, located at the interface, are harvested and washed three times with PBS (centrifugation at 208g for 10 min at ambient temperature).
5. Cells are then transferred to a polypropylene tube and processed according to **Subheading 3.2., step 2**.

3.6. Extraction of RNA from Infected Monocytes

1. From step 4 of 3.5, the cells are seeded at 1.8×10^8 into a T-150 polystyrene flask in 50 mL of Monocyte media (*see* **Note 10**).

2. The flasks are incubated for 1 to 2 d in a 37°C incubator, 5% CO_2, 97% humidity.
3. The cell monolayer is then washed three times with PBS (centrifugation at 208g for 10 min at ambient temperature.).
4. Lyse and process the cells in the flask starting from **Subheading 3.2., step 2** but transfer lysed cells to a screw-capped polypropylene tube.

3.7. Extraction of RNA from Infected T-Lymphocytes

1. From **step 4** of **Subheading 3.4.**, the cells are seeded at 1×10^7 into T-25 polystyrene flask containing 10 mL of T-lymphocyte media (*see* **Note 10**).
2. The flasks are incubated for 1 d in a 37°C incubator, 5% CO_2, 97% humidity.
3. Transfer the supernatant to anther T-25 flask and repeat **steps 1** and **2**.
4. The supernatant is transferred to a 50 mL conical tube and centrifuged at 208g for 10 min at ambient temperature.
5. Proceed to **Subheading 3.2., step 2**.

3.8. HIV-1 RNA Genome Extraction

In extracting the HIV genome from virions, it is critical to have the centrifuge in an appropriate hood. Also, safety glasses should be worn, as well as a face shield, double gloves, disposable sleeves, and lab coat.

1. From the cell culture (*see* **Note 11**) centrifuge at 208g for 20 min at 4°C in a polypropylene tube. Keep supernatant and viral pellet on ice at all times.
2. Pour the supernatant into two tubes, balance them and mark the outer side of the tubes (to mark the position of the virion pellet). Centrifuge at appropriate speed and time (*see* **Note 12**).
3. After pelleting, pour off supernatant and carefully stand the bottles (or tubes) upright onto a gauze and let drain off for 2 to 3 min.
4. Use a cotton-tip applicator to wipe off remaining fluid in bottle (tube).
5. Proceed to **Subheading 3.2., step 2**.

3.9. Electrophoresis

The following procedures for electrophoresis and transfer are the most widely used for separation, immobilization, and detection of RNA species by Northern blot process. Electro- or "dry" blotting of RNA gels is also prevalent but because of the wide variety of commercial equipment for this method, only the more common method of capillary transfer will be described. If the electroblot apparatus is available, then the manufacturer's instructions should be closely followed.

3.9.1. Formaldehyde Gels

1. Gel preparation (in fume hood because formaldehyde in toxic): For every 100 mL volume of gel solution required, dissolve the appropriate amount of agarose to give a 1 to 1.5% (w/v) solution in 60 mL sterile distilled water by heating in a microwave or over a hotplate. Allow the solution to cool to approx 50–60°C, add

10 mL of 10X GRB, 16 mL formaldehyde and water to 100 mL. Mix thoroughly and pour into gel tray with well-forming comb fitted. Allow the gel to cool and set or at least one hour at ambient temperature (or 30 min at at 4°C).

2. Fit gel tray into electrophoresis cell, overlay with 1X GRB, and remove comb. Wash out sample wells carefully with buffer.

3. Sample preparation: to 4 µL (10–20 µg) of RNA sample add 16 µL of sample buffer and incubate at 68°C for 10 min. Cool on ice, add 2 µL of tracking dye, and load samples into wells.

4. Prepare a sample of appropriately sized RNA or DNA molecular weight markers and apply them to the outside lanes of the gel.

5. Subject samples to electrophoresis at a constant voltage of 6–8 V/cm of gel length, until the bromophenol blue dye (fastest running) has migrated to two thirds or three quarters of the length of the gel.

6. After electrophoresis, rinse the gel for 10 minutes in transfer buffer, and excise one of the lanes containing the molecular weight markers. This gel segment can then be stained with 0.5 µg/mL ethidium bromide and the marker bands visualized by UV transillumination. Photograph the stained gel fragment with a fluorescent ruler to determine the migration distance of molecular weight markers and other RNA species.

3.9.2. Glyoxal Gels

1. Gel preparation: same as for formaldehyde gels except the agarose content is varied between 1 and 2% final, and a 1/10 vol of 100 mM Na$_2$HPO4/NaH$_2$PO$_4$ (pH 6.5) is added after the gel is cooled to 50°C and the gel is overlaid and electrophoresed in 10–15 mL Na$_2$HPO$_4$/NaH$_2$PO$_4$ (pH 6.5) running buffer.

2. Prepare each 4 µL RNA sample for electrophoresis by adding 16 µL glyoxal sample buffer, incubation at 50°C for 15 min, cool on ice, and add 2 mL tracking dye.

3. Subject samples to electrophoresis with circulation of buffer, at 3–5 V/cm gel length for the appropriate time.

3.10. Capillary Transfer to Membrane

1. Soak membrane for 20 min in transfer buffer.

2. Soak transfer wick, and gently place on the gel tray. See figure for transfer system.

3. Lay the gel face down, and ensure no air bubbles are present between the membrane and the gel (roll bubbles out with sterile cell culture pipet). Fill the tray with transfer buffer (*see* **Note 13**), and complete transfer system as in Fig. 1 in Chapter 9.

4. Allow the transfer to proceed for 12–14 h, changing blotting paper when needed.

5. When transfer is complete, carefully remove the stack of papers, and gently peel membrane away from the gel.

6. Rinse the membrane in transfer buffer to remove any pieces of gel, air dry and then irreversibly bind the RNA to the membrane by UV-crosslinking or by baking in an oven at 80°C for 2 h prior to hybridization (after crosslinking membrane can be stored at 4°C).

7. Stain the remaining gel with ethidium bromide to assess transfer efficiency.

3.11. Hybridization of RNA Blots (Northern Blotting)

If studies with deletions are being examined then general probes can be utilized, because size differences in the RNA species will be apparent. Oligonucleotide or oligoribonucleotide probes can be used to differentiate between RNA subtypes or splicing patterns. However, hybridization conditions will have to be varied to detect such differences efficiently.

1. Prewet the membrane with 5X SSC, and carefully place the wet membrane in a heat-sealable plastic bag.
2. Add 1 mL of pre-hybridization buffer per 20 cm^2. Seal bag, and incubate at 42°C for 4–8 h with constant agitation (*see* **Note 14**).
3. Remove the pre-hybridization solution, and replace with an equal volume of hybridization solution containing an appropriately labeled probe (50 ng/mL) (*see* **Note 15**). Continue incubation at 42°C with constant agitation for a further 16–24 h (*see* **Note 14**).
4. Remove the membrane (*see* **Note 16**) from the bag and wash twice with 200 mL of wash solution at ambient temperature for 10 min with constant agitation.
5. Wash the membrane twice with was solution 2 at 50–65°C for 10–15 min with constant agitation.
6. Wash the membrane twice with wash solution 3 at 50–65°C for 10–15 min with constant agitation (*see* **Note 17**).
7. If dsDNA probe was used, rinse with antibody wash buffer and add 0.5 mL/cm^2 blocking agent (0.5%) and incubate, with gentle agitation, for 60 min at ambient temperature. Rinse with antibody wash buffer and incubate, with gentle agitation and at ambient temperature, with 0.25 mL/cm^2 antibody wash buffer containing 0.5% BSA with 1000-fold HRP. Rinse several times with antibody wash buffer and incubate, with gentle agitation at ambient temperature, twice in an excess of antibody wash buffer for 10 min. followed by two washes in an excess of antibody wash buffer containing 0.1% Tween-20. In the dark room (red light on), transfer the membrane to a dry flat-bottom plastic box (*see* **Note 18**). Add equal volumes of reagent 1 and 2 (0.125 mL/cm^2). Incubate and swirl for 1 min. Drain off excess solution, and wrap the membrane (*see* **Note 18**) with plastic wrap. Expose the membrane to film at ambient temperature (*see* **Note 19**).
8. If an oligonucleotide probe was used, rinse with excess Buffer 1 and incubate for 30 min, with gentle agitation at ambient temperature, with the liquid blocking buffer (0.5 mL/cm^2). Follow this incubation with another incubation, with gentle agitation at ambient temperature with buffer 2 (0.25 mL/cm^2), supplemented with 1X (1000-fold dilution) HRP- conjugate and 0.5% BSA fraction for 30 min at ambient temperature. In the dark room (red light on), transfer the membrane to a dry flat-bottom plastic box (*see* **Note 18**) add equal volumes of reagent 1 and 2 (0.125 mL/cm^2). Incubate and swirl for 1 min. Drain off any excess solution, and wrap the membrane (*see* **Note 18**) with plastic wrap. Expose the membrane to film at ambient temperature (*see* **Note 19**).

9. The position of the RNA bands produced on the autoradiograph can be compared with the position of the molecular weight markers in the gel obtained by ethidium bromide staining (**Subheading 3.9.**). In addition, any marker lanes transferred to the membrane can be cut off and stained for comparison.

4. Notes

1. An additional method can be used including dextran sulfate, which is known to enhance hybridization and reduce background. Under these conditions the 20X SSC in the prehybridization and hybridization should be omitted and replaced with the following: 50 mM Tris-HCl (pH 7.5), 1 M sodium chloride, 10% (w/v) dextran sulfate, and 1% (w/v) sodium pyrophosphate.
2. More success has been achieved in Northern detection when DNA, rather than RNA, has been utilized as a probe.
3. At times, labeling DNA or RNA by standard radioactive methods (nick translated or random primer labeling with ^{32}P nucleotides, or end labeling with ^{32}P) may be necessary due to signal strength; though, it is slowly becoming unnecessary because of changes in nonradioactive technology.
4. Prior to labeling the dsDNA must first be heated in a boiling water bath for 5 min and snap cool on wet ice. A dsDNA of at least 2.5 kb in size has been successfully labeled and hybridized to RNA.
5. Although manufacturer's probe life stability is 6 mo, probes that have been stored at –20°C in aluminum foil for over two years have been used successfully.
6. Assuming 100% labeling efficiency and using 10 μL of probe, without any dilutions, is saves time and works very well.
7. If phase separation is not achieved, add a further half volume of TAE buffer mix and re-centrifuge as before.
8. If the 260/280 ratio is below 1.8 then the RNA preparation may be contaminated with proteins and should be treated with Proteinase K by standard methods, and re-extracted with phenol/chloroform and re-precipitated.
9. As HIV RNA species and HIV genome are not polyadenylated then there is no requirement for selection of mRNA species by oligo dT cellulose or poly U sepharose affinity chromatography.
10. If cells are less than 1.8×10^8, which is likely in patients with a depressed immune system, the amount of media and flask can be proportionally reduced. When exact number is not known, error on the smaller amount.
11. HIV genome isolation from the HIV-infected cells, blood or tissue, is also possible. This is achieved by first growing the peripheral blood mononuclear cells in culture either in Monocyte media or in T lymphocyte media for 7 to 14 d followed by centrifugation process in **Subheading 3.7.** For tissue, after the homogenizing the tissue in either media, grow in media used in the homogenizing step (either for T-cell or monocyte growth) for 7–14 d and the proceed as in **Subheading 3.7.** with the supernatant.
12. For a rotor that holds 200–250-mL bottles, centrifuge at 16,500g for 3 h at 4°C; and for a rotor that holds 25–30-mL tubes (polycarbonate), centrifuge at 105,000g for 45 min at 4°C.

13. The sodium phosphate transfer buffer can be replaced by 10–20X SSC transfer buffer if required. Some laboratories find that SSC has a higher transfer efficiency for large molecular weight RNAs, so it may be of particular use in considering the size of the RNA signal.

14. After prehybridization or hybridization, the sealable bag containing the buffer, and membrane may be stored at –20°C.

15. The dsDNA probe must first heated in a boiling water bath boiled for 5 min, then snap cooled on wet ice.

16. The solution containing the nonradioactive probe has been successfully reused (stored at –20°C).

17. If a ^{32}P-labeled probe is used, periodically monitor the membrane with a Geiger counter to check the relative position and strength of the radioactive signal during the final wash. When the background is minimal, the wash can be terminated. The dry, plastic box can be a pipet tip box, just be enough for the membrane to fit.

18. Leaving the membrane moist prior to exposure allows for the efficient removal of the probe if rehybridization is planned. Probes can be removed by treating the membrane with 100–200 mL of 5 mM Tris-HCl (pH 8.0), 0.2 mM EDTA, 0.1X Denhardt's solution at 65°C for 2 h. This wash can be repeated if necessary.

19. The exposure time depends on the intensity of the band (from 5 s to 1 min is a good starting point). In some cases, if a band is present but not visible by ethidium bromide staining, after an 8-min exposure to film the band will be clearly present.

References

1. Alwine, J. C., Kemp, D. J., and Stark, G. R. (1977) Method for detection of specific RNAs in agarose gels by transfer to diazobenzylozxymethyl-paper and hybridization with DNA probes. *Proc. Natl. Acad. Sci. USA* **74,** 5350–5354.

2. Junker, U., Bevec, D., Barske, C., Kalfoglou, C., Escaich, S., Dobrovnik, M., Hauber, J., and Bohnlein, E. (1996) Intracellular expression of cellular eif-5a mutants inhibits HIV-1 replication in human T cells: a feasibility cells. *Hum. Gene Ther.* **7(15),** 1861–1869.

3. Cagnon, L., Cucchiarini, M., Lefebvre, J. C., and Doglio, A. (1995) Protection of a T-cell from human immunodeficiency virus replication by the stable expression of a short antisense RNA sequence carried by a shuttle RNA molecule. *J. Acquir. Immune. Defic. Syndr. Hum. Retroviol.* **9(4),** 349–358.

4. Dyhr-Mikkelsen, H. and Kjems, J. (1995) Inefficient spliceosome assembly and abnormal branch site selection in splicing of an HIV-1 transcript in vitro. *J. Biol. Chem.* **270(41),** 24,060–24,066.

5. Zhang, D., Zhang, N., Wick, M. M., and Byrn, R. A. (1995) HIV type 1 protease activation of NF-kappa B within T lymphoid cells. *AIDS Res. Hum. Retroviruses.* **11(2),** 223–230.

6. Naif, H., Ho-Shon, M., Chang, J., and Cunningham, A. L. (1994) Molecular mechanisms of IL-4 effect on HIV expression in promonocytic cell lines and primary human monocytes. *J. Leukoc. Biol.* **56(3),** 335–339.

7. Weissman, D., Poli, G., and Fauci, A. S. (1995) IL-10 synergizes with multiple cytokines in enhancing HIV production in cells of monocytic lineage. *J. Acquir. Immune. Defic. Syndr. Hum. Retroviol.* **9(5),** 442–449.

8. Berkhout, B. and van Wamel, J. L. (1995) Inhibition of human immunodeficiency virus expression by sense transcripts encoding the retroviral leader RNA. *Antiviral. Res.* **26(2),** 101–105.

9. Biswas, P., Smith, C. A., Goletti, D., Hardy, E. C., Jackson, R. W., and Fauci, A. S. (1995) Cross-linking of CD30 induces HIV expression in chronically infected T cells. *Immunity* **2(6),** 587–596.

10. Harrington, R. D. and Geballe, A. P. (1996) Human immunodeficiency virus type-1 susceptible whole cell and microcell hybrids. *Ann. Clin. Lab. Sci.* **26(6),** 522–530.

11. Radding, W., Pan, Z. Q., Hunter, E., Johnston, P., Williams, J. P., and McDonald, J. M. (1996) Expression of HIV-1 envelope glycoprotein alters cellular calmodulin. *Biochem. Biophys. Res. Commun.* **218(1),** 192–197.

12. Schroder, H. C, Ushijima, H., Theis, C., Seve, A. P., Hubert, J., and Muller, W. E. (1995) Expression of nuclear lectin carbohydrate-binding protein 35 in human immunodeficiency virus type 1-infected Molt-3 cells. *J. Acquir. Immune. Defic. Syndr. Hum. Retroviol.* **9(4),** 340–348.

11

Rapid Identification of Cloned HIV-1 Fragments

Wei Dong, Anindita Kar Roy, and Yen Li

1. Introduction

Genetic analysis of HIV-1 frequently involves molecular cloning. The general laboratory approach of identifying a desired molecular clone after a successful transformation includes picking colonies, growing stationary-phase bacterial cultures, isolating plasmid DNA using any number of DNA isolation protocols, and, finally restriction endonuclease mapping of the molecular clones *(1,2)*. The approach is time-consuming and labor-intensive. It may take several days before the correct clone can be identified. An alternative but equally time-consuming approach is the procedure of colony filter hybridization *(1,2)*. This procedure includes transferring bacterial colonies to a nitrocellulose or nylon membrane, denaturing plasmid DNA *in situ*, hybridizing to a radioactive or chemiluminescent labeled probe, washing off the excess probe, and, finally, exposing the filter to X-ray film. To simplify clone identification, vectors containing the lacZ promoter and a partial *lacZ* gene encoding the α-fragment of β-galactosidase were developed (pUC vectors) *(3,4)*. Upon induction by IPTG (isopropyl-β-D-thio-galactopyranoside), the expressed β-galactosidase could cleave X-gal (5-bromo-4-choloro-3-indoyl-β-D-galactopyranoside) and turn the colonies blue. Colonies were white when an insert interrupted the reading frame of the β-galactosidase. However, the blue/white color selection was not absolute due to the leakiness of the *lacZ* gene expression. Furthermore, damaged restriction endonuclease ends or dimerization of the cloning vector might give rise to white colonies as well. In addition, when a single restriction endonuclease site is used for cloning and if the

From: *Methods in Molecular Medicine, Vol. 17: HIV Protocols*
Edited by: N. L. Michael and J. H. Kim © Humana Press Inc., Totowa, NJ

orientation of the insert is important, additional restriction endonuclease mapping might be needed.

A simple method that allows rapid identification of molecular clones is highly desirable and such a method was developed and used routinely in our laboratory to identify correct molecular clones of HIV-1 without the necessity of isolating plasmid DNA. The method, termed colony polymerase chain reaction (cPCR) *(5)*, uses oligonucloetides that flank the multiple-cloning sites. A major advantage of cPCR is its rapidilty and versatility in that it is not limited to plasmid cloning. With slight modification, phage cloning is also applicable. cPCR is especially useful in identifying clones using the commercially available TA cloning of PCR products (Invitrogen Corp., San Diego, CA). Cloning the HIV-1 long-terminal repeat (LTR) from patient clinical samples into a green fluorescence protein (GFP)-containing vector (pEGFP-1; CLONTECH, Palo Alto, CA) is used as an example. GFP from the jellyfish *Aequorea victoria* has been used as a reporter gene to monitor gene expression and protein localization in a number of systems including: *C. elegans,* dictyostelium, drosophila, *E. coli*, xenopus, yeast, zebrafish, mammalian cells and plants. GFP emits green fluorescence light when exposed to ultraviolet (UV) light. No additional protein, substrates, or cofactors are required for light emission.

2. Materials and Methods

2.1. Vectors

1. pEGFP was genetically engineered from its wild-type GFP to exhibit brighter fluorescence and higher expression in mammalian cells and was purchased from CLONTECH. It has excitation maxima at 488 nm and emission maxima at 507 nm. Upstream from the enhanced GFP coding sequence is the multiple-cloning site (MCS). LTRs from patients' HIV-1 provirus were cloned into the MCS.
2. Numerous commercial plasmid or phagemid vectors are suitable for cloning and are employed in this method. Many of these vectors are pUC derived and contain M13 and β-galactosidase sequences.

2.2. Reagents and Buffers

1. Testing LTRs were obtained from N. Michael (Walter Reed Army Institute of Research, Rockville, MD) *(7)*. They were obtained by PCR amplification of HIV-1 provirus from seropositive individuals using primers (position 128–148 and position 783–763 of HIV-1HXB2) with built-in restriction endonuclease recognition sequences (Xba I and Xho I).
2. Thermal stable DNA polymerases such as Taq (Perkin Elmer, Promega), recombinant exo⁻ Pfu (Stratagene, La Jolla, CA), and VentR(exo⁻) DNA polymerase (New England Biolabs, Beverly, MA) were tested and were comparable for cPCR. One-half unit of the enzyme per tube was sufficient for the amplification reaction. A Perkin-Elmer PCR kit is used as an example here. Tenfold dilution of

supplier's 10× PCR buffer was used in the reaction. The final concentration of the 1× reaction buffer contains 1.5 mM MgCl$_2$, 50 mM KCl, 10 mM Tris-HCl, pH 8.3 and 0.001% (w/v) gelatin. Other ingredients in the reaction included 200 μM each of the primers.

2.3. Primers

1. M13 universal (5'-TGACCGGCAGCAAAATG-3') and β-galactosidase reverse (5'-GGAAACAGCTATGACCATG-3') primers were used if the DNA fragments were short (**Note 1**) and utilized different restriction endonuclease sites. Other promoter primers such as SP6 (5'-TTTAGGTGA CTATAGAATAC-3'), T3 (5'-AATTAACCCTCACTAAAGGG-3'), and T7 (5'-GTAATACGACTCACTATA GGGC-3') might also be used. These primers were either purchased from a commercial vendor or synthesized by an oligonucleotide synthesizer without special purification (**Note 2**). Because most of the pUC-based plasmid vectors contain the M13 sequence and *lacZ* gene, the universal and reverse primers may have a wider usefulness than the single-strand phage promoter primers.

2. To identify the orientation of the insert of a clone, an internal primer and an external primer were needed. An internal primer was the primer that could anneal to the sequence located in the insert; an external primer was the primer that could anneal to the vector. Examples of external primers are listed above. When designing the internal primer, it should be located at least 100 basepairs (bp) away from the external primer in order to distinguish the PCR product from the primer dimer in the agarose gel electrophoresis analysis. However, the internal primer is not recommended to be more than 3 kbp away from the external primer because the efficiency of PCR amplification of a long DNA fragment is low and therefore reduces the possibility of identifying positive clones.

3. Methods

1. Well-separated colonies were picked with sterile toothpicks one at a time. The colony was first streaked on a fresh agar plate with appropriate antibiotics. The remaining bacteria on the toothpick were resuspended in 25 μL of 1× PCR buffer. Label the streak on the plate and the PCR tube identically so that one would have a stock of bacteria for liquid culture later. Seventy microliters of mineral oil was added to each tube (**Note 3**).

2. DNA was heat denatured *in situ* at 94°C for 10 min. A 2× PCR master mixture in 1× PCR reaction buffer containing 400 μM dNTPs, 3 mM MgCl$_2$, 2 μM of the primers, and 0.5 unit/tube of Taq DNA polymerase was prepared. Twenty-five microliters of the 2× reaction mixture were added to the 25 μL of the denatured DNA solution beneath the mineral oil. The PCR was carried out under the following conditions: denaturing at 94°C for 1 min, annealing at 55°C for 1 min (**Note 4**), and polymerizing at 72°C for 1 min. (**Note 5**). This was repeated for 35 cycles.

3. At the end of the PCR, 10 μL of the reaction product were loaded on a 0.7% agarose gel for gel electrophoresis separation (**Note 6**). Hae III-cut ϕχ174 repli-

cation form DNA (**Note 7**) was used as the molecular weight marker to measure the size of the PCR product. The number of colonies that can be screened by the cPCR is only limited by the number of available positions in the thermal cycler.

4. Like all PCRs, controls are important for the cPCR method. The reagent and buffer without exogenous DNA is the required negative control. The cloning vector may be used as a positive control for the universal and reverse primers. Otherwise, it may be used as a negative control for the internal primer. The vector control should be derived from a colony on an agar plate. For an internal primer positive control, we generally use a clone to which the internal primer can also anneal. For example, to identify HIV-1 LTR clones derived from patient samples, we used existing HIV-1 LTR clones (NL4-3 or HXB2). The positive control clone should be prepared similarly (i.e., from a colony on an agar plate). Similar procedures has been employed for DNA sequencing *(8,9)*.

4. Notes

1. Fragments less than 3 kbp long have been successfully characterized using this method. For fragments longer that 3 kpb, we recommend an internal primer and an external primer like the M13 universal and reverse primers so that the amplified fragment is less than 3 kpb to ensure the successful application of the method.

2. The oligonucleotide primers may be purified by high-performance liquid chromatography, simple polyacrylamide gel electrophoresis, or oligo purification cartridge. All of these procedures will remove the n-1 oligonucleotides. For identification of positive clones, the primers need not be highly purified.

3. A regular 0.5-mL eppendorf centrifuge tube is sufficient for the procedure. Thin-walled PCR tubes should work with this procedure.

4. The annealing temperature should be determined empirically or estimated by the GC content of the primer in the PCR salt concentration. There are several computer software programs available that empirically derive the annealing temperature. We have tested Oligo (v. 4.0) and MacVector (v. 4.5, Oxford Molecular Group, Beaverton, OR). They both gave satisfactory results.

5. The extension rate of Taq DNA polymerase at 72°C is 2–4 kb/min. Extension rates of recombinant exo⁻ Pfu (Stratagene) and VentR(exo⁻) DNA polymerase have not been established by manufacturers. We generally used the same extension rate for Pfu and Vent DNA polymerase and obtained satisfactory results.

6. To analyze a 0.5–3-kpb DNA fragment, 0.7% agarose gel electrophoresis is sufficient. For DNA size outside this range, a different percentage gel should be used. Please consult **ref. *1***.

7. One hundred to 200 ng of the marker DNA should be used for sizing. A 1-kbp ladder from Bethesda Research Laboratory (Life Technology, Inc., Bethesda, MD) or Hind III digested λ DNA may also be used as the size marker, depending on the expected size of the product.

References

1. Sambrook, J., Fritsch, E. F., and Maniatis, T. (eds.) (1989), in *Molecular Cloning, A Laboratory Manual 2nd Edition*. Cold Spring Harbor Laboratory Press, Cold Spring Harbor, New York.
2. Ausubel, F. M., Brent, R., Kingston, R. E., Moore, D. D., Seidman, J. G., Smith, J. A., and Struhl, K. (1987) *Current Protocols in Molecular Biology*, Green Publishing Associates/Wiley–Interscience, New York.
3. Vieira, J. and Messing, J. (1982) The pUC plasmids, an M13mp7-derived system for insertion mutagenesis and sequencing with synthetic universal primers. *Gene* **19,** 259–268.
4. Yanisch-Perron, C., Vieira, J., and Messing, J. (1985) Improved M13 phage cloning vectors and host strains: Nucleotide sequences of the M13mp18 and pUC19 vectors. *Gene* **33,** 103–119.
5. Saiki, R. K., Gelfand, D. H., Stoffel, S., Scharf, S. J., Higuchi, R., Horn, G. T., Mullis, K. B., and Erlich, H. A. (1988) Primer-directed enzymatic amplification of DNA with a thermostable DNA polymerase. *Science* **239,** 487–491.
6. Wang, S. and Hazelrigg, T., (1994) Implications for bcd mRNA localization from spatial distribution of exu protein in Drosophila oogenesis. *Nature* **369,** 400–403.
7. Michael, N. L., D'Arcy, L., Ehrenberg, P. K., and Redfield, R. R. (1994) Naturally occurring genotypes of the human immunodeficiency virus type 1 long terminal repeat display a wide rage of basal and Tat-induced transcriptional activities. *J Virol.* **68,** 3163–3174.
8. Hoffman, M. A. and Brian, D. A., (1991) Sequencing PCR DNA amplified directly from a bacterial colony. *Biotechniques* **11,** 30,31.
9. Frothingham, M. A., Allen, R. L., and Wilson, K. H. (1991) Rapid 16S ribosomal DNA sequencing from a single colony without DNA extrction or purification. *Bioechniques* **11,** 40–44.

12

PCR Amplification and Cloning
of Virtually Full-Length HIV-1 Provirus

Mika Salminen

1. Introduction

Molecular analyses of HIV-1 variation, and its impact on the biological properties of the virus have by necessity been restricted by the scarcity of cloned proviruses. Only a handful of full-length clones exist *(1)*, and of these, even a smaller fraction are infectious upon transfection into cell lines. Furthermore, the available infectious clones only represent subtypes B and D *(1)*. The main reasons for the lack of infectious clones are related to the relatively low copy number of proviral DNA especially in primary cultures *(8)*.

HIV-1 isolates that have been adapted to growth in established cell lines usually reach higher proviral copy numbers in cell culture, and most infectious HIV-1 proviral clones have been cloned from such sources *(3,4)*. However, not all HIV-1 primary isolates can be adapted for growth in immortalized cell lines, and, even if they can, the virus may change so that it will no longer represent the original isolate in all biological aspects. Some HIV-1 proviruses have been cloned from primary PBMC cultures enriched for CD4+ cells and, in one case, brain tissue from a patient who died with fulminant HIV-1 related encephalitis *(5,6)*. The method used to clone the proviruses in all the cases above has been λ phage cloning, which involves a very laborious and time-consuming screening process. Frequently, relatively few clones can be found, especially when primary cultures were used. Clearly, a more efficient method for generation of proviral clones from primary PBMC cultures would be desirable. Polymerase chain reaction (PCR), with its million-fold amplification potential, would seem to be the obvious choice of method. However, until recently, the method has not been successful, and reproducibly has been applicable only to amplification of pieces smaller than approx 5-kb *(2)*.

From: *Methods in Molecular Medicine, Vol. 17: HIV Protocols*
Edited by: N. L. Michael and J. H. Kim © Humana Press Inc., Totowa, NJ

The development of more efficient amplification procedures relying on mixtures of processive and proofreading thermostable polymerases has resulted in amplification of more than 40-kb-long stretches of DNA, which opens up the possibility of amplifying the complete genome of HIV-1 in a single reaction. As the HIV-1 provirus carries identical LTR-sequences in both ends of the genome, it is not possible to simply choose the amplification primers from the beginning and the end of the genome. Furthermore, abundant sequence variation makes it difficult to find conserved regions in the genome to choose primers from.

The procedure for amplification presented here relies on the careful choice of primers from two conserved regions, the tRNA primer binding site (located on the boundary of the 5' LTR and the gag leader region) and the mRNA polyadenylation signal site (in the R/U5 junction of the 3' LTR). This PCR strategy amplifies a 9 kb stretch of DNA which contains all of the coding regions of the provirus and the U3 and R regions of the 3' LTR *(7)*. The amplicon can be easily cloned into commercially available vectors by utilizing the propensity of the *Taq* polymerase to add extra, unpaired A-residues to the 3' end of the DNA strands. Clones are screened by hybridization to specific HIV-1 probes and size. The cloning strategy does not by itself produce infectious proviruses, but those can be regenerated by separate amplification of the missing LTR regions. X can Be used

2. Materials

2.1. PCR

2.1.1. Isolation of Total PBMC DNA

Blood and Cell Culture Kits (Qiagen, Inc., Chatsworth, CA, cat. 13349, 13323, 13343, and 13362). Alternate: Isolation of DNA from Mammalian Cells: Protocol I *(9)*.

2.1.2. Amplification Kit

Expand Long Template PCR System Kit (Boehringer Mannheim, Indianapolis, IN cat no. 1681-842).

2.1.3. PCR Primer Sequences

1. msF12b 5'-AAATCTCTAGCAGTggcgccCGAACAG.
2. msR5b 5'-GCATGCgccCTCAAggcAAGCTTTATTGAGGCT.

2.2. TA Cloning

2.2.1. Ligation

TA cloning kit (Invitrogen Corp., Sorrento, CA. cat. no. K2000-01).

2.2.2. Transformation

1. STBL-2 Max Efficiency competent cells (Gibco-BRL Life Technologies, Frederick, MD, cat. no. 10268-019)
2. SOC media: 2% Tryptone (w/v), 0.5% yeast extract (w/v), 10 mM NaCl, 2.5 mM KCl, 10 mM MgSO$_4$, 10 mM MgCl$_2$. Sterilize by autoclaving, then add sterile-filtered glucose to a final concentration of 20 mM.

2.2.3. Screening for Clones

1. TB/Ampicillin media: 11.8 g peptone 140, 23.6 g yeast extract, 9.4 g K$_2$HPO$_4$, 2.2 g KH$_2$PO$_4$. Bring to 1 L with distilled water and sterilize by autoclaving. For plates, add 15 g/L bacto agar before autoclaving. Cool media to 50°C before adding sterile-filtered ampicillin (in H$_2$O) to a final concentration of 150 μg/mL.
2. 96-Well microplate replicator (The Lab Mart, J & H Berge, Inc., Plainfield, NJ, cat no. V373420).
3. Falcon standard Petri dishes, 150 × 15 mm (Falcon #1058).

2.2.4. Hybridization/Autoradiography

1. 20X SSPE: 3.6 M NaCl, 0.2 M NaH$_2$PO$_4$, pH 7.4, 0.02 M ethylenediamine tetra-acetic acid (EDTA).
2. Hybridization buffer: 6X SSPE, 0.5% sodium dodecyl sulfate (SDS), 0.02% bovine serum albumin (BSA), 0.02% Ficoll, 0.02% polyvinylpyrrolidone.
3. Whatman 3MM paper.
4. Oligodeoxynucleotide probe MSGAG8: 5' AGACAGGCTAATTTTTTAGGG AAGATCTGGCCTTCC.
5. Polynucleotide kinase and 10X kinase buffer (Boerhinger Mannheim #174645).
6. Gamma-[^{32}P]-adenosine triphosphate, triethylammonium salt, aqueous solution, 3000Ci/mmol (Amersham PB.10168).
7. Select-D, Sephadex G-25 spin column (5 Prime-3 Prime, Inc., # 5301-233431).
8. Liquid scintillation counter.
9. Beckman GPR-5 centrifuge or equivalent.

2.3. Consumables

1. 0.5-mL Thin-walled reaction tubes.
2. 1.5-mL Microfuge tubes.
3. DynaWax phase separation wax (FINNZYMES OY, Espoo, Finland, cat. no. F-600).
4. 1000-, 200-, and 20-μL ART filter pipet tips (Continental Laboratory Products, San Diego, CA, cat. no. 2079, 2069, and 2149).
5. 20 μL Positive displacement tips (Fisher Scientific, Pittsburgh, PA, cat. no. 22 35 415-9).

3. Methods

3.1. Isolation of Total PBMC DNA from Infected Cell Culture

Since the amplified fragment is long, a crucial factor to success is the quality of the input template DNA. It must be of high mol-wt (>50 kb on average) and clean (ratio of absorbance at 260–280 nm ≥ 1.8). It is also necessary to try to maximize the number of infected cells in the culture. Therefore, DNA must be isolated from cells that do not show extensive cytopathic effects, but do produce peak levels of p24 antigen production. Many methods for DNA isolation exist, but we have found that gentle phenol/chloroform extraction *(9)* or Qiagen-column purification usually perform well (Qiagen). The latter method is very rapid and provides the advantage of avoiding the use of highly toxic chemicals. The final DNA should be resuspended to a concentration of 0.1–1 μg/μL in 1X TE, pH 8.0, and stored at –20°C until used.

3.2. PCR

3.2.1. PCR setup

PCR is performed in thin walled tubes in a final volume of 50 μL. To achieve a hot start, crucial reagents are separated into two layers by a phase separation wax (DynaWax), (*see* **Note 1**). All setup can be done at room temperature.

1. Bring out templates to thaw in a template hood.
2. Change to a new pair of disposable gloves.
3. Bring out PCR reagents (except enzyme), primers, and sterile water to thaw in a clean reagent hood. Vortex reagents after thawing.
4. While thawing reagents, put DynaWax bottle in water bath in Decca-beaker on a hot plate to melt and label PCR tubes 1–10 and R, – and +.
5. Prepare Master mix A (**Table 1**) in 1.5-mL microfuge tubes (*see* **Note 2**).
6. Vortex and aliquot 25 μL of Master mix A into each thin-walled sample tube.
7. Aliquot 2 drops of melted Dynawax into each tube, making sure that the drops fall into the middle of the tube forming a separating meniscus on top of Master mix A. Let wax solidify for 1 min.
8. Prepare Master mix B (**Table 1**) in 1.5-mL microfuge tubes.
9. Put reagents away, and take a new pair of disposable gloves.
10. Vortex Master mix B, and layer 23 μL each in three PCR tubes on top of solidified wax and label tubes R, – and + (for controls).
11. Transfer Master mix B and PCR tubes to template hood
12. Add 2 μL sterile water into PCR tube R (reagent control), and close the tube.
13. Add 2 μL of 100 ng/mL uninfected PBMC genomic DNA into the PCR tube labeled "–" (negative DNA control), and close the tube.
14. Add 24 μL (12 × 2 μL) 100 ng/μL infected cell genomic DNA template into Master mix B tube with positive displacement pipet.
15. Vortex Master mix B for 10 s.
16. Aliquot 25 μL each of Master mix B on top of wax into tubes 1–10 and close the tubes.
17. Remove all tubes from clean area.
18. Add 2 μL of a positive control to tube +, and close tube (*see* **Note 4**).
19. Close the tubes, and transfer to the thermal cycler.

Table 1
Master Mixes[a]

| | Master mix A | | |
	15X	1X	
10X Expand Buffer #1	75	5	
Taq/Pwo enzyme	15	1	
(*see* **Note 3**)			
Sterile water	285	19	
Total volume	375	25	
	Master mix B		
	15X	1X	Final concentration
1.25 m*M* dNTP (each)	210	14	350 µ*M* (each)
5 µ*M* msF12/R5 (each)	75	5	0.5 µ*M* (each)
Sterile water	60	4	
Total volume	345	23	

[a]All volumes are in µL.

3.2.2. PCR Program

1. Perform a single cycle of 94°C for 2 min followed by 10 cycles of 94°C for 10 s, 60°C for 30 s, 68°C for 8 min, followed by 20 cycles of 94°C for 10 s, 55°C for 30 s, 68°C for 8 min, followed by 1 cycle of 72°C for 30 min and then hold at 4°C.
2. After PCR, store samples frozen at –20°C.

3.3. TA Cloning of Amplicons

3.3.1. PCR Product Gel Purification

1. Pool the products of ten 50 µL amplification reactions.
2. Load on a 1% Seaplaque Low Melt agarose/TAE (Tris-acetate-EDTA) gel and run at 80 V, +4°C until fully separated.
3. Cut out a 9-kb band using sterile razor blade, with minimum exposure to UV light to reduce nicking. UV transilluminators with long-wave filters are helpful in this regard.
4. Purify amplified fragment with Qiaquick (Qiagen) gel purification kit, and elute in 30 µL of sterile water. Keep product on ice while analyzing 5 µL of the product by gel electrophoresis (*see* **Note 5**).

3.3.2. Ligations

1. Combine the following reagents (as supplied in the TA-cloning kit) in a sterile 1.5 mL microfuge tube held on ice: 10 µL gel purified DNA, 2 µL pCRII TA-vector, 2 µL 10X ligation buffer, 4 µL sterile water, 2 µL T4 DNA ligase enzyme.

2. Ligate at 15°C overnight.
3. Inactivate ligation by heating to 70°C for 10 min.

3.3.3. Transformations

1. Combine the following reagents in a sterile 1.5-mL microfuge tube held on ice: 2.5 µL ligation reaction, 50 µL STBL2 Max Efficiency cells (Gibco-BRL).
2. Keep on ice for 30 min.
3. Transfer tubes into a 42°C water bath for 35 s.
4. Immediately place on ice for 2 min.
5. Add 1 mL of SOC media and recover for 30 min at 37°C, 225 rpm agitation.
6. Plate 250 µL on each of four amp/TB plates (150-mm diameter circular plates or 30 × 30-cm square plates).
7. Incubate plates 16–24 h at 32°C.

3.3.4. Screening Transformations

1. Pick 400–600 transparent colonies with sterile toothpicks (*see* **Note 7**) individually into sterile microtiter wells containing 200 µL Amp/TB media and grow overnight at 32°C.
2. Using sterile technique, lay down a single nylon transfer membrane filters on agarose/Amp/TB plates, generating one such plate for each microtiter plate.
3. Using a microtiter replicator, stamp replicates of each microtiter plate on the filter/agarose/Amp/TB plate. Next, stamp replicates of each microtiter plate on agarose/Amp/TB plate without filters.
4. Incubate plates overnight at 32°C.
5. Store microtiter cultures as masters at 4°C (maximum two weeks). Make sure to label plates carefully so that they can be correctly oriented with their cognate filters.
6. Lift filters with replicated colonies off plates, and proceed with denaturation and fixing of DNA. Store plates without filters at 4°C as secondary master plates (2 wk max).

3.3.5. Fix DNA to Filters

1. Set up four Whatman 3MM papers in a row, and soak them in the following reagents: A, 10% SDS; B, 0.5 M NaOH; C, 1 M Tris-HCl, pH 7.5; D, 2 X SSC.
2. Incubate filters with bacteria side up on each filter for 5 min, transferring in sequence A–B–C–D.
3. Air dry filters at room temperature for 1 h or until completely dry.

3.3.6. Hybridization

1. Thaw the radioisotope behind a lucite shield.
2. To a 0.5-mL microfuge tube held on wet ice, add 0.5 µL of a 20 µM solution of oligonucleotide, 2.0 µL of 10X polynucleotide kinase buffer, 11.5 µL of sterile water, 5.0 µL (50 µCi) of γ-[^{32}P]-adenosine triphosphate, and 1.0 µL (8 U) of polynucleotide kinase. Mix gently with a pipet tip.

3. Incubate in a 37°C water bath for 30 min.
4. Place the reaction on ice.
5. Invert the G-25 column enough times so that the matrix inside is well mixed.
6. Remove the upper and then the lower caps. Let the buffer drain out for about 10 min.
7. Place the column into a 1.5-mL centrifuge tube. Place this assembly into the large tube that was just used for draining the column. Seal with a cap.
8. Spin this setup in the Beckman GPR centrifuge at 1100g for 2 min. Remove the dried column with forceps. Place it into a fresh 1.5-mL centrifuge tube, and discard the first one. The column is now prepared for a sample.
9. Pipet the entire 20 µL volume of the kinase reaction onto the dried column bed. Place this assembly back into the large centrifuge tube. Cap it and seal it with parafilm.
10. Spin at 1100g for 4 min in the Beckman GPR centrifuge.
11. Break the cap seal. Remove the column with forceps and discard it into radioactive waste. Remove the approx 25 µL in the small centrifuge tube directly with a pipetman. Place this into a fresh 1.5-mL centrifuge tube.
12. Remove 1 µL of the purified sample, and count in a liquid scintillation counter.
13. Prehybridize membranes in designated plastic hybridization container (Tupperware with lid) in 50 mL hybridization buffer, containing 10 µg denatured herring sperm DNA (boiled in 1 mL hybridization buffer for 5 min), at 55°C for 1 h.
14. Combine 1×10^6 cpm-labeled probe in a screw cap tube to 1 mL of hybridization buffer.
15. Put in 100°C heat block (with water) for 5 min.
16. Incubate 5 min on ice.
17. Microcentrifuge for 30 s at 10,000g.
18. Using an ART tip, transfer the solution from the previous step to the prehybridization box.
19. Incubate in designated water bath at 42°C overnight.
20. On the next morning, pour off hybridization solution into high-activity radioisotope waste container.
21. Wash once with 200 mL 2X SSC, 0.1% SDS at room temperature.
22. Pour washing solution into low-activity waste container.
23. Wash once with 200 mL 1X SSC at 37°C for 1 h.
24. Pour washing solution into low-activity waste container. Let hybridized, washed membranes dry on Whatman 3MM filter paper before autoradiography.

3.3.7. Autoradiography

1. Cover the dry nylon membranes with saran-wrap or enclose in a sealable plastic bag.
2. Transfer the covered nylon membranes into autoradiography cassettes.
3. In darkroom, apply Kodak XAR-5 film or equivalent film to covered nylon membrane, and close into autoradiography cassette. Attach to membrane with paperclips on each side. Punch holes in film to be able to orient it after autoradiography.
4. After autoradiography, develop films.

3.3.8. Identification of Clones with the Appropriate Insert

1. Restreak hybridization-positive clones twice and pick several single colonies for overnight 3-mL cultures (*see* **Note 8**).
2. Screen pure cultures from overnight 3-mL miniprep cultures by restriction enzyme analysis (*see* **Note 9**).

3.3.9. Maxipreps of Clones for Sequencing/Long-Term Atorage

1. Attempt a standard maxiprep.
2. If the yield is low or if the insert is unstable, a chloramphenicol amplification step might prove useful (*see* **Note 8**) as given in **steps 3** to **6**.
3. In the afternoon, start a 50-mL overnight culture (TB/Amp) from a single colony of fresh (<1 wk) pure culture plate.
4. Add 20 mL of the overnight culture to 250 mL of TB/Amp, and grow at 32°C for **exactly** 5 h with agitation.
5. Add chloramphenicol to final concentration of 170 μg/mL, and allow culture to continue incubating at 32°C overnight.
6. Process in the standard fashion.

4. Notes

1. To prevent PCR contamination, all pipeting should be done with strictly dedicated pipets, filter pipets, and contamination-free prepared reagents. It is essential to use disposable gloves, which must be changed if reagents are touched after handling template DNAs. Template is added last to prevent contamination (preferably with a positive displacement pipet). The author also highly recommends using two different (dedicated) hoods for template addition and PCR master mix assembly. Always include reagent controls and negative DNA controls in these experiments.
2. This protocol is designed for ten replicates of the same template plus positive, negative, and reagent controls (two extra reactions are also included). Before doing such a preparative amplification, it is good practice to run a single reaction to verify that the template is amplifiable.
3. This enzyme (which comes with the Boehringer-Mannheim kit) may be substituted by a 6:1 mixture of *Taq* (Perkin-Elmer) and *Pfu* (Stratagene). However, the author doesn't know if it will be as sensitive in PCR and what fraction of the amplicons will contain A-overhangs. *Pfu* is a proofreading enzyme and may remove the overhangs over time, especially if the product is stored at 4°C.
4. Since PCR is so sensitive to carryover contamination, it is best to use a low copy number control, such as a DNA from infected cell culture. However, if such material is not available, an infectious clone, such as the widely available pNL4-3 clone can be used. In this case, use no more than 50 pg of plasmid (approx 5×10^6 copies). Never bring plasmid clones into clean areas.
5. Check the purified fragment on a gel to make sure that the fragment has not degraded during purification (as evidenced by excessive smearing) and that

enough DNA is present. The ligation reaction has been optimized for a concentration of 50–100 ng/µL of DNA after purification. If more is needed, scale-up the ligation, concentrate the DNA, or run more preparative PCRs.

6. The STBL2 cells are β-galactosidase negative, therefore cannot inserts cannot be distinguished from the background by color selection on X-gal plates. Growth at 32°C produces colonies more slowly, but with a higher yield of full-length inserts (*see* **Note 8**).

7. Clones are more transparent and frequently grow poorly, whereas background colonies, which are yellowish and tend to grow faster and form denser colonies. Expect very low cloning efficiencies. The author has usually recovered between 1 and 20 full-length clones/100 screened colonies.

8. Cloned HIV-1 proviral DNA sequences are frequently toxic to *Escherichia coli* (maps to at least the gp41 region of the *env* gene; author's unpublished observations) which can lead to their elimination from cultures over time. On a plate this may be evidenced by the appearance of denser foci of fast growth particularly in the first streak of a pure culture. In large overnight cultures, it is manifested by the emergence of smaller plasmids. This can be prevented by not allowing the culture to grow to high density and by growing the culture at lower than usual temperatures (32°C). Since lower cell density results in less plasmid in the final preparation, a chloramphenicol enrichment procedure is added which stops cell growth and division, but allows the plasmid replication to continue, leading to large increase in copy numbers per cell. Using this method, relatively small-scale cultures can yield several hundreds of micrograms of plasmid. A drawback of chloramphenicol amplification is the insertion of ribonucleotides into plasmid DNA which are more liable to degradative enzymes. Sometimes the apparent "poison" sequences in the HIV-1 genome also lead to insertional inactivation by bacterial IS sequences. This is especially troublesome, since the insertions are frequently accompanied by a simultaneous deletions, leading to difficulty in detecting the IS sequence before sequencing. The author has encountered IS insertions in plasmids grown in several different commercially available *E. coli* strains, some of which were supposedly IS negative.

9. Use 0.7% agarose gels for best resolution. *Eco*RI cuts in the vector on both sides of the 9-kb insert. Most HIV-1 genomes have no *Eco*RI sites or a single site which frequently results in two DNA fragments of 4 and 5 kb. Since the vector is 4 kb, only these two bands will be seen on an ethidium bromide stained agarose gel given this stoichiometry.

References

1. Myers, G., Korber, B., Hanhn, B. K., Jeang, K.-T., Mellors, J. W., McCutchan, F. E., et al. (eds.) (1995) *Human Retroviruses and AIDS Theoretical Biology and Biophysics*, Group T-10, MS K710, Los Alamos National Laboratory, Los Alamos, NM.
2. Edmonson, P. F. and Mullins, J. I. (1992) Efficient amplification of HIV half-genomes from tissue DNA. *Nucleic Acids Res.* **20,** 4933.

3. Hahn, B. H., Gonda, M. A., Shaw, G. M., Popovic, M., Hoxie, J. A., Gallo, R. C., and Wong-Staal, F. (1985) Genomic diversity of the acquired immune deficiency syndrome virus HTLV-III: different viruses exhibit greatest divergence in their envelope genes. *Proc. Natl. Acad. Sci. USA* **82,** 4813–4817.
4. Hahn, B. H., Shaw, G. M., Arya, S. K., Popovic, M., Gallo, R. C., and Wong-Staal, F. (1984) Molecular cloning and characterization of the HTLV-III virus associated with AIDS. *Nature* **312,** 166–169.
5. Li, Y., Hui, H., Burgess, C. J., Price, R. W., Sharp, P. M., Hahn, B. H., and Shaw, G. M. (1992) Complete nucleotide sequence, genome organization, and biological properties of human immunodeficiency virus type 1 in vivo: evidence for limited defectiveness and complementation. *J. Virol.* **66,** 6587–6600.
6. Li, Y., Kappes, J. C., Conway, J. A., Price, R. W., Shaw, G. M., and Hahn, B. H. (1991) Molecular characterization of human immunodeficiency virus type 1 cloned directly from uncultured human brain tissue: identification of replication-competent and -defective viral genomes. *J. Virol.* **65,** 3973–3985.
7. Salminen, M. O., Koch, C., Sanders-Buell, E., Ehrenberg, P. K., Michael, N. L., Carr, J. K., et al. (1995) Recovery of virtually full-length HIV-1 provirus of diverse subtypes from primary virus cultures using the polymerase chain reaction. *Virology* **213,** 80–86.
8. Simmonds, P., Balfe, P., Peutherer, J. F., Ludlam, C. A., Bishop, J. O., and Brown, A. J. (1990) Human immunodeficiency virus-infected individuals contain provirus in small numbers of peripheral mononuclear cells and at low copy numbers. *J. Virol.* **64,** 864–872.
9. Isolation of DNA from mammalian cells: Protocol I (1989) in, *Molecular Cloning: A Laboratory Manual* (Sambrook, J., Fritch, E. F., and Maniatis, T., eds.), 2nd ed., Cold Spring Harbor Laboratory Press, Cold Spring Harbor, N.Y.

13

Quantitation of HIV-1 *gag* DNA and RNA From Single Frozen Cell Pellets

Maryanne Vahey, Sandra C. Barrick, and Martin Nau

1. Introduction

The assessment of viral load in the blood, tissues, and bodily fluids of persons infected with human immunodeficiency virus is fundamental to defining the stage of disease *(1–3)*, the effect of antiviral treatments to abate disease *(4, 5)*, disease progression *(6–8)*, and propensity for the transmission of disease *(9, 10)* as well. Now accepted as a surrogate for all of these features of HIV-1 disease, specific guidelines have been adopted for the use of viral load measures in the clinical management of the disease *(11)*.

We present here a method for the assessment of HIV-1 *gag* DNA and RNA from a single frozen pellet of cells. These cells can be obtained from the conventional isolation of peripheral blood mononuclear cells (PBMC) or from other body compartments such as semen or cervical secretions. The pelleted cells are snap frozen in liquid nitrogen after the liquid has been carefully decanted from the pellet. Frozen cells prepared in this manner and stored at −80°C are stable indefinitely for the assays we describe here.

The protocols that follow detail the extraction of nucleic acids, polymerase chain reaction (PCR), and mini-gel separation and detection of the PCR products. The number of cell equivalents used in the PCR assay for the determination of HIV-1 *gag* DNA and RNA is standardized by the use of the quantitation of β–globin DNA. Quantitation of the β–globin DNA and HIV-1 *gag* DNA PCR assays use iterations of unknowns with standard curves consisting of dilution series of plasmids *(12, 13)*, referred to in the procedures as PEC or "plasmid external control." For HIV-1 *gag* RNA quantitation, complementary RNA transcripts prepared from the PEC plasmid serve as the external standard template.

From: *Methods in Molecular Medicine, Vol. 17: HIV Protocols*
Edited by: N. L. Michael and J. H. Kim © Humana Press Inc., Totowa, NJ

2. Materials

2.1. Nucleic Acid Extraction

1. Diethylpyrocarbonate solution (Sigma, D5758).
2. RNasin, 40 U/μL (Promega, #N2514).
3. Dithiothreitol (DTT), 0.1 M solution (Boehringer-Mannheim, #100-032).
4. RNA STAT-60 (Teltest, #TL-4110).
5. DNA STAT-60 (Teltest, #TL-4110).
6. DNase I, RNase-free, 10 U/μL (Boehringer Mannheim, #776785).
7. TM buffer (100 mM Tris-HCl, pH 7.4, 40 mM MgCl$_2$).

2.2. β-Globin Standards and Amplification

The materials are given in two parts. The first part lists the materials needed for preparation of the β–globin external standards, and the second part lists the materials needed for β–globin PCR amplification.

2.2.1. β-Globin External Standard Preparation

1. β–Globin external standard plasmid (β–globin PEC) *(13)* (*see* **Note 8**).
2. Diluent I buffer: 4 μg/mL carrier tRNA in DEPC-treated distilled water (*see* **Subheading 3.1.**).
3. 1.5-mL microfuge tubes.
4. Spectrophotometer.

2.2.2. β-Globin Amplification

1. β–Globin external standards (*see* **Subheading 3.2.1.**).
2. Deoxynucleotide triphosphates (dNTPs), 25 mM (Promega, #U1240).
3. Sterile deionized water.
4. 10X PCR buffer (Perkin Elmer, #N808-0006).
5. *Taq* DNA polymerase (Perkin Elmer, #N801-0060).
6. Mineral oil (Perkin Elmer, #186-2302).
7. β–Globin primers, 20 μM β–globin sense primer: 5' GAA GAG CCA AGG ACA GGT AC; β–globin antisense primer: 5' CAA CTT CAT CCA CGT TCA CC.
8. DNA Thermal Cycler (Perkin-Elmer).

2.3. HIV-1 gag DNA standards and amplification

The materials are given in two parts. The first part lists the materials needed for preparation of the HIV-1 *gag* DNA external standards and the second part lists the materials needed for HIV-1 *gag* DNA PCR amplification.

2.3.1. HIV-1 gag PEC DNA Standards

1. HIV-1 *gag* external standard plasmid (HIV-1 *gag* PEC) *(13)* (*see* **Note 9**).
2. Carrier tRNA, 10 mg/mL solution (Boehringer-Mannheim, #109495).

3. Diluent I buffer: 4 µg/mL carrier tRNA in DEPC-treated distilled water (*see* **Subheading 3.1.**).
4. 1.5-mL microfuge tubes.
5. Spectrophotometer.

2.3.2. HIV-1 gag DNA Amplification

1. HIV-1 *gag* DNA external standards (*see* **Subheading 3.2.1.**)
2. Deoxynucleotide triphosphates (dNTPs), 25 m*M* (Promega, #U1240).
3. Sterile deionized water.
4. 10X PCR buffer (Perkin Elmer, #N808-0006).
5. *Taq* DNA polymerase (Perkin Elmer, #N801-0060).
6. Mineral oil (Perkin Elmer, #186-2302).
7. HIV-1 *gag* DNA primers, 20 µ*M* HIV-1 *gag* DNA sense primer: 5' CAA TGA GGA AGC TGC AGA ATG GGA TAG; HIV-1 *gag* DNA antisense primer: 5' CAT CCA TCC TAT TTG TTC CTG AAG G.
8. DNA Thermal Cycler (Perkin-Elmer).

2.4. HIV-1 gag RNA Standards and Amplification

The materials are given in five sections. The first three list materials needed for preparation of the *gag* cRNA external standard and the fourth and fifth list those needed for reverse transcription and PCR amplification of HIV-1 *gag* RNA.

2.4.1. Linearization of the HIV-1 gag PEC DNA

1. Acetylated bovine serum albumin (BSA), 10 mg/mL (New England Biolabs #145S).
2. Ethanol.
3. HIV-1 *gag* PEC DNA.
4. *Xba* I restriction enzyme and 10X restriction buffer 2 (New England Biolabs, #145S).
5. Phenol (Gibco, #550UA).
6. Chloroform (Baxter Scientific, #4445).
7. Spectrophotometer.
8. 10X TBE: 108 g Tris base, 55 g boric acid, 40 mL 0.5 *M* EDTA, pH 8.0, distilled water in quantity sufficient to bring volume to G< 1 L.
9. 5X oligonucleotide loading buffer: 5 mL 10 TBE, 2 mL 1% xylene cyanol FF, 3 mL 100% glycerol.
10. TE buffer: 1 mL 1 *M* Tris-HCl, pH 8.0 (0.01 *M*), 0.2 mL 0.5 *M* EDTA, pH 8.0 (0.001 *M*), 98.8 mL sterile water.
11. TEN buffer: 2 mL 5 *M* NaCl (0.1 *M*), 1 mL 1 *M* Tris-HCl, pH 8.0 (0.01 *M*), 0.2 mL 0.5 *M* EDTA, pH 8.0 (0.001 *M*), 96.8 mL sterile water.

2.4.2. In vitro Transcription of HIV-1 gag cRNA

1. 5X transcription buffer (in Promega, #P2075); 200 m*M* Tris-HCl, pH 7.5, 30 m*M* MgCl$_2$, 10 m*M* spermidine, 50 m*M* NaCl.
2. Linearized HIV-1 *gag* PEC DNA.
3. 0.1 *M* DTT (in Promega #P2075).

4. RNasin, 40 units/μL (Promega N2514).
5. 2.5 m*M* rNTPs (Promega #P1221, 10 m*M* each of four mixed in equal volumes).
6. T7 RNA polymerase (in Promega #P2075).
7. DNase I, RNase-free (Boehringer-Mannheim, #776785).
8. RNA marker I (Boehringer-Mannheim, #1062611).
9. Chloroform (Baxter Scientific, # 4443).
10. TE buffer: 1 mL 1 *M* Tris-HCl, pH 8.0 (0.01 *M*), 0.2 mL 0.5 *M* EDTA, pH 8.0 (0.001 *M*), 98.8 mL sterile water.
11. Formamide loading buffer: 10 mL formamide, 0.2 mL 0.5 *M* EDTA, pH 8.0, 20 mg bromphenol blue.
12. Phenol: chloroform: isoamyl alcohol (25:24:1).
13. Ammonium persulfate (Bio-Rad, #161-0200), 1.0 mL 10% aqueous solution, made freshly.
14. Gel-Mix 6 (Gibco).
15. Vertical mini-gel electrophoresis system (Bio-Rad).
16. Speed-Vac system (Savant Instruments).
17. Ethidium bromide, 5 μg/mL, in 1X TBE buffer.

2.4.3. Preparation of HIV-1 gag cRNA External Standard Dilutions

1. HIV-1 *gag* cRNA (*see* **Subheading 2.4.2.**).
2. Carrier tRNA, 10 mg/mL solution (Boehringer-Mannheim, #109495).
3. Dithiothreitol (DTT), 0.1 *M* solution (in Promega #P2075).
4. RNasin, 40 units/μL (Promega N2514).
5. Diluent I buffer: 4 μg/mL carrier tRNA.
6. Diluent II buffer: 5 m*M* DTT, 1 U/μL RNasin, 4 μg/mL carrier tRNA.

2.4.4. HIV-1 gag cDNA Preparation by Reverse Transcription

1. Mineral oil (Perkin Elmer, #186-2302).
2. *gag* antisense primer: 5.0 μ*M*.
3. HIV-1 *gag* cRNA standard dilutions (*see* **Subheading 2.4.3.**).
4. Sterile water.
5. Reverse transcriptase enzyme, 200 U/μL (Gibco-BRL, SuperScript II RNase H-, #18064-014).
6. 5X reverse transcriptase buffer (shipped with the enzyme).
7. 0.1 *M* dithiothreitol solution (Gibco-BRL, #8053A).
8. dNTPs, 25 m*M* (Promega, #U1240).
9. RNasin, 40 U/μL (Promega, #N2514).
10. Heat block, 45°C.

2.4.5. HIV-1 gag cDNA Amplification

1. Mineral oil (Perkin Elmer, #186-2302).
2. *gag* sense primer, 20 μ*M* solution.
3. *gag* antisense primer, 20 μ*M* solution.
4. dNTPs, 25 m*M* (Promega, #U1240).

5. *Taq* DNA polymerase, 5 U/μL (Perkin Elmer, #N808-0006).
6. 10X PCR buffer (Perkin Elmer, #N801-0060).
7. Thermal cycler.
8. Sterile water.

2.5. Liquid Hybridization Assay

The materials for the liquid hybridization (LH) assay will be listed in two sections. The first lists materials needed to 5'-end label the hybridization probe with ^{32}P, while the second lists items needed for the LH reaction itself.

2.5.1. 5'-End Labeling of the Oligonucleotide Probe

1. Oligonucleotide probes: *gag* probe, 5' ATG AGA GAA CCA AGG GGA AGT GAC ATA GCA; β–globin probe, 5' AAG TCA GGG CAG AGC CAT CTA TTG CTT ACA.
2. Polynucleotide kinase and 10X kinase buffer (Boerhinger Mannheim, #174645).
3. Gamma-[^{32}P]-adenosine triphosphate, triethylammonium salt, aqueous solution, 3000 Ci/mmol (Amersham, PB.10168).
4. Select-D, Sephadex G-25 spin column (5 Prime-3 Prime, Inc., # 5301-233431).
5. Liquid scintillation counter.
6. Beckman GPR-5 centrifuge or equivalent.

2.5.2. Liquid Hybridization Reaction

1. 1.1X OH Buffer: 667 μL 1 *M* NaCl, 888 μL 0.5 *M* EDTA, pH 8.0, 8.445 mL distilled H_2O.
2. 5X DNA loading buffer: 5.0 mL 10X TBE, 0.5 mL 1% w/v bromophenol blue, 3.0 mL 100% glycerol, 1.5 mL sterile distilled water.
3. 1X TBE (1:10 dilution of 10X TBE).

2.6. Polyacrylamide Gel Electrophoresis of Hybridized PCR Products

1. Acrylamide/bis-acrylamide (19:1), 40% solution (Sigma, #A2917 or Bio-Rad).
2. 1X TBE (1:10 dilution of 10X TBE) (Sigma, #A2917 or Bio-Rad).
3. TEMED (Gibco-BRL, #5524UB).
4. Ammonium persulfate (Bio Rad, #161-0200), 10% freshly prepared aqueous solution.
5. ATTO Dual Mini Slab Gel System or any other mini-gel system (Serva Biochemicals, #92222).
6. Power supply (such as Gibco-BRL, #250).

2.7. Signal Detection and Analysis

1. Molecular Dynamics Phosphorimager or similar device employing storage phosphor technology.
2. Computer with Microsoft Excel or similar spreadsheet program.

3. Methods

3.1. Simultaneous Extraction
of DNA and RNA from Frozen Cell Pellets

This procedure will result in the extraction of both DNA and RNA from the same frozen cell pellet. These nucleic acid templates are used in the PCR assays to quantitate HIV-1*gag* DNA and RNA and to standardize assay input for cell equivalents using β–globin DNA quantitation.

1. Prepare DEPC-treated distilled water by adjusting 1 L of distilled water to 0.1% (v/v) with DEPC, let stand overnight at 37°C, and then autoclave at 121°C for ≥ 15 min.
2. Remove frozen cell pellets from the –80°C freezer.
3. Working in a clean laminar flow hood, add the appropriate amount of RNA STAT-60 to the cell pellet in each tube. Ensure that the cells have been lysed by repetitive pipetting. Use 0.8 mL of RNA STAT-60 for 5 x 10⁶ cells (*see* **Note 1**).
4. Allow the lysate to stand at room temperature for 10 min. Transfer lysate to 1.5 mL microcentrifuge tube. Tubes may now be brought to a standard BL-2 laboratory. The rest of this procedure is carried out at the bench top.
5. Add 0.2 mL of chloroform per 1 mL of the RNA STAT-60 used.
6. Vortex vigorously for 15 s. Let samples stand at room temperature for 2 to 3 min.
7. Centrifuge samples for 15 min at 12,000*g*, 4°C.
8. The upper aqueous phase contains the RNA. Transfer this phase to new, labeled 1.5 microcentrifuge tube (*see* **Note 2**). Save the organic phase for use in step 20.
9. Add 0.5 mL of isopropanol per 1 mL of RNA STAT-60. Vortex samples and precipitate for 10 min at room temperature (*see* **Note 1**).
10. Centrifuge samples for 10 min at 12,000*g*, 4°C.
11. Decant supernate and wash the pellet with 0.5 mL cold 75% ethanol. Centrifuge for 5 min at 12,000*g* at 4°C.
12. Decant supernatant and siphon excess liquid from the cell pellet using a disposable tip taking care to avoid the pellet. Air dry the samples for 15 min. Do not use a vacuum centrifuge to dry samples.
13. Resuspend pellet in 86 µL of DEPC-treated H₂0. Heat to 95°C for 5 min then vortex vigorously in order to resuspend the RNA.
14. Repeat 95°C incubation for another 5 min. Vortex and quick-chill in ice water for 5 min.
15. Place the samples on ice and add the following to each: 1 µL 0.1 *M* DTT, 2.5 µL, RNasin (40 U/µL), 2.5 µL of TM buffer, and 5.0 µL DNase I (RNase-free) (10 U/µL).
16. Incubate at 37°C for 1 h.
17. Heat to 95°C for 15 min to inactivate the DNase I enzyme.
18 Chill on ice and add 3 µL RNasin (40 U/µL) to each sample.
19. The RNA template is now ready for reverse transcriptase reactions and can be stored in appropriately labeled 1.5-mL microfuge tubes at –80°C.
20. After removing the RNA in the upper aqueous phase in **step 8**, add the appropriate amount of DNA STAT-60 reagent to each tube containing the organic phase.

21. Use 0.8 mL of DNA STAT-60 for 5×10^6 cells (*see* **Note 3**).
22. Add 0.16 mL of chloroform per 1.0 mL of DNA STAT-60, vortex vigorously for 15 s. Let stand at room temperature for 2–3 min.
23. Centrifuge the extract at 12,000*g* for 15 min at 4°C.
24. The extract should separate into two phases: a lower organic phase and an upper aqueous phase (DNA remains in the aqueous phase) (*see* **Note 4**).
25. Transfer the aqueous phase to a new tube and precipitate with isopropanol. Add 0.5 mL of isopropanol per 1.0 mL of DNA STAT-60 used for homogenization (*see* **Note 5**).
26. Let the samples stand at room temperature for 10 min and then centrifuge at 12,000*g* for 10 min at 4°C. A small clear to white pellet should appear on the bottom of the tube.
27. Decant supernatant and add 800 µL of 75% ethanol per 1 mL of the DNA STAT-60 used in the initial extraction to the tube.
28. Centrifuge samples at 12,000*g* at 4°C for 5 min.
29. Decant supernatant and siphon excess liquid from the pellet using a pipetman and disposable tip taking care to avoid the pellet. Air dry the samples for 15 min. Do not use a vacuum centrifuge to dry samples.
30. Dissolve the DNA pellet in 0.1 mL of DEPC-treated H_2O by gently pipetting the mixture. Place samples into a 95°C heat block for 15 min to ensure complete resuspension of the DNA. Place samples on ice to chill.
31. The DNA is now ready for use as PCR template. Store samples at –80°C.

3.2. Amplification of β–Globin DNA by PCR

This protocol gives the details of an assay for the amplification of β–globin sequences by PCR to determine the levels of this housekeeping gene as a means of standardizing the cell equivalents assessed in the subsequent HIV-1 *gag* DNA and RNA assays. The number of cell equivalents is arrived at by interpolation of values obtained for the clinical specimens with a standard curve of known copy numbers of a plasmid containing the β–globin target sequence (β–globin PEC). The protocol is given in two parts. The first part describes the preparation of the β–globin external standard curve and the second part describes the β–globin PCR amplification.

3.2.1. Preparation of β–Globin External Standards

1. Turn on the spectrophotometer, set the wavelength to 260 nm, and allow it to warm-up according to the manufacturer's instructions.
2. Add 300 µL of distilled water (*see* **Note 7**) to a 1.5 mL microfuge tube labeled "blank" and 292.5 µL to a tube labeled "sample".
3. Add 7.5 µL of β–globin PEC DNA to the sample tube and vortex briefly to mix.
4. Blank the spectrophotometer with the water in the "blank" tube.
5. Read the sample OD at 260 nm.
6. Change the wavelength to 280 nm, re-blank, and read the sample OD at 280 nm.

Table 1
Dilution of β-Globin PEC DNA Standards

Tubes	Diluent I	Copies/10 μL
No dilution	0	50,000
200 μL from tube 1	800 μL	10,000
500 μL from tube 2	500 μL	5,000
200 μL from tube 3	800 μL	1,000
500 μL from tube 4	500 μL	500
200 μL from tube 5	800 μL	100

7. Calculate the ratio of OD_{260}/OD_{280}. This number should be ≥ 1.8 if the DNA is pure.
8. Calculate the β–globin PEC concentration by the following formula: concentration of PEC (μg/mL) = OD_{260} × 40 (dilution factor) × 50 μg/mL (double-stranded DNA correction factor).
9. The β–globin PEC DNA template is diluted into aliquots to provide 100, 500, 1,000, 5,000, 10,000, and 50,000 copies per 10 μL. Given that β–globin PEC DNA is 3.47 × 10^{-18} g/copy (*see* **Note 8**), 50,000 copies per 10 μL equates to 1.74 × 10^{-11} g/mL (or 17.5 pg/mL). Dilute the β–globin PEC stock in step 8 in diluent buffer I to this concentration using several large, serial dilution steps. For the remaining β–globin PEC standards, use the serial dilution scheme given in **Table 1**.
10. These standards should be aliquoted in 50 μL amounts and stored at –20°C.

3.2.2. β–Globin Amplification

1. Prewarm the thermocycler block to 95°C.
2. Assemble reagents from freezers and allow them to thaw on ice.
3. In a clean laminar-flow hood, assemble and label PCR (0.5 mL) tubes and place them in a rack. Tubes to be labeled are one for the assay blank (H_2O) and each clinical specimen and the β–globin PEC dilution series. Tubes are placed in the rack left to right. In addition, label a 1.5 mL or larger tube for your PCR master mix.
4. Determine the number of reaction tubes to be run and add two. Make a master-mix by multiplying this number by the values given in **Table 2**. Hold the master mix on ice.
5. To the tube labeled as the assay blank, add 10 μL of sterile H_2O.
6. To the tubes labeled as clinical specimens, add 8 μL of H_2O and 2 μL of clinical specimen DNA to the appropriate corresponding tube (*see* **Note 6**).
7. To tubes appropriately labeled for ß-globin DNA PEC curve dilution series, add 10 μL of each dilution working from the low dilution to the high dilution.
8. Starting with the assay blank tube, continuing with the clinical specimen tubes, and finally with the β–globin PEC curve tubes, aliquot 90 μL of PCR master-mix to each tube to bring the final volume of each reaction to 100 μL.
9. Add 60 μL of mineral oil to all samples using a pipetman and a disposable pipet tip, changing tips between each tube.

Table 2
β-Globin PCR Set-up

Component	Volume (μL/reaction)	Final concentration
DI water	68.7	
10X buffer	10.0	$[Mg^{2+}] = 1.50$ mM
β-Globin Sense, 20 μM	5.0	1.0 μM
β-Globin Antisense, 20 μM	5.0	1.0 μM
dNTPs, 25 mM each	0.8	200 μM each
Taq polymerase, 5 U/μL	0.5	0.025 U/μL
Master-mix volume/reaction	90 μL	
Template volume	10 μL	
Final volume	100 μL	

10. Vortex each tube briefly and centrifuge at 12,000g for 5 s.
11. Place tubes into the preheated thermocycler and initiate the following program: 95°C for 30 s, 50°C for 30 s, 72°C for 3 min for 22 cycles followed by a single incubation at 72°C for 10 min followed by 4°C until tubes are removed for storage.
12. Store tubes at 4°C.

3.3. Amplification of HIV-1 gag DNA by PCR

This protocol gives the details of PCR for HIV-1 *gag* DNA. The number of copies of *gag* DNA is arrived at by interpolation of values obtained for the clinical specimens with a standard curve of known copy numbers of a plasmid containing the HIV-1 *gag* target sequence (HIV-1 *gag* PEC). This protocol is essentially the same as the one used for β–globin PCR with changes made in the volume of material used in the assay and the use of HIV-1 *gag* specific primers instead of β–globin primers. The protocol is given in two parts. The first part describes the preparation of the HIV-1 *gag* external standard curve and the second part describes the HIV-1 *gag* DNA PCR amplification.

3.3.1. Preparation of HIV-1 gag DNA External Standards

1. Determine the OD$_{260}$ and OD$_{280}$ of the HIV-1 *gag* DNA PEC as given in **Subheading 3.2.1., steps 1–8** for the β–globin PEC.
2. The HIV-1 *gag* DNA template is diluted into aliquots to provide 5, 10, 50, 100, 500, 1,000, and 5,000 copies per 10 μL. Given that the HIV-1 *gag* DNA PEC DNA is 4.31×10^{-18} g/copy (*see* **Note 9**), 5,000 copies per 10 μL equates to 2.16×10^{-12} g/mL (or 2.16 pg/mL). Dilute the HIV-1 *gag* DNA stock in diluent buffer I to this concentration using several large, serial dilution steps. For the remaining H IV-1 *gag* DNA standards, use the serial dilution scheme given in **Table 3**.
3. These standards should be aliquoted in 50 μL amounts and stored at –20°C.

Table 3
Dilution of HIV-1 *gag* DNA PEC DNA Standards

Tubes	Diluent I	Copies/10 μL
No dilution		5,000
200 μL from tube 1	800 μL	1,000
500 μL from tube 2	500 μL	500
200 μL from tube 3	800 μL	100
500 μL from tube 4	500 μL	50
200 μL from tube 5	800 μL	10
500 μL from tube 5	500 μL	5

Table 4
HIV-1 *gag* DNA PCR Set-up

Component	Volume (μL/reaction)	Final concentration
Distilled water	48.7	
10X buffer	10.0	$[Mg^{2+}] = 1.50$ mM
gag Sense, 20 μM	5.0	1.0 μM
gag Antisense, 20 μM	5.0	1.0 μM
dNTPs, 25 mM each	0.8	200 μM each
Taq polymerase, 5 U/μL	0.5	0.025 U/μL
Master-mix volume/reaction	70 μL	
Template volume	30 μL	
Final volume	100 μL	

3.3.2. HIV-1 gag DNA Amplification

1. Prewarm the thermocycler block to 95°C.
2. Assemble reagents from freezers and allow them to thaw on ice.
3. In a clean laminar-flow hood, assemble and label PCR (0.5 mL) tubes and place in a rack. Label one tube each for the assay blank (H$_2$O), each clinical specimen, and each dilution of the HIV-1 DNA PEC external standards. Tubes are placed in the rack left to right. In addition, label a 1.5 mL or larger tube for your PCR master mix.
4. Determine the number of reaction tubes to be run and add two. Make a master-mix by multiplying this number by the values given in **Table 4**. Hold the master mix on ice.
5. To tube labeled as the assay blank, add 30 μL of sterile H$_2$O.
6. To the tubes appropriately labeled for HIV-1 *gag* DNA PEC curve dilution series, add 20 μL of H$_2$O.
7. To the tubes appropriately labeled for the DNA clinical specimens, add 30 μL (1.5 × 106 cell equivalents) of the corresponding DNA clinical specimens.

8. Aliquot 10 µL of HIV-1 *gag* DNA PEC curve dilution series into the appropriate corresponding tubes working from the low dilution to the high dilution.
9. Starting with the assay blank tube, continuing with the clinical specimen tubes, and finally with the *gag* DNA PEC curve tubes, aliquot 70 µL of PCR master-mix to each tube to bring the final volume of each reaction to 100 µL.
10. Add 60 µL of mineral oil to all tubes using a pipetman and a disposable pipet tip, changing tips between each sample.
11. Vortex each tube briefly and centrifuge at 12,000g for 5 s.
12. Place tubes into the preheated thermocycler and initiate the following program: 95°C for 30 s, 55°C for 30 s, 72°C for 3 min for 25 cycles followed by a single incubation at 72°C for 10 min followed by 4°C until tubes are removed for storage.
13. Store tubes at 4°C.

3.4. Amplification of HIV-1 gag RNA by Reverse Transcriptase–PCR (RT-PCR)

This protocol gives the details of the amplification of HIV-1 *gag* RNA by a linked RT-PCR assay. The RNA extracted from the frozen cell pellet must first be converted to complementary DNA (cDNA) by the enzyme reverse transcriptase as only DNA is a template for the *Taq* DNA polymerase used in the subsequent PCR assay. The number of copies of *gag* RNA is arrived at by interpolation of values obtained for the clinical specimens with a standard curve of known copy numbers of a complementary RNA (cRNA) transcribed in vitro from the HIV-1 *gag* PEC DNA plasmid. The protocol is given in five sections. The first three sections describe the preparation of the HIV-1 *gag* cRNA external standard curve and the fourth and fifth sections describe the HIV-1 *gag* RNA reverse transcription and PCR amplification, respectively.

3.4.1. Linearization of the HIV-1 gag PEC DNA

1. Add to a 1.5 mL microfuge tube 50 µg of HIV-1 *gag* PEC DNA, 10 µL of 10X restriction buffer 2, 1 µL acetylated BSA, and a volume of water sufficient to bring the volume to 95 µL.
2. Add 5 µL (100 U) of *Xba* I restriction enzyme and gently mix.
3. Incubate for 4 h in a 37°C water bath.
4. Remove a 1 µL aliquot of the restriction digest and add 4 µL of water and 1 µL of 5X oligonucleotide loading buffer.
5. Aliquot 0.2 µg of undigested PEC DNA into another tube, bring the volume to 5 µL with water, and add 1 µL of 5X oligonucleotide loading buffer.
6. Electrophorese the DNAs in adjacent wells, along with molecular weight standards, through a 0.8% agarose mini-gel with 1X TBE running buffer and 0.5 µg/mL ethidium bromide at 8 Vcm^{-1} for 50 V-h, and visualize with UV light.
7. Ensure that all of the DNA in the digested sample shows delayed migration compared with the position of the major band in the undigested sample. This delayed band should size at 4 kb.

8. To the remaining 99 μL of PEC DNA, add 200 μL of TEN buffer, 150 μL of phenol solution, and 150 μL of chloroform.
9. Vortex briefly.
10. Centrifuge at 12,000g for 5 min at room temperature in a microcentrifuge.
11. Carefully remove the upper, aqueous phase to a fresh 1.5 mL microfuge tube.
12. Add 300 μL of chloroform to the aqueous phase, vortex, centrifuge again, and remove the upper, aqueous phase to a fresh 1.5 mL microfuge tube.
13. Add 300 μL of cold, 100% ethanol and mix by inversion 10 times.
14. Incubate at –20°C for 1 h.
15. Centrifuge at 12,000g for 15 min at 4°C in a microcentrifuge.
16. Carefully remove the supernatant and discard without disturbing the pellet.
17. Add 500 μL of cold, 70% ethanol and centrifuge at 12,000g for 5 min at 4°C in a microcentrifuge.
18. Carefully remove the supernatant and discard without disturbing the pellet.
19. Air-dry for 15 min.
20. Resuspend the pellet in 50 μL TE buffer.
21. Store the purified, linearized PEC DNA at 4°C.

3.4.2. In vitro Transcription of HIV-1 gag cRNA

1. Prepare water baths at 37°C and 40°C.
2. Add, in the precise order given, the reagents listed in **steps 3–8** to a 1.5 mL microfuge tube held at room temperature.
3. 20 μL of 5X transcription buffer.
4. 10 μL of 0.1 M DTT.
5. 4 μL of 40 U/μL RNasin.
6. 20 μL of 2.5 mM rNTPs.
7. 2 μL (≈ 1 μg) of Xba I linearized PEC DNA.
8. 2 μL (20 units) of T7 RNA polymerase.
9. Bring the total reaction volume to 100 μL with DEPC-treated water.
10. Incubate in a 40°C water bath for 2 h.
11. Remove the tube and add 2.5 μL of DNase I.
12. Incubate in a 37°C water bath for 15 min.
13. Remove the tube and add 100 μL of the phenol: chloroform:isoamyl alcohol to the sample and vortex briefly.
14. Centrifuge the tube at 12,000g for 5 min in a microfuge.
15. Carefully remove the upper, aqueous phase to a fresh microfuge tube.
16. Add 100 μL of chloroform, vortex, recentrifuge, and remove the upper, aqueous phase to a fresh microfuge tube.
17. Add 200 μL of cold, 100% ethanol and mix by inversion 10 times.
18. Place in a –20°C freezer for 1 h.
19. Centrifuge at 12,000g for 15 min at 4°C in a microcentrifuge.
20. Carefully remove the supernatant and discard without disturbing the pellet.
21. Add 500 μL of cold, 70% ethanol and centrifuge at 12,000g for 5 min at 4°C in a microcentrifuge.

22. Carefully remove the supernatant and discard without disturbing the pellet.
23. Air-dry for 15 min.
24. Resuspend the pellet in 50 μL TE buffer and place on ice.
25. Store at –80°C in 10 μL aliquots.
26. Determine the OD_{260} and OD_{280} of the HIV-1 *gag* cRNA as given in **Subheading 3.2.1., steps 1–8**, for the β–globin PEC with the following modifications: concentration of cRNA (μg/mL) = (OD_{260}) x (40, dilution factor) x 40 (RNA constant). The OD_{260}/OD_{280} ratio for pure RNA should be ≥ 2.0.
27. The integrity of the cRNA product should be analyzed on a denaturing 6% polyacrylamide gel as given in **steps 28–41**.
28. Set-up a vertical mini-gel form.
29. Warm 10 mL of Gel-Mix 6 to room temperature, add 60 μL of 10% ammonium persulfate, and swirl to mix.
30. Draw the gel solution up into a pipet, fill the gel form, add the comb, and allow to polymerize for 1 h.
31. Withdraw the comb, flush the wells of unpolymerized acrylamide gel solution, and prerun the gel at 200 V for 15 min in 1X TBE.
32. Place 300 ng of cRNA into a 0.5 mL microfuge tube and 5 μg of RNA markers into another 0.5 mL microfuge tube.
33. Dry down the RNAs in a Speed-Vac for 5 min.
34. Add 5 μL of formamide loading buffer to each tube and place in a 95°C heat block for 5 min.
35. Vortex briefly, microfuge for 10 s to collect the fluid in the bottom of the tubes, and return to the heat block for 1 min.
36. Place the tubes directly onto wet ice.
37. Turn-off the power to the gel apparatus, re-flush the wells, and load samples in adjacent wells.
38. Electrophorese at 200 V for 30 min.
39. Stain the gel for 10 min at room temperature in 5 μg/mL ethidium bromide TBE buffer.
40. Visualize the gel with UV light.
41. A single band should be visualized at 1,300 nucleotides in the cRNA, lane which migrates between the adjacent 1,600 and 1,000 nucleotide RNA markers.

3.4.3. Preparation of HIV-1 gag cRNA External Standard Dilutions.

1. The HIV-1 *gag* cRNA template is diluted into aliquots to provide 5, 10, 100, 500, 1,000, 5,000, 10,000, 50,000, and 100,000 copies per 8 μL. Given that the HIV-1 *gag* cRNA is 7.36×10^{-19} g/copy (*see* **Note 10**), 100,000 copies per 8 μL equates to $9.20 \times 10\text{-}12$ g/mL (or 9.20 pg/mL). Dilute the HIV-1 *gag* cRNA stock in diluent buffer I to a 100-fold higher concentration (920 pg/mL) using several large, serial dilution steps. Then dilute to 9.20 pg/mL and to subsequent concentrations for the HIV-1 *gag* cRNA standards using the serial dilution scheme given in **Table 5**.
2. These standards should be aliquoted in 10 μL amounts and stored at –80°C.

Table 5
Dilution of HIV-1 *gag* cRNA Standards

Tubes	Diluent II	Copies/8 μL
No dilution		100,000
500 μL from tube 1	500 μL	50,000
200 μL from tube 2	800 μL	10,000
500 μL from tube 3	500 μL	5,000
200 μL from tube 4	800 μL	1,000
500 μL from tube 5	500 μL	500
200 μL from tube 6	800 μL	100
100 μL from tube 7	900 μL	10
500 μL from tube 8	500 μL	5

3.4.4. HIV-1 gag cDNA Preparation by Reverse Transcription

1. Prewarm the thermocycler to 45°C.
2. Assemble the appropriate reagents from freezers and allow them to thaw at room temperature for 5–10 min. Place tubes on wet ice outside the hood. Do not remove enzymes from freezer until required.
3. Determine the amount of RT+ and RT- (*see* **Note 11**) master mixes required.
4. In a clean laminar-flow hood, label PCR (0.5 mL) tubes and place them in a rack. Tubes to be labeled are two assay blanks (one RT+ H_2O and one RT- H_2O); one set of *gag* RNA PEC dilution series; one set of clinical specimen RNAs; and RT- for desired number of clinical specimens. (RT+, RT-). Tubes are placed in the rack left to right. In addition, label two 1.5 mL or larger tubes: one for the RT+ master-mix and one for the RT- master-mix.
5. To the tubes labeled as the assay blanks (RT+, RT-), add 10 μL of H_2O. Add 2 μL of H_2O to each *gag* cRNA PEC dilution tube.
6. Make separate master-mixes for reverse transcriptase reactions (RT+) and control reactions without the enzyme (RT-) by determining the number of reactions to be run and then adding two. Multiply these numbers by the respective volumes given in **Table 6**.
7. Add 11.9 μL of either RT + or RT- master mix to each tube.
8. Add 60 μL of mineral oil to all tubes using a pipetman and a disposable tip, changing tips between each sample.
9. Add 10 μL sterile water to water tubes and 2 μL to each PEC tube.
10. Aliquot 8 μL of each *gag* PEC cRNA standard into each standard curve tube working from the low to the high copy number dilution.
11. To tubes labeled as RNA clinical specimens (RT+/RT-), add 10 μL (5×10^5 cell equivalents) of the corresponding RNA clinical specimens.
12. Vortex the tubes briefly and centrifuge the tubes at 12,000*g* for 5 s.
13. Place the tubes into the preheated thermocycler and soak as follows: 45°C for 15 min. 95°C for 10 min to heat kill RT enzyme. Soak at 4°C, approximately 2–3 min.

Table 6
HIV-1 *gag* cDNA Set-up

Per RT+ reaction add		Per RT- reaction add	
5X RT Buffer	4.0 μL	5X RT Buffer	4.0 μL
0.1 *M* DTT	2.0 μL	0.1 M DTT	2.0 μL
RNasin (40 U/μL)	0.5 μL	RNasin	0.5 μL
dNTP mix (25.0 m*M*)	0.4 μL	dNTP mix (25.0 m*M*)	0.4 μL
HIV *gag* AS primer[a]	4.0 μL	HIV-1 *gag* AS primer[a]	4.0 μL
RT enzyme (200 U/μL)	1.0 μL	H_2O	1.0 μL
Total	11.9 μL	Total	11.9 μL

[a]*gag* AS primer, antisense primer.

Table 7
HIV-1 *gag* cDNA PCR Set-up

Component	Volume (μL/Reaction)	Final concentration
Deionized water	56.8	
10X PCR Buffer	10.0	$[Mg^{2+}] = 1.64$ m*M*
HIV^{-1} *gag* sense, 20 μ*M*	5.0	1.0 μ*M*
HIV^{-1} *gag* antisense, 20 μ*M*	5.0	1.0 μ*M*
dNTPs, 25 m*M* each	0.8	200 μ*M* each
Taq polymerase, 5 U/μL	0.5	0.025 U/μL
Master-mix volume/reaction	78.1 μL	
Template volume	21.9 μL	
Final volume	100 μL	

3.4.5 HIV-1 gag cDNA Amplification

1. Samples are now ready for PCR amplification. Prewarm the thermocycler to 95°C.
2. Set up and label a 1.5 mL or larger tube in the hood to contain PCR master-mix.
3. Determine the number of reaction tubes to be run and add two. Make a master-mix by multiplying this number by the volumes given in **Table 7**.
4. In a clean laminar-flow hood, place the previously transcribed samples from the *gag* RNA reverse transcriptase reaction in a rack.
5. Aliquot 78.1 μL of PCR master-mix to each of the RT reaction tubes (21.9 μL) to bring the final volume of each reaction to 100 μL. Vortex each tube briefly and centrifuge at 12,000*g* for 5 s.
6. Place tubes into the preheated thermocycler and initiate the following program: 95°C for 30 s, 50°C for 45 s, 72°C for 2 min for 4 cycles followed 24 cycles of 94°C for 30 s, 55°C for 30 s, and 72°C for 1 min followed by a

single incubation at 72°C for 10 min followed by 4°C until tubes are removed for storage.

7. Store RT-PCR reactions at 4°C until subjected to the liquid hybridization (LH) assay. The LH assay should be performed no later than the next day.

3.5. Liquid Hybridization Reaction

This protocol describes procedures for the specific detection of PCR products by the hybridization of radiolabeled oligonucleotide probes complimentary to the internal sequence of the PCR product. The probes are 5'-end labeled with ^{32}P using the polynucleotide kinase enzyme. Precautions for the use of ^{32}P must be followed throughout and waste disposed according to the local radiation safety guidelines. The protocols for the liquid hybridization (LH) reaction will be given in two sections. The first section describes the 5'-end labeling reaction, while the second describes the LH reaction itself. The β-globin amplifications will be hybridized to the β–globin probe, while both the HIV-1 *gag* DNA and cDNA amplifications will be hybridized with the *gag* probe.

3.5.1. 5'-End Labeling of the Oligonucleotide Probe

1. Thaw the radioisotope behind a lucite shield.
2. To a 0.5 mL microfuge tube held on wet ice, add 0.5 μL of a 20 μ*M* solution of oligonucleotide (either the β–globin or HIV-1 *gag* probe), 2.0 μL of 10X polynucleotide kinase buffer, 11.5 μL of sterile water, 5.0 μL (50 μCi) of gamma-[^{32}P]adenosine trisphosphate, and 1.0 μL (8 U) of polynucleotide kinase. Mix gently with a pipet tip.
3. Incubate in a 37°C water bath for 30 min.
4. Place the reaction on ice.
5. Invert the G-25 column enough times so that the matrix inside is well mixed.
6. First remove the upper, then the lower caps. Let the buffer drain out for about 10 min.
7. Place the column into a 1.5 mL centrifuge tubes. Place this assembly into the large tube that you just used for draining the column. Seal with a cap.
8. Spin this set-up in the Beckman GPR centrifuge at 2,300 rpm for two minutes. Remove the dried column with forceps. Place it into a fresh 1.5 mL centrifuge tube and discard the first one. Now your column is prepared for a sample.
9. Pipet the entire 20 μL volume of the kinase reaction onto the dried column bed. Place this assembly back into the large centrifuge tube. Cap it and seal it with parafilm.
10. Spin at 2,300 rpm for 4 min, in the Beckman GPR centrifuge.
11. Break the cap seal. Remove the column with forceps and discard it into radioactive waste. Remove the approximately 25 μL in the small centrifuge tube directly with a pipetman. Place this into a fresh 1.5 mL centrifuge tube.
12. Remove 1 μL of the purified sample and count in a liquid scintillation counter.

3.5.2. Liquid Hybridization Reaction

1. Warm the thermocycler to 95°C. Label fresh 0.5 mL tubes to correspond to each PCR reaction.
2. Obtain PCR product tubes from storage. If removing samples from the freezer, allow the tubes to thaw at room temperature for 5–10 min. Place tubes on wet ice within 10 min.
3. Transfer 30 μL of PCR reactions to appropriately labeled 0.5 mL microfuge tubes.
4. Determine the number of reactions to be run and add two. Each hybridization reaction will require 1 μL of the appropriate ^{32}P-probe diluted to 5.0 x 10^4 cpm/ μL in H$_2$O and 10 μL of 1.1X OH Buffer. Multiply the number of reactions by the volumes above to develop the master-mix.
5. Add 10 μL of the master mix into each specimen tube containing 30 μL of PCR product and mix.
6. Centrifuge at 12,000g for 5 s.
7. Place samples into thermocycler and incubate at 94°C for 5 min, 55°C for 10 min, and arrive at a 4°C soak.
8. Add 4 μL of 5X DNA Loading Buffer to each sample. Vortex and centrifuge at 12,000g for 5 s.

3.6. Miniacrylamide Gel Electrophoresis of Hybridized PCR Products

This is a protocol for the rapid separation of hybridized PCR products from unincorporated reactants using miniacrylamide gels. Precautions for the use of ^{32}P must be followed throughout and waste disposed according to the local radiation safety guidelines.

1. Assemble mini-gel plates and apparatus according to the manufacturer's instructions.
2. Prepare a 10% polyacrylamide gel mix by adding the following reagents to a 50 mL tube: 5 mL of 40% acrylamide/bisacrylamide solution, 2 mL of 10X TBE, 13 mL distilled water, 125 μL 10% ammonium persulfate solution. This formula will make enough for two gels for the Serva Dual Mini Slab apparatus.
3. Mix gently by inverting the tube several times.
4. Add 20 μL of TEMED and mix again.
5. Pour the gels using a pipet-aid with a disposable pipet, and deliver the gel solution to each gel sandwich, taking care not to introduce bubbles. Insert the comb and allow gels to polymerize (at least 30 min).
6. Fill the gel apparatus with 1X TBE.
7. Carefully place the gel sandwich into the rig by inserting it at an angle to avoid introducing any bubbles under the gel.
8. Assemble the gel apparatus as per manual's instructions. Fill the upper buffer tank with 1X TBE.
9. Prerun the gels for at least 5 min at 200 V.
10. Load 10 μL of sample in alternate wells in order to avoid bleed over signal.

11. Run the gel(s) for 35 min at 200 V for HIV-1 *gag* reactions and 45 min for β–globin reactions.
12. When the dye front is 60% through the gel for HIV-1 *gag* or 80% for β–globin, the gel run is completed.

3.7. Detection and Analysis of the Hybridized PCR Products

The acrylamide gels containing electrophoresed liquid hybridization products are analyzed using either storage phosphor technology or conventional autoradiography for the quantitation specific PCR signals. We employ a Molecular Dynamics Phosphorimager to quantitate the ^{32}P signal in the PCR bands *(12)*. The advantages of this system include a 5-log dynamic range of quantitation, no threshold effects, and the ability to electronically store gel images and data files. Gels are imaged according to the manufacturer's instructions.

3.7.1. Detection and Analysis of the β–globin PCR Signals

1. The size of the β–globin band is 278 bp.
2. First, determine the signal intensity for the water blank reactions.
3. For each β–globin DNA PEC reaction, the signal intensity of the water reaction is subtracted from the PEC signal. The $\log_{10}$ transformation of these signal intensities is then plotted as the dependent variable against the $\log_{10}$ transformation of the copy number input.
4. For each experimental β–globin DNA reaction, determine the β–globin copy number by interpolation of the standard curve.
5. Derive the median β–globin copy number.
6. For each experimental β–globin DNA reaction, determine the ratio of (β–globin copy number)$_{median}$/(β–globin copy number)$_{experimental}$. This number is the β–globin correction factor (*see* **Note 12**).

3.7.2. Detection and Analysis of HIV-1 gag DNA PCR signals

1. The size of the HIV-1 *gag* band is 136 bp.
2. First, determine the signal intensity for the water blank reactions.
3. For each HIV-1 *gag* DNA PEC reaction, the signal intensity of the water reaction is subtracted from the PEC signal. The $\log_{10}$ transformation of these signal intensities is then plotted as the dependent variable against the $\log_{10}$ transformation of the copy number input.
4. For each experimental HIV-1 *gag* DNA reaction, determine the raw HIV-1 *gag* DNA copy number by interpolation of the standard curve.
5. For each experimental HIV-1 *gag* DNA reaction, multiply the raw HIV-1 *gag* DNA copy number by the β–globin correction factor to obtain the corrected HIV-1 *gag* DNA copy number.
6. Divide corrected HIV-1 *gag* DNA copy number by 15 to obtain the corrected HIV-1 *gag* DNA copy number per 100,000 cell equivalents.

3.7.3. Detection and Analysis of HIV-1 gag cDNA PCR Signals

1. Determine the corrected HIV-1 *gag* cDNA copy number for each experimental HIV-1 *gag* cDNA reaction as given in **Subheading 3.7.2., steps 1–5,** for HIV-1 *gag* DNA reactions.
2. Divide the corrected HIV-1 *gag* cDNA copy number by 5 to obtain the corrected HIV-1 *gag* cDNA copy number per 100,000 cell equivalents.

4. Notes

1. If RNA is being extracted from a smaller number of cells, the precipitation in **step 8** should be carried out for 30 min at 4°C.
2. If the phases are not sharply defined, repeat the chloroform extraction, and transfer the aqueous phase to new tubes.
3. If DNA is being extracted from a smaller number of cells, the precipitation in **step 25** should be carried out for 30 min at 4°C.
4. If the phases are not sharply defined, repeat the chloroform extraction, and transfer the aqueous phase to fresh tubes.
5. The isopropanol used in this procedure is stored at room temperature.
6. The 2 μL input (1×10^5 cell equivalents) used here has been optimized for PBMC applications. This input can be increased to 10 μL and the volume of water changed appropriately if there are fewer cells in a sample and more signal is needed in the PCR assay.
7. Do not use DEPC-treated water as this will interfere with the accuracy of these measurements.
8. The β–globin PEC contains 268 bp of the human β–globin gene cloned into the Sma I site of pBluescript II KS- for a total size of 3,229 bp *(13)*. Given the formula weight of DNA as 648 g/mol-bp, the β–globin PEC formula weight is 2.09×10^6 g/mol. When divided by Avogadro's number (6.022×10^{23}), a single copy of β–globin PEC weighs 3.47×10^{-18} g.
9. The HIV-1 *gag* DNA PEC contains a 1,266 bp insert of HIVLAI DNA (sequence positions 44–1309 to include partial 5' LTR and partial *gag* coding sequences) cloned into the Sma I site of pGEM-3Z for a total size of 4,009 bp *(13)*. Using the same logic as given in **Note 8**, a single copy of HIV-1 *gag* DNA PEC weighs 4.31×10^{-18} g.
10. The HIV-1 *gag* cRNA is a 1,300 nucleotide RNA. Given the formula weight of RNA as 341 g/mol-nucleotide, the HIV-1 *gag* cRNA formula weight is 4.43×10^5 g/mol. When divided by Avogadro's number (6.022×10^{23}), a single copy of HIV-1 *gag* cRNA PEC weighs 7.36×10^{-19} g.
11. The RT- is a mock reaction in which the reverse transcriptase enzyme is omitted from the reaction. This is a control for contaminating levels of DNA in the sample, which would be detected in the subsequent PCR. The absence of signal following the PCR for the RT- control reactions confirms the lack of DNA sequences contaminating the RNA preparation.
12. The β–globin amplifications correct for the amount of amplifiable DNA input in each reaction.

References

1. Mellors, J.W., Kingsley, L.A., Rinaldo, C.D., et al. (1995) Quantitation of HIV-1 RNA in plasma predicts outcome after seroconversion. *Ann. Intern. Med.* **122,** 573–579.
2. Coombs, R.W., Collier, A.C., Allain, J.P., et al. (1989) Plasma viremia in human immunodeficiency virus infection. *N. Engl. J. Med.* **321,** 1626–1631.
3. Wei, X., Ghosh, S.K., Taylor, M.E., et al. (1995) Viral dynamics in human immunodeficiency virus type 1 infection. *Nature* **373,** 117–122.
4. Molina, J.M., Ferchal, R., Chevret, S., Barateau, V., Poirot, C., Morinet, F., and Modai, J. (1994) Quantification of HIV-1 virus load under zidovudine therapy in patients with symptomatic HIV-1 infection: relation to disease progression. *AIDS* **8,** 27–33.
5. Schooley, R.T. (1995) Correlation between viral load measurements and outcome in clinical trials of antiviral drugs. *AIDS* **9,** S15–S19.
6. Michael, N.L., Mo, T., Abderrazzak, M., et al. (1995) Human immunodeficiency virus type 1 cellular RNA load and splicing patterns predict disease progression in a longitudinally studied cohort. *J Virol.* **69,** 1868–1877.
7. O'Brien, W.A., Hartigan, P.A., Martin, D., et al. (1996) Changes in plasma HIV-1 RNA and CD4+ lymphocyte counts and the risk of progression to AIDS. *N. Engl. J. Med.* **334,** 426–431.
8. Wong, M.T., Dolan, M., Kozlow, R., et al. (1996) Patterns of viral load and T-cell phenotype are established early and are correlated with the rate of disease progression in HIV-1 infected persons. *J. Infec. Dis.* **173,** 877–887.
9. Dickover, R.E., Garratty, E.M., Herman, S.A., et al. (1996) Identification of levels of maternal HIV-1 RNA associated with risk of perinatal transmission. *JAMA* **275,** 599–610.
10. Connor, E.M., Sperling, R.S., Glebe, R., et al. (1994) Reduction in maternal-infant transmission of human immunodeficiency virus type 1 with zidovudine treatment. *N. Eng. J. Med.* **331,** 1174–1180.
11. Saag, M.S., Holodiny, M., Kuritzkes. D.R., et al. (1996) HIV viral load markers in clinical practice. *Nature Med.* **2,** 625–629.
12. Vahey, M. and Wong, M.T. (1995) A quantitative liquid hybridization polymerase chain reaction methodology employing storage phosphor technology. In the Cold Spring Harbor Laboratory Manual for PCR (Diffenbach, C.W. and Dveksler, G.S., ed.) Cold Spring Harbor Press, NY, pp. 313–338.
13. Michael, N.L., Vahey, M., Burke, D.S., and Redfield, R.R. (1992) Viral DNA and mRNA expression correlate with the stage of human immunodeficiency virus (HIV) type 1 infection in humans: evidence for viral replication in all stages of HIV disease. *J. Virol.* **66,** 310–316.

14

Quantitative PCR for HIV-1 Proviral DNA

Davide Zella and Paola Secchiero

1. Introduction

A salient feature regarding the HIV (and all the retroviruses in general) replicative cycle is the retrotranscription of the RNA genome to DNA (provirus), followed by its integration in the genome of the host cell.

Although serologic analyses play a major role in the diagnosis of HIV-1 infection, direct detection of HIV proviral DNA in peripheral blood monocuelar cells (PBMC) is a useful diagnostic tool in several situations. These include children born to seropositive mothers, because the maternal immunoglobulins (IgG) are transplacentally acquired, and adults at risk of AIDS prior to seroconversion (mainly partners of seropositives).

Quantification of HIV-1 proviral DNA can provide important information such as the number of infected cells in clinical samples (PBMC and/or tissues). In in vitro experiments, quantification of proviral DNA measures the efficacy of chemical compounds in restricting viral entry into target cells.

By virtue of its ability to amplify minute amounts of viral DNA from small samples, the polymerase chain reaction (PCR) technique is the molecular method most commonly employed for detection and quantification of HIV-1. Several quantitative PCR methods are currently used (reviewed in **ref. _1_**) and may be classified into semi-quantitative and quantitative competitive methods.

In this chapter we describe a different approach based on noncompetitive PCR for HIV-1 DNA quantification. This method uses a nonhomologous internal standard (IS) which is coamplified with the wild-type target sequence in the same vial and with the same pair of primers. This assay allows the identification of false negative results due to the presence of inhibitors of Taq poly-

From: _Methods in Molecular Medicine, Vol. 17: HIV Protocols_
Edited by: N. L. Michael and J. H. Kim © Humana Press Inc., Totowa, NJ

merase and is suitable for bona fide quantitative analysis. Quantification of HIV proviral DNA is obtained by using an external standard curve in which known increasing amounts of the viral target are amplified in parallel with test samples. A small number of copies (n = 100–200) of the IS molecule is coamplified with HIV-1 DNA in both the external standards and test samples to detect the presence of PCR inhibitors and/or to correct for differences in efficiency of amplification among the different tubes/samples. Densitometric analysis of hybridization products obtained from the external standards allows construction of a standard curve from which the amount of HIV proviral DNA in test samples is interpolated.

The protocol described can be divided into four general steps: (1) preparation of the samples (DNA extraction), (2) PCR amplification, (3) analysis of the PCR products and construction of the standard curve, (4) quantification of HIV-1 proviral DNA in the test samples.

2. Materials and Reagents
2.1. Primers, Plasmids, and Probes

The primers SK38/39 *(2)* used to amplify the gag region of the HIV-1 proviral sequence (**Table 1**) and the positive control template, the recombinant HIV-1 DNA "Gene-Amplimer HIV-1 control reagent," are commercially available (Perkins Elmer Cetus, Norwalk, CT). The synthetic non-homologous internal standard has been synthesized as described in **Note 1**. Stocks of (IS) plasmid are prepared using the Plasmid Midi Kit (Quiagen, Chatsworth, CA); following linearization by BamHI digestion, the plasmid is stored in aliquots at –20°C (stable for approx 6–8 mo). The sequences of the oligonucleotide probes used for hybridization of the amplification products (viral target and IS molecule) are reported in **Table 1**.

2.2. Solutions and Reagents

1. Lysis buffer: 0.5% Nonidet P-40, 0.5% Tween 20, 1.5 mM MgCl$_2$, 50 mM TrisHCl pH 8.3, and 50 mM KCl.
2. Stoffel Taq polymerase (10 U/µL), 10× Stoffel buffer, and dNTP (10 mM each) are from Perkin Elmer. Stock solution (20 µM) of primers are prepared in H$_2$O.
3. Hybridization solution (for oligonucleotide hybridization): 6× SSC (1× SSC is 0.15 M NaCl plus 0.015 M sodium citrate), 5× Denhardt's solution, 0.1% sodium dodecyl sulfate (SDS), and 100 µg of tRNA per milliliter.
4. Probe labeling: DNA 5'-end-labeling kit (Boehringer Mannheim, Indianapolis, IN) and [γ-^{32}P]dCTP (Amersham, Arlington Heights, IL). Alternatively, kits for a nonradioactive oligonucleotide and detection system may be used (e.g., ECL 3'-oligolabeling and detection system from Amersham).

Table 1
Sequence of the Oligonucleotide Primers and Probes Used for HIV-1
Quantitative PCR

Primer SK 38:	5'-ATAATCCACCTATCCCAGTAGGAGAAAT-3'
Primer SK 39:	5'-TTTGGTCCTTGTCTTATGTCCAGAATGC-3'
Primer SK 19:	5'-ATCCTGGGATTAAATAAAATAGTAAGAATGTATAGCCCTAC-3'
Primer IS:	5'-ATATATGAGTAAACTTGGTCTGACAGTTACCAATGCTTAAT-3'

3. Methods

1. Sample preparation. For small samples (containing between 5×10^3 and 1×10^6 cells), we suggest resuspending the cells in 20–100 μL of lysis buffer supplemented with 100 μg of proteinase K (Boehringer Mannheim) per milliliter. After incubating the cells at 56°C for 2 h, heat the tube at 98°C for 30 min to inactivate the proteinase K and immediately move it to wet ice. Before use, vortex and centrifuge briefly, at maximum speed in a microcentrifuge. Use the clarified supernatant as template for the PCR reaction.

2. PCR reaction. For DNA amplification, add 1 μg of purified DNA or an aliquot of crude lysate (1 μg of DNA corresponds to approximately 1.5×10^5 diploid cells) to a mixture containing 1× Stoffel buffer (10 m*M* KCl, 10 m*M* TrisHCl [pH8.3]), 5 m*M* MgCl$_2$), 0.2 m*M* (each) dNTPs, 0.5 μ*M* (each) primers SK38 and SK39 and 5 U of ampliTaq DNA polymerase Stoffel fragment, in a total volume of 100 μL. Overlay the samples with 75–100 μL of mineral oil. Keep the samples on ice, and eventually perform a hot start in a prewarmed thermal cycler at 92°C.
   The PCR conditions are as follows: 1 min at 92°C, 1 min at 55°C, and 2 min at 72°C for the first 5 cycles, and then 1 min at 92°C, 1 min at 55°C, and 3 min at 72°C with an increase of 3 s/cycle for the subsequent 26 cycles (**Fig. 1**).

3. Analysis of the amplification products. After the PCR reaction, analyze the amplification products by agarose gel elctrophoresis, Southern blot transfer, and hybridization *(3)* with a mix of two [^{32}P]-labeled, specific oligonucleotide probes, SK19 and IS for the HIV-1 gag and the IS amplified regions, respectively (**Table 1**). Alternatively, immobilize two identical aliquots of each amplification product on nylon filters in duplicate by using a slot blot apparatus (Schleicher and Schuell, Keene, NH). Two separate hybridizations are then performed, each with one or the two labeled probes. Hybridization is performed at 55°C. Washes are for 30–45 min in 2X SSC–0.1% SDS at room temperature.

4. Construction of the standard curve. To quantitate the proviral DNA in the samples analyzed, a standard curve is constructed for each amplification experiment following the principles previously described *(4,5)*. To generate the standard curve, known numbers of molecules of the wild-type target (GeneAmplimer HIV-1 control reagent; at least 4 concentrations from 10 to 10^4 molecules) are coamplified with a constant number (between 100 and 200) of IS molecules (**Fig. 1**). To ensure a homogenous distribution of the IS molecules in each tube, add the IS to the

1. PCR reaction

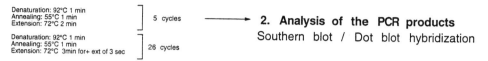

3. Construction of the Standard curve

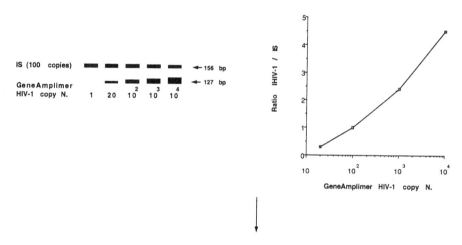

4. Quantification of HIV-1 DNA in the test samples

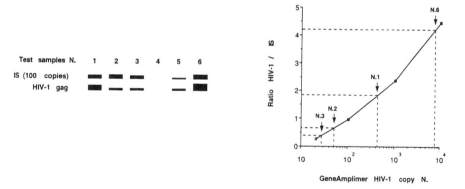

Fig. 1. Schematic representation of the method.

PCR mixture immediately before it is divided into aliquots into the individual reaction vials.

5. Proviral DNA quantification. After hybridization of the PCR products with the probes (**Table 1**), determine the intensities of the bands corresponding to the target sequence and to the IS by densitometric analysis using appropriate software (e.g., Image 1.59 for Apple Macintosh; National Institutes of Health, Bethesda, MD). The densitometric analysis of hybridization products obtained from the "standard curve samples" is used to construct a standard curve by plotting, on a logarithmic scale, the HIV-1/IS ratio against the initial number of HIV-1 recombinant molecules (**Fig. 1**).

The amount of HIV-1 DNA present in a test sample is then interpolated from the standard curve, by plotting the HIV-1/IS value calculated for the sample, following hybridization of the PCR products (**Fig. 1**).

4. Comments

1. Potential results that may be obtain by analyzing clinical samples, according to the procedure described above, are schematically exemplified in the last panel of Fig. 1. Clinical specimens that are partially or totally noncompetent for amplification, as demonstrated by a drastic reduction (test sample N 5) or lack (test sample N 4) of amplification of the internal control (IS) are shown. In this case, an additional procedure for DNA purification should be used.

2. Variations in the IS amplification signal, as compared to the mean value of the IS controls, are frequently observed (i.e., test samples N 1–3, and N 6). However this variability, inherent to the PCR technique, particularly when it is used to test clinical specimens, does not affect the HIV DNA quantification, because only the relative proportions (ratio HIV/IS) and not the absolute amount of target and IS products are measured in each tube.

5. Notes

1. The synthetic nonhomologous IS molecule was obtained by amplification of a portion of PGEM4Z DNA with chimeric primers consisting of the SK38 and SK39 HIV-1 sequences at the 5' ends and 20 bases complementary to a region of the plasmid at the 3' ends. The plasmid region was chosen on the basis of the percent G + C composition similar to that of the HIV-1 wild-type target sequence. The 156-bp PCR product was cloned in the PCRII vector and was designated IS. The sequences of the oligonucleotide probes used for hybridization of the amplification products (**Table 1**) were chosen to have a similar percent G + C composition, and therefore, a similar efficiency of hybridization for the wild-type target (HIV-1 DNA) and IS.

2. To avoid the problems of PCR contamination, we recommend that samples be handled and DNA be isolated in a hood with laminar airflow, preferably in an area not used for the preparation of DNA template-free PCR cocktails or for the analysis and cloning of PCR products.

References

1. Clementi, M., Menzo, S., Manzin, A., and Bagnarelli, P. (1995) Quantitative molecular methods in virology. *Arch. Virol.* **140,** 1523–1539.

2. Ou, C. Y., Kwok, S., Michell, S. W., Mack, D. H., Sninsky, J. J., Krebs, J. W., Feorino, P., Warfield, J., and Schochetman, G. (1988) DNA amplification for direct detection of HIV-1 in DNA of peripheral mononuclear cells. *Science* **239,** 295–297.

3. Sambrook, J., Fritsch, E. F., Maniatis, T., Ford, N., Nolan, C., and Ferguson, M. (eds.) (1989) *Molecular cloning: a laboratory manual,* 2nd ed., Cold Spring Harbor Press, Cold Spring Harbor, New York.

4. Gerna, G., Baldanti, F., Sarasini, A., Furione, M., Percivalle, E., Revello, M. G., Zipeto, D., Zella, D., and the Italian Foscarnet Study Group (1994) Effect of foscarnet induction treatment on quantitation of human cytomegalovirus (HCMV) DNA in peripheral blood polymorphonuclear leukocytes and aquenous humor of AIDS patients with HCMV retinitis. *Antimicrob. Agents Chemother.* **38,** 38–44.

5. Secchiero, P., Zella, D., Crowley, R. W., Gallo, R. C., and Lusso, P. (1995) Quantitative PCR for human herpesviruses 6 and 7. *J. Clinical Microbiol.* **33,** 2124–2130.

15

Diagnosis and Direct Automated Sequencing of HIV-1 From Dried Blood Spots (DBS) Collected on Filter Paper

Sharon A. Cassol, Stanley Read, Bruce G. Weniger, Richard Pilon, Barbara Leung, and Theresa Mo

[handwritten: Probably not EMP. difficult to synthesize novo → 1-2 kb]

1. Introduction

Since its discovery in 1981, human immunodeficiency virus type 1 (HIV-1) has rapidly emerged as one of the most devastating infectious pathogens of this century *(1–3)*. The World Health Organization (WHO) estimates that, as of 1995, there were at least 15 million HIV- infected men, women, and children worldwide, with the vast majority of infections occurring in developing countries and isolated rural regions where specimen collection, preparation and shipment are difficult *(4)*. Simple and improved sampling methods that can be widely applied under difficult field conditions are needed to effectively monitor the changing dynamics of the HIV-1/AIDS pandemic, track the spread of HIV-1 variants among different population groups, and ensure that research and interventive activities are directed against biologically important variants of the virus. To date, at least eight major HIV-1 subtypes, designated A through H, have been identified *(5,6)*. More recently, a ninth subtype, I, has been detected *(7)*, as well as several highly divergent, or "outlying" variants of HIV-1 that have been tentatively classified as group O *(8,9)*. This subtyping is based on a relatively small number of specimens collected from a few geographic areas and the full range and distribution of HIV-1 variants remains to be established. The collection of whole blood on filter paper provides an innovative and powerful approach for the systematic and unbiased collection of large numbers of field specimens for diagnostic and surveillance purposes *(10–19)*. These specimens, commonly known as Guthrie cards or dried blood spots

From: *Methods in Molecular Medicine, Vol. 17: HIV Protocols*
Edited by: N. L. Michael and J. H. Kim © Humana Press Inc., Totowa, NJ

(DBS), are collected by carefully applying a few drops of fresh blood, drawn by venipuncture, or by finger- or heel-prick with a lance, onto an absorbent filter paper matrix. After the blood has saturated the filter, it is simply air-dried, placed in a high-quality bond envelope *(20)*, and shipped to a centralized reference laboratory for analysis (**Table 1**). This chapter describes a reliable protocol for obtaining consistent yields of high quality HIV-1 proviral DNA from small amounts of dried blood and outlines some of the more important applications of this technology for the polymerase chain reaction (PCR)-based diagnosis and genetic characterization of HIV-1 (**Table 2**).

2. Materials
2.1. Reagents and Suppliers

1. Amicon Division, W.R. Grace & Co., Beverly, MA, 01915-1065. Tel: 1-800-343-0690; Products—Centricon 100 columns, Catalog No. 4211.
2. BioRad Laboratories, Hercules, CA, 94547; Tel: 1-800-424-6723; Product—Chelex-100, 100–200 mesh, Catalog No. 142-2832
3. Boehringer-Mannheim Corporation, Indianapolis, IN. Tel. 1-800-428-5433; Product—Expand Long Template PCR System containing 10X concentrated PCR buffer (22.5 mM MgCl$_2$, 500 mM Tris-HCl, 160 mM (NH$_4$)$_2$SO$_4$) and 2.6 U of Expand enzyme consisting of a mix of *Pwo* and *Taq* DNA polymerases. 190 reactions, Catalog No. 1681-842.
4. FMC BioProducts, Rockland, MD 04841; Product—NuSieve Agarose, Catalog No. 50084.
5. Millipore Corporation, Bedford MA 01730-9125, Tel. 1-800-645-5476; Product—Ultrafree-MC Filters, Catalog No. UFC3LTKOO.
6. Perkin-Elmer Corporation, Applied Biosystems Division, Foster City, CA 94404-1128 Tel: (415) 570-6667. Products—Uracil *N*-glycosylase, Catalog No. N808-0096; ABI Prism DNA Sequencing, Chemistry Guide, Catalog No. 903563, Version A, May 1995; Dye Terminator Cycle Sequencing Kit with AmpliTaq DNA Polymerase Catalog No. 401384; Dye Terminator Cycle Sequencing, Kit with FS DNA Polymerase, FS.
7. Pharmacia, Piscataway, NJ. Tel: 1-800-526-3593; Products—100 base-pair ladder, Catalog No. 27-4001-01; dATP, Catalog No. 27-2050; dCTP, Catalog No. 27-2060; dGTP, Catalog No. 27-2070; dTTP, Catalog No. 27-2080.
8. Princeton Separations, Inc., Adelphia, NJ. Tel: 908-431-3338; Fax: 908-431-3768. Product—Centri-Sep Spin Column, 100 pack, catalog No. CS-901.
9. Quiagen Inc., 9600 Chatsworth, CA 91311. Tel: 1-800-426-8157 or 800-362-7737 (Technical): Product—QIA Quick Gel Extraction Kit, 250 columns, Catalog No. 28704.
10. Roche Diagnostic Systems, Inc., Branchburg, NJ 08876-1760. Tel: 1-800-526-1247. Products—Specimen Wash Buffer from the Amplicor Whole Blood Specimen Preparation Kit, Catalog No. US:87253; Amplicor HIV-1 Amplification and Detection Kits, Catalog Numbers. US:87260 and US:87271, respectively.

Table 1
Advantages and Disadvantages of DBS-Based Genetic Screening[a]

Advantages:
- Ease and economy of sample collection, storage and shipment
- Noninfectious transport medium
- Stability of sample—no need for refrigeration or on-site sample processing
- Allows for centralization of testing facilities
- Facilitates systematic, unbiased surveillance
- Widely applicable—facilitates follow-up of migratory and hard-to-reach populations

Disadvantages:
- Cannot provide live virus for study in culture
- May be more difficult to obtain long PCR fragments (>1.2 kb)

[a]Table taken from **ref. 19**.

Table 2
Current and Potential Applications of DBS
to Clinical Diagnosis and Field Surveillance of HIV-1[a]

Perinatal
- Early differential diagnosis of infected vs uninfected infants
- Precise determination of perinatal transmission rates in specific populations over time
- Assessment of interventive strategies
- Genetic characterization of vertically transmitted strains

Therapeutic
- Screening for drug resistant mutations
- Evaluating the risk for mother-to-child transmission of resistant genotypes

International
- Determining frequency and distribution of HIV-1 subtypes
- Tracking the spread of HIV-1 subtypes between continents
- Assessing the rate of virus evolution at the individual and population levels
- Initial screening for genetic recombinants

[a]Table taken from **ref. 19**.

11. Schleicher & Schuell, Keene, NH, 03431. Tel. 1-800-245-4024. Product—#903 Blood Collection Paper; Catalog No. 58370.
12. Sigma Chemical Co., St. Louis, MO, 63178. Tel. 1-800-325-30130. Products—ethidiunn bromide, Catalog No. E8751; bromophenol blue/xylene cyanol, Catalog No. B3269.

2.2. Reagents Not Included in Diagnostic and Sequencing Kits

1. 0.5X TBE gel electrophoresis buffer: 44 m*M* Tris-borate; 44.5 m*M* boric acid, 1 m*M* EDTA. One liter of 10X stock is prepared by dissolving in deionized H$_2$O: 54 g of Tris base, 27.5 g of boric acid and 20 mL of 0.5 *M* EDTA.
2. 5X Ficoll/loading dye: 25% Ficoll, 1% bromophenol blue/xylene cyanol.

3. Methods

3.1. Preparation of DBS

Universal precautions should be followed during the collection and preparation of DBS for shipment. The following protocol provides sufficient DNA for at least two diagnostic and 12 sequencing reactions.

1. Collect approximately 2 mL of whole blood by venipuncture in an acid–citrate–dextrose Vacutainer tube (Becton Dickinson) (*see* **Notes 1** and **2**).
2. Using a micropipetor and sterile plugged tips, apply 50 μL aliquots of the blood to the back of a standard newborn screening blotter (Schleicher & Schuell, #903) in a dropwise fashion (*see* **Note 3**).
3. Air dry for at least 3 h, and place each filter in an individual bond envelope. Seal the envelope, and enclose in a second, outer bond envelope for storage or shipment (*see* **Notes 4** and **5**).

3.2 Removal of Hemoglobin, Elution, and Concentration of DNA

The procedure described below is rapid and efficient. The eluted DNA can be concentrated and amplified directly, obviating the need for phenol/chloroform extraction (*see* **Note 6**).

1. If the DNA is to be used for diagnostic purposes, a single 50-μL blood spot will suffice. For sequencing applications, we routinely process and pool the DNA from three 50-μL spots.
2. Excise each circle of dried blood (approx 1 cm^2) with clean, acid depurinated scissors (*see* **Note 7**), cut in half, and place each half in a 1.5-mL sterile screw-cap microfuge tube (*see* **Note 8**). Use a different pair of scissors for each patient and each control specimen.
3. Add 1.0 mL of specimen wash buffer (Amplicor Whole Blood Specimen Preparation Kit; Roche Diagnostic Systems) to each tube.
4. Incubate at 25°C for 30 min on an Eppendorf Thermomixer™ set at 1000 revolutions/min to lyse the red cells and release hemoglobin.
5. Aspirate the hemoglobin-containing supernatant, taking particular care to remove as much solution as possible (*see* **Note 9**).
6. Combine the two halves of each filter in the same microfuge tube, and add 200 μL of a 5% slurry of Chelex-100 (BioRad) in H$_2$0.
7. Incubate at 95°C for 1 h on Thermomixer at 1000 revolutions/min to elute the DNA from the filter (*see* **Note 10**).
8. Spin the tubes (14,000*g* for 5 min) to bring down the Chelex resin.

Table 3
Frequently Used Oligonucleotide Primers[a]

PCR primer	Orientation	Sequence (5'–3')	Location
Outer MK603-F	→	CAAAAATTGTGGGTCACA GTCTATTATGGGGTACCT	89–126
Outer CD4XBO-R2	←	gttctgagTATAATTCACTTT TCCAATTGTCC	1426–1439
Inner MK650iF	→	AATGTCAGCACAG TACAATGTACAC	715–739
Inner V3iR	←	ACAATTTCTGGGTC CCCTCCTGAGCA	1078–1103

[a]Sequence and map locations of oligonucleotides used as nested primers in PCR reactions. Numbered according to the gp120 sequence of HIV-1$_{LAI}$ (GenBank accession no. K02013). The first nine nucleotides of the CD4XBO-R2 pruner consists of a *gttctcgag* clamp that is not HIV-1 specific.

9. Remove and pool Chelex supernatants for each patient (i.e., from 1 to 3 DBS).
10. Concentrate the pooled supernatant to approx 40 μL in an Ultrafree-MC centrifugal filtration unit as specified by the manufacturer (Millipore) (*see* **Note 11**).
11. Collect the DNA concentrate from filter cup and use directly in PCR amplification reactions.

3.3. Diagnosis of HIV-1 Infection

1. For large-scale diagnostic screening using the Roche microwell system, adjust the DNA concentrate to 50 μL with sterile water and make to 7.5 mM MgCl$_2$. Amplify and detect the viral DNA exactly as specified in the Amplicor HIV-1 Amplification and Detection kits (*see* **Note 12**).
2. Alternatively, a 40 μL aliquot of the DNA can be amplified in a standard nested PCR reaction using dUTP and uracil N-glycoslase (Perkin Elmer) to prevent carryover contamination and guard against false-positive results (*see* **Note 13 and 14**).
3. Check second round reactions for amplification product by loading 8 μL of the PCR product, mixed with 2 μL of 5X loading dye on a 1.5% agarose gel in 0.5X TBE buffer. Electrophorese at 100 V for 30–60 min (*see* **Note 14**).
4. Stain the gel with ethidium bromide (0.5 μg/mL in H$_2$O), and detect the product by UV transillumination. Photograph and record the results.

3.4. Sequencing of the HIV-1 Genome

For sequence analysis, the authors routinely use a two-step, nested PCR protocol and conserved primers, such as the C2V3 env primer sets shown in **Table 3** (*see* **Note 15**).

1. For the first amplification, add 40 μL of the DNA concentrate to a thin-walled 0.5-mL GeneAmp reaction tube (on ice) containing 500 μM each of dATP, dCTP,

dGTP and dTTP (*see* **Note 16**); 500 n*M* of each outer PCR primer (MK603-F and CD4XBO-R2; **Table 1**), and H$_2$0 (to 50 µL final volume).

2. While still on ice, add 10 µL of cold master mix 2, system 2 (Expand Long Template PCR System; Boehringer Mannheim, Cat. No. 1661-842) (*see* **Note 17**).

3. Place the cold PCR tubes in a 9600 GeneAmp Perkin-Elmer thermocycler set at a 94°C soak cycle. Begin cycling immediately, as follows: 94°C for 2 min to denature template (once), 94°C for 10 s, 50°C for 30 s, 68°C for 2 min (repeat 37 times), 68°C for 7 min (once), and 4°C overnight, or until required for amplification 2.

4. For amplification 2, transfer 3–5 µL of the first PCR product into a second GeneAmp tube and amplify for 40 cycles using the inner primer set (MK650iF and V3iR). Use the same reaction components and cycling parameters.

5. Add loading dye to 8 µL of PCR product and electrophorese on a 1.5% NuSieve as described above (*see* **Notes 18** and **19**).

6. Photograph the gel, record the results, and cut out the PCR product band using a UV transilluminator and a clean scalpel blade.

7. Place the gel slice in a microfuge tube, solubilize, and purify the DNA using a QIA Quick Gel Extraction kit (Quiagen) (*see* **Note 20**).

8. Quantify the DNA by reanalyzing on NuSieve gel using 300 ng of a 100 bp ladder (Pharmacia, Cat. No. 27-4001-01) as the reference standard (*see* **Note 21**).

9. Sequence directly using a Dye Terminator Cycle Sequencing Kit with Amplitaq, or preferably, Amplitaq DNA Polymerase, FS as specified by the manufacturer (ABI).

10. Remove the excess dye on a Centri-sep spin column (Princeton Separations) according to manufacturer's instructions and electrophoresis sequencing reaction for 10 h on a 373A Fluorescent DNA Sequencer (ABI).

11. Assemble, align, and edit the data for the forward and reverse strands (*see* **Note 22**).

4. Notes

1. A wide range of clinical specimens can be applied to filter paper and used as a source of material for HIV-1 genetic analysis. Some examples are fresh capillary blood, collected by heel-stick or venipuncture, anticoagulated whole blood (citrate, EDTA), peripheral blood mononuclear cells, and cultured cell lines. Although most work with DBS has been done on specimens collected from pediatric patients *(15,16)*, adult DBS specimens have included patients from different risk categories (persons attending sexually-transmitted disease clinics, prostitutes, injecting drug users, homosexual and bisexual men, and spouses of HIV-1-infected individuals) and at various stages of disease (ranging from asymptomatic infection to AIDS) *(17)*. In the pediatric setting, the sensitivity of the DBS PCR method is comparable to conventional PCR and better than virus isolation in culture, and approaches 100% in infants older than 16 d of age *(16)*. As in other diagnostic tests, the sensitivity of DBS PCR in neonates under 15 d of age is significantly lower, in the range of 26%. To reduce test error in the neonatal period and achieve earliest possible definitive diagnosis, it is recommended that all neonates be tested by repeat DBS PCR of independent samples collected at birth, and at 30 and 60 d of life.

2. In addition to clinical specimens, it is recommended that at least one positive and two negative DBS controls be included in each PCR assay. As with any laboratory method, additional controls may be useful in startup protocols to ensure that the procedure is reproducible and achieving its maximum sensitivity. Negative controls can be prepared from uninfected, HIV-1 seronegative blood donors, while positive controls of known HIV-1 copy number can be prepared by progressively diluting cultured 8E5 cells *(21)*, containing a single integrated copy of HIV-l_{LAV} proviral DNA per cell with normal seronegative donor blood. DNA extracted from DBS containing these dilution mixtures can then be used to construct a standard curve and assess DNA recovery. The HIV-1 copy number in positive controls should be kept at the lowest possible concentration to avoid the risk of PCR product carryover to clinical samples. The 8E5 HIV-l_{LAV} cell line (which can be obtained from the NIH Reference Reagent Program, Cat. No. 95) is also an excellent positive control for sequence analysis of the V3-envelope region since it contains a highly characteristic QR amino acid insert immediately upstream of the hexameric V3-tip sequence. This insert readily distinguishes 8E5 from most clinical variants of the virus and serves as a control for carryover contamination.

3. The authors have routinely used Schleicher & Schuell #903 paper, originally designed for neonatal metabolic screening, as the absorbent matrix *(13–19)*. This collection device consists of a blotter containing five-1 cm^2 circles for blood application and a sturdy paper overlay that covers the absorbent blotter and the dried blood. The precise method of applying the blood to the blotter is not critical, provided that the blood is fresh and not clotted. In the case of heel-pricks, care should be taken to avoid diluting the sample with extracellular fluid. A standardized method for the collection and preparation of blood spot specimens has been published by the National Committee for Clinical Laboratory Standards *(22)*. In most of the author's studies, we have simply applied 20–40 drops of whole blood to the back of the filter paper using a syringe or pipeting device.

4. The blood spots must be thoroughly dried at room temperature (in a biocontainment hood when possible), before covering them with the attached paper overlay and sealing them in a high-quality sturdy bond envelope, preferably one that is air-permeable and water-resistant *(20)*. When the back of the filter is used, the dried blotter should be double-enveloped to ensure safe shipping. The plastic bags used in some early studies are to be avoided since they release undesirable chemicals and cause heat buildup and moisture accumulation, leading to degradation of the DNA. In regions where the humidity is excessively high, inclusion of a pack of desiccant may be desirable to prevent moisture accumulation and microbial contamination. A recently described modification, designed to ensure that the sample remains "sterile" is to use blotters that have been preimpregnated with 2M guanidine thiocyanate *(23)*. Although this matrix has been successfully used for PCR-based studies of human genomic sequences, its applicability to low abundancy HIV-1 sequences has not yet been demonstrated.

5. When double-packaged using either an inner envelope or the filter paper overlay as the inner container, and a high-quality, extra-strong bond envelope as the outer

container, as recommended by the Centers for Disease Control in Atlanta *(20)*, DBS specimens can be safely shipped or transported by mail or courier. Upon arrival at the reference or research laboratory, DBS are routinely stored at −20°C to ensure optimal specimen integrity Although not recommended, the authors were able to obtain high-quality V3-loop sequence data from a series of DBS that were inadvertently left at room temperature for 6 mo *(17)*. In other studies, we found that repeat freeze-thawing and storage of DBS for up to 15 wk at room temperature had no adverse effect on the ability to detect HIV-1 DNA in DBS *(14)*.

6. To obtain high yields of amplifiable DNA from whole blood, heme and inhibitory substances must be removed from the preparation and the DNA must be effectively released and collected from the nucleated cells. The earliest DBS protocols *(11,13)* were geared towards obtaining highly purified nucleic acid and involved lengthy organic extraction, followed by DNA precipitation, amplification, and detection of the PCR product by solution hybridization with radiolabeled probes. These methods were tedious, labor intensive, and did not lend themselves to large-scale screening and throughput. In addition, the DNA was frequently lost during the precipitation step, leading to false-negative results.

7. To depurinate and prevent cross-contamination between specimens, scissors are routinely washed in 0.25 *N* HCl for 10 min followed by a thorough rinsing in sterile water.

8. If screw-cap tubes are not used, the lids will pop open during Chelex treatment.

9. If carefully performed, this step removes >95% of the hemoglobin. If not removed, residual heme will act as a potent inhibitor of PCR.

10. The DNA remains bound to the filter and can be efficiently recovered by heating at >95°C for one hour at pH 10.0 in a suspension of 5% Chelex-100, a polyvalent resin that chelates metal ions and prevents the breakdown of DNA during subsequent processing *(24)*. Alkaline lysis at high temperature also significantly enhances the PCR amplification signal by ensuring the mononuclear cell membranes are disrupted and that the DNA is completely denatured. One of the most common causes of PCR failure is incomplete denaturation of the DNA. Care must be taken to remove all of the Chelex resin, or metal ions will leach back into solution.

11. Although not always necessary, a quick concentration step using a Centricon-100 (Amicon) or Ultrafree-MC filter (Millipore) leads to more reliable detection of low copy HIV-1 sequences. In both of these systems, the DNA-containing solution is simply poured into a filter cup and concentrated (five- to tenfold) by centrifugal force. The DNA is retained in the cup, while small-mol-wt substances such as salts and PCR inhibitors pass through the filter and are collected in the filtrate collection tube. These concentration devices are used according to manufacturer's specifications, but some "in-house" experimentation with times and speeds of centrifugation may be required to achieve optimal DNA yields. Recent studies in the authors' laboratory suggests that the Millipore filter may give the most reproducible results (unpublished data), but the system has not been rigorously tested in different population cohorts. Further scale-up of this part of the protocol would be highly beneficial, especially for longer PCR prod-

ucts and large-scale sequencing efforts. In theory, it should be possible to extract and purify large amounts of high-quality DNA from filter supports. The challenge is to recover large amounts of DNA in an intact and concentrated form, free of whole-blood inhibitors.

12. One of the most promising applications of DBS PCR, has been its adaptation to newborn screening using a rapid microwell plate assay developed by Roche Diagnostic Systems, Somerville, NJ, USA. The use of this standardized, quality controlled ELISA-type kit broadens the applicability of DBS technology and renders it suitable for large-scale, population-based screening in clinical and public health laboratories. In the microwell detection system, an aliquot of the concentrated Chelex supernatant is amplified with biotinylated gag primers as specified by the manufacturer (Amplicor HIV-1 Amplification and Detection Kit, Roche Diagnostic Systems). After amplification, the PCR product is denatured and hybridized to individual wells of a plate coated with the appropriate HIV-1-specific oligonucleotide probe. The plate is then washed and incubated with avidin–horseradish peroxidase conjugate. Following further washing and incubation with the chromogen, the labeled amplicon is detected colorimetrically by reading the reaction on a microwell plate reader at a wavelength of 450 nm. Details of the procedure, its controls, interpretation and performance in the perinatal setting have been described previously *(16)*. Studies to assess the assay's performance on specimens collected internationally, and in adult populations, to screen for new HIV-1 infections in incidence cohorts, are ongoing.

13. For diagnostic applications, all amplifications are performed using uracil-N-glycosylase (UNG) to reduce the risk of false-positive results due to PCR carryover contamination *(25)*. In this method, dUTP is substituted for dTTP in the PCR reaction mixture, and all subsequent PCR reactions are pretreated with UNG for 10 min at room temperature to cleave and excise uracil from any dU-containing PCR product that has been inadvertently carried over from a previous reaction. This is followed by a heat inactivation step to remove residual UNG and prevent degradation of the desired product. Provided that UNG digestion is carried out to completion, and that the residual UNG enzyme is completely inactivated prior to thermocycling, this method is highly effective in controlling against minute amounts of contamination. It is not, however, a substitute for the extreme care that is required of all PCR-based techniques. For a discussion of the stringent laboratory precautions required for accurate diagnosis, *see* **ref. 26**. In diagnostic applications requiring nested PCR, dUTP can be used in both the first and second PCR reactions, but UNG is added to the first reaction only. A wide range of different primer sets can be used (gag, pol, env) provided that they recognize and bind efficiently to the HIV-1 strains under study.

14. An efficient nested PCR using conserved gag or pol primers, provides reliable detection of HIV-1 from as few as five DBS copies of the HIV-1 provirus/100,000 nucleated cells (*14*, unpublished data). Following amplification and electrophoretic separation on agarose, the PCR product is visualized directly by staining the gel with ethidium bromide. This approach is highly sensitive, ensures that the

correct size of DNA fragment has been amplified in sufficient amounts, and serves as a simple, low-cost method in regions where budgets and resources are limited. In our hands, nested PCR of the pol gene region, combined with agarose electrophoretic analysis, has been particularly valuable for confirming the presence of proviral DNA in DBS containing highly divergent strains of HIV-1. Once the presence of HIV-1 has been documented using conserved pol primers, a panel of envelope primers can be used to fish out new variants that are not easily recognized by conventional env primer sets.

15. Sequencing of DBS specimens provides a rapid screening system to monitor the global spread and emergence of newly identified and previously recognized HIV-1 subtypes (unpublished data, *17*). The method is particularly well-suited to large-scale epidemiological studies of migratory, isolated, or hard-to-reach populations and should facilitate routine surveillance of breakthrough infections in vaccine field trials. The steps involved in DBS sequencing are common to all applications that employ sequencing techniques to classify, compare, and differentiate between HIV-1 subtypes. When performing sequencing applications, a number of choices must be made with respect to the selection of the target sequence, the purification of the PCR and sequencing product, the selection of the sequencing chemistry, the fidelity and accuracy of the sequencing enzyme, as well as the overall cost and potential for automation and high volume throughput. No matter what choices are made, the PCR should be fully optimized and both the forward and reverse strands of the DNA should be sequenced, aligned, and edited. Since the authors' laboratory is interested in large-scale epidemiological studies, we have focused primarily on cycle sequencing using dye-labeled primers *(17)*. This sequencing strategy requires the least amount of DNA and the chemistry is robust, versatile, and can be easily applied to the direct population sequencing of a wide range of PCR products. These features of cycle sequencing render the technology suitable for automation and mass screening applications.

16. Although the authors have successfully sequenced dUTP-containing PCR products, most of sequence work has been performed on products generated with dTTP. Since the potential for carryover contamination is great in the absence of dUTP and UNG, extreme care must be taken to avoid false-positive results and all studies should be stringently controlled to rule out this possibility. In particular, sequencing studies with dTTP should be restricted to regions of the genome that are not amplified for diagnostic purposes, and all new sequences should be extensively compared and screened against current and previous PCR products sequenced in the investigator's laboratory. Some of the most common indicators of laboratory contamination are extensive divergence between linked specimens and identity, or "near-identity" between unlinked specimens or with specimen sequences, molecular clones and/or PCR products previously studied. Reasonable precautions to guard against tube-to-tube carryover of PCR product include performing each step in the amplification and analysis process (sample processing, pre-PCR, first round PCR, nest PCR, and sequencing) in a separate laboratory or containment hood, using designated pipetors and plugged tips, cleaning

work areas with bleach after each assay, using disposable gloves that are changed frequently, aliquoting reagents in small volumes suitable for a single PCR assay, and performing first and second round PCR reactions in clean, designated thermocyclers housed in separate rooms.

17. In recent studies, the authors have successfully replaced *Taq* polymerase with Expand, a new polymerase system that exhibits increased fidelity and enhanced processivity. Using the improved amplification system, outer DBS PCR products of 1.2 kb are now attainable on a regular basis.

18. It is extremely important that PCR reactions be optimized so that only a single bright band is detectable by agarose electrophoresis. If multiple bands are detected, high-quality sequence data is unlikely, even if the specific band of interest is excised and purified. Although seemingly homogeneous, these bands frequently contain heteroduplexes or artifact PCR products generated by primer oligomerization. If the same primers are used for sequencing, these bands give rise to multiple sets of fragments, rendering the sequencing pattern complex and uninterpretable. Well-designed primers and the use of "hot start" methods that minimize oligomerization and secondary priming are important factors to consider when optimizing PCR reactions. A complete discussion of potential difficulties is beyond the scope of this chapter, but an excellent overview of problems encountered during automated fluorescent sequencing is presented in **ref. 27**.

19. For successful analysis of PCR products using dye terminator cycle sequencing, it is important to clean up the PCR reaction by removing excess primers and residual nucleotides, even if the same primers are to be used for the sequencing reaction. Although a variety of different methods exist for purifying PCR products, the authors routinely separate our reactions on 1.5% agarose to determine the size and quality of the product. High-quality sequence grade agarose is required to avoid carryover of fluorescent contaminants that are often present in lower grades of agarose.

20. Following electrophoresis, the PCR product band is excised on a UV transilluminator and further purified using a QIA Quick Gel Extraction kit according to manufacturer's recommendations. The band should be cut out as quickly as possible under long wave UV light to avoid damaging the DNA. With respect to the QIA columns, some adjustments of the time and speed of centrifugation may be required for optimal purification.

21. After purification, the DNA needs to be accurately quantified. A simple method is to reanalyze by agarose electrophoresis using a reference standard to quantify the PCR product. The amount of PCR product added to the sequencing reaction is critical. Too little product will lead to weak signal strength, while too much product results in off-scale data and short sequence reads.

22. A wide range of different software programs are available to assist in the analysis and interpretation of the data. Many of these procedures are well described in the ABI user manuals accompanying the software packages *(27)* and in the literature relating to phylogenetic analysis *(28,29)*. In the authors' hands, direct sequencing of the PCR product amplified from DBS has been particularly successful in

the pediatric setting and in seroconverters and early-stage asymptomatic patients where the viral repertoire is relatively homogeneous. Using this approach, minor variants are also detected provided that they represent >10% of the total virus populations. However, in patients dually infected with different HIV-1 subtypes, and in patients infected with more than one major variant of the virus, where one of the variants contains an insertion or deletion, cloning of the PCR product may be required prior to sequencing. The authors have found that, in the vast majority of HIV-1-infected patients, most gag, pol and C2V3 env gene regions give can be sequenced directly from the PCR product. In contrast, the V1V2 env region of HIV-1 frequently contains large insertions, and, as in other sequencing applications, successful analysis of this region may require molecular cloning of the PCR product, followed by sequencing of individual clones.

23. Recent studies in our laboratory, and others, indicate that accurate quantification *(30)* and sequencing of HIV-1 RNA from dried whole blood and dried plasma is also feasible and reliable (manuscript in preparation).

References

1. Lederberg, J., Shope, R. E., and Oaks, S., Jr., (eds.) (1992) *Emerging Infections: Microbial Threats to Health in the United States.* National Acadermy of Sciences, Washington, DC.
2. Hu, D. J., Dondero, T. J., Rayfield, M. S., George, J. R., Schochetman, G., Jaffe, H. W., et al. (1996) The emerging genetic diversity of HIV. The importance of global surveillance for diagnostics, research and prevention. *JAMA* **275,** 210–215.
3. Weniger, B. B., Takebe, Y., Ou, C-Y., and Yamazaki, S. (1994) The molecular epidemiology of HIV in Asia. *AIDS* **8 (Suppl 2),** S13–S28.
4. Nowak, R. (1995) Staging ethical AIDS trials in Africa. *Science* **269,** 1332–1335.
5. Myers, G., Korber, B., Wain-Hobson, S., Smith, R. F., and Pavlakis, G. N. (1993) *Human Retroviruses and AIDS.* Los Alamos National Laboratory, Los Alamos, New Mexico.
6. Louwagie, J., McCutchan, F. E., Peeters, M., Brennen, T. P., Buell, E., Eddy, G. A., et al. (1993) Phylogenetic analysis of gag genes from 70 international HIV-1 isolates provides evidence for multiple genotypes. *AIDS* **7,** 769–780.
7. Kostrikis, L. G., Bagdades, E, Cao, Y, Zhang, L., Dimitriou, D., and Ho, D. D. (1995) Genetic analysis of human immunodeficiency virus type 1 strains from patients in Cyprus: identification of a new subtype designated subtype I. *J Virol.* **69,** 6122–6130.
8. Gurtler, L. G., Hauser, P. H., Eberle, J., von Brunn, A., Knapp, S., Zekeng, L., Tsague, J. M., and Kaptue, L. (1994) A new subtype of human immunodeficiency virus type 1 (MVP-5180) from Cameroon. *J. Virol.* **68,** 1581–1585.
9. DeLeys, R., Vanderborght, B, Vanden Haesevelde, M., van Geel, A., Wauters, C., et al. (1990) Isolation and partial characterization of an unusual human immuno-deficiency retrovirus from two persons of West-Central African origin. *J. Virol.* **64,** 1207–1216.
10. Garrick, M. D., Dembure, B. S., Cuthrie, R. (1973) Sickle-cell anemia and other

hemoglobinopathies: procedures and strategy for screening employing spots of blood on filter paper as specimens. *N. Engl. J. Med.* **288,** 1256–1268.

11. McCabe, E. R. B., Huang, S. -Z., Seltzer, W. K., and Law, M. L. (1987) DNA microextraction from dried blood spots on filter paper blotters: potential applications to newborn screening. *Hum. Genet.* **75,** 213–216.

12. Hoff, R., Berarde, V. P., Weiblen, B. J., Mahoney-Trout, L, Mitchell, M., and Grad, G. (1988) Seroprevalence of human immunodeficiency virus among child-bearing women: estimation by testing samples of blood from newborns in New York State. *N. Engl. J. Med.* **318,** 525–530.

13. Cassol, S., Salas, T., Arella, M., Neumann, P., Schechter, M., and O'Shaughnessy, M. (1991) Use of dried blood spot specimens in the detection of human immunodeficiency virus type 1 by the polymerase chain reaction. *J. Clin. Microbiol.* **29,** 667–671.

14. Cassol, S., Salas, T., Gill, M. J., Montpetit, M., Rudnik, J., Sy, C. T., et al. (1992) Stability of dried blood spot specimens for detection of human immunodeficiency virus DNA by polymerase chain reaction. *J. Clin. Microbiol.* **30,** 3039–3042.

15. Cassol, S. A., Lapointe, N., Salas, T., Hankins, C., Arella, M., Fauvel, M., et al. (1992) Diagnosis of vertical HIV-1 transmission using the polymerase chain reaction and dried blood spot specimens. *J. Acq. Immun. Defic. Syndr.* **5,** 113–119.

16. Cassol, S., Butcher, A., Kinard, S., Spadoro, J., Sy, T., Lapointe, N., et al. (1994) Rapid screening for the early detection of mother-to-child transmission of HIV-1. *J. Clin. Microbiol.* **32,** 2641–2545.

17. Cassol, S., Weniger, B. G., Babu, P. G. Salminen, M., Zheng, X., Htoon, M. T., et al. (1996) Detection of HIV-1 env subtypes A, B, C and E in Asia using dried blood spots: a new surveillance tool for molecular epidemiology. *AIDS Res. Hum. Retrovir.* **12,** 1435–1441.

18. Cassol, S., Read, S., Weniger, B G., Gomez, P., Lapointe, N., Ou, C-Y., et al. (1996) Dried blood spots collected on filter paper: an international resource for the diagnosis and genetic characterization of HIV-1. Mem. Inst. Oswaldo Cruz, Rio de Janeiro, **91,** 351–358.

19. Cassol, S. (1996) Applications of dried blood spots to the diagnosis and field surveillance of HIV-1. *Benchmark* **3,** 7–9.

20. Knudsen, R. C., Slazyk, W. E., Richmond, J. Y., and Hannon, W. H. (1993) Guide-lines from the Centers for Disease Control and Prevention (Atlanta) for the shipment of dried blood spot specimens. *Infant Screening* **16,** 1–3. FAX Information Service (404-332-4565). Document no. 101011, 13 October.

21. Folks, T. M., Powell, D., Lightfoote, M., Koenig, S., Fauci, A. S., Benn, S., et al. (1986) Biological and biochemical characterization of a cloned Leu-3-cell surviving infection with the acquired immune deficiency syndrome retrovirus. *J. Exp. Med.* **164,** 280–290.

22. National Committee for Clinical Laboratory Standards. NCCL Approved Standard LA4-A2. (1992) Blood collection on filter paper for neonatal screening programs. National Committee for Laboratory Standards, Villanova, PA.

23. Harvey, M. A., King, T. H., and Burghoff, R. (1996) Impregnated 903 blood col-

lection paper. A tool for DNA preparation from dried blood spots for PCR amplification. A technical Bulletin from the Research and Development, Schleicher &
Schuell, Inc., Keene, NH 03431; Fax (603) 357-3627.

24. Singer-Sam, J., Tanguay, R. L., and Riggs, A. D. (1989) Use of Chelex to improve the PCR signal from a small number of cells. *Amplifications* **3,** 11.

25. Longo, M. C., Beringer, M. S., and Hartley, J. L. (1990) Use of uracil DNA
glycosylase to control carry-over contamination in polymerase chain reactions.
Gene **93,** 125–128.

26. Kwok, S. (1990) Procedures to minimize PCR-product carry-over, in *PCR Protocols: A Guide to Methods and Application*, (Innis, M. A., Gelfand, S. H., Sninsky,
J. J., and White, T. J. eds), Academic Press, San Diego, CA, pp. 142–145.

27. Perkin Elmer Corporation, Applied Biosystems Division. (1995) *Comparative PCR
Sequencing: A Guide to Sequencing-Based Mutation Detection.* Foster City, CA.

28. Smith, S., Overbeek, R., Woese, C. R. Gilbert, W., and Gillevet, P. (1994) The
genetic Data environment: an expandable GUI for multiple sequence analysis.
Comp. Appl. Biol. Sci. **10,** 671–675.

29. Olsen, G. J., Matsude, H., Hagstrom, R., and Overbeek, R. (1994) FastDNAml: A
tool for construction of phylogenetic trees of DNA sequences using maximum
likelihood. *Comput. Appl. Biosci.* **10,** 41–48.

30. Cassol, S., Gill, M. J., Pilon, R., Cormier, M., Voight, R. F., Willoughby, B., and
Forbes, J. (1997) Quantification of human immunodeficiency virus type 1 RNA
frim dried plasma spots collected on filter paper. *J. Clin. Microbiol.* **35,** 2795–2801.

16

Quantification of HIV-1 RNA in Dried Plasma Spots (DPS)

A Field Approach to Therapeutic Monitoring

Sharon A. Cassol, Francisco Diaz-Mitoma, Richard Pilon, Michelle Janes, and D. William Cameron

1. Introduction

The ability to accurately measure viral RNA in the plasma *(1–3)* and intracellular *(4–7)* compartments of HIV-1-infected persons has led to a dramatic improvement in the understanding of the natural history of HIV-1 and AIDS. A number of recent studies have convincingly demonstrated that high levels of viral replication occur at all stages of disease *(8–10)*, and that changes in viral RNA load are predictive of disease outcome *(11,12)*, and response to therapy *(13,14)*. These findings, combined with the introduction of potent new antivirals *(15,16)*, have stimulated a growing interest in viral load monitoring, both as a function of disease status, and as a predictor of disease progression and therapeutic efficacy.

The most commonly used quantification methods measure HIV-1 virion RNA levels in plasma either by the reverse transcriptase-polymerase chain reaction (RT-PCR) *(17–19)* or the branched DNA (bDNA) signal amplification assay *(20,21)*. As currently formatted, both assays are performed on fresh plasma processed within 4–6 h of collection, or on cryopreserved plasma that has been separated and frozen immediately after collection, at –20°C or colder. If in-house quantification is not available, the frozen plasma is then shipped on dry ice to a designated reference laboratory for analysis. These specialized handling requirements render the technology unsuitable for use in developing countries, where dry ice is unavailable and facilities and resources are limited.

From: *Methods in Molecular Medicine, Vol. 17: HIV Protocols*
Edited by: N. L. Michael and J. H. Kim © Humana Press Inc., Totowa, NJ

Simple and improved methods that eliminate the need for cryopreservation and extensive on-site processing and analysis would be highly advantageous.

The collection of blood specimens on filter paper blotters (Guthrie cards) provides an innovative and powerful approach for the PCR-based analysis of HIV-1 *(22,23,25–29)*. Using this technique, large numbers of difficult field specimens can be systematically collected, dried, and shipped without cryopreservation *(29)* or biosafety hazard *(30)*. Since first introduced for HIV-1 genetic testing in 1991 *(22)*, dried whole blood specimens, in combination with DNA PCR and sequencing, have been used to rapidly screen for the presence of virus in newborns *(23–25,31)*, monitor the emergence drug resistant mutations *(26)*, characterize the genotype of transmitted virus *(26)*, and track the spread of HIV-1 subtypes in Asia *(27)*.

In this chapter, the extension of filter paper technology to the quantification of HIV-1 RNA in dried plasma is described. After the plasma has saturated the filter, it is simply air-dried, placed in a high-quality bond envelope *(30)*, and shipped at ambient temperature to a suitable reference or research laboratory for RNA extraction and analysis using modifications of a commercially available RT-PCR kit. When evaluated under a variety of different environmental conditions and across the spectrum of HIV-1 disease, the results of dried plasma testing were biologically equivalent to those obtained using more conventional HIV-1 RNA quantification methods (**Fig. 1**). It is anticipated that dried plasma spots (DPS) will prove particularly valuable for monitoring therapeutic efficacy among isolated and hard-to-reach populations and assessing viral replication kinetics in patients infected with different HIV-1 subtypes.

2. Materials
2.1. Consumables and Suppliers

1. Becton Dickinson, Rutherford, NJ: Vacutainer blood collection tubes, EDTA (BD #367665 or equivalent).
2. Roche Molecular Systems, Inc., Somerville, NJ: Amplicor HIV monitor kit.
3. Sarstedt, St. Laurent, Quebec, Canada: 2.0 mL polypropylene, screw cap microcentrifuge tubes, Cat. no. 72.693.005.
4. Schleicher & Schuell, Keene, NH: #903 blood collection paper, Cat. no. 58370.
5. Fisher Scientific, Nepean, Ottawa, Ontario, Canada: Isopropanol, reagent grade, Cat. no. A416-500; ethanol, Cat. no. A962-4.
6. Consumables (tubes, caps, micropetors, plugged tips, and tray) as specified in the package insert of the Amplicor HIV RNA kit (Roche).

2.2. Equipment

In addition to the equipment needed for RT-PCR analysis (Perkin-Elmer GeneAmp 9600 thermocycler, microcentrifuge, multi-channel pipetor, vortex

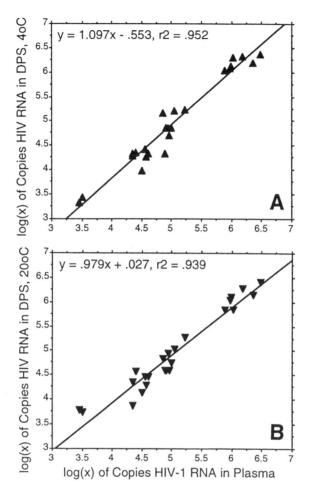

Fig. 1. Regression analysis of viral RNA measurement in paired DPS and fresh frozen plasma. DPS were refrigerated **(A)**, or stored at room temperature (20°C) **(B)** for 7–16 d prior to analysis. Linear regression analysis of $\log_{10}$ transformed HIV-1 *gag* RNA levels are shown for 24 paired patients, representing all stages of HIV-1 infection (asymptomatic through AIDS). The formula for the curve fit is given (y = intercept + slope [x] along with the square of the correlation coefficient [r^2]). (Figure taken from **ref. 38**.)

mixer, 37°C incubator, microwell plate washer and reader and computer (see Amplicor HIV-1 Monitor package insert), DPS requires multiple pairs of scissors and an Eppendorf Thermomixer, model 5436 (Brinkman, Cat. no. #3514-32 with transfer rack, Cat. no. #3515-19).

3. Methods
3.1. Preparation of DPS

Manipulation of infected blood specimens should be performed under strict biosafety precautions (*see* **Note 1**) *(32)*, and in an environment that is free of contaminating PCR amplicons and cloned viral sequences (*see* **Note 2**) *(33)*. A variety of different techniques is acceptable for the preparation of plasma, provided that there is no substantial inhibition of subsequent PCR amplification reactions and that the same procedure is used throughout an entire study (*see* **Note 3**). The following protocol is routinely used in our laboratory.

1. Collect whole blood by venipuncture in "lavender-top" vacutainer tubes (Becton Dickinson) containing EDTA as the anticoagulant (*see* **Note 4**).
2. Transport tube to the virology laboratory at room temperature.
3. Centrifuge tube at 1200g for 20 min at room temperature to separate plasma from whole blood. For reliable results, plasma separation should be completed within 6 h of blood collection (*see* **Notes 3** and **5**).
4. Remove the separated plasma, and transfer to a new sterile tube.
5. Using a micropipetor and sterile plugged tips, apply 50-μL aliquots of the clarified plasma to individual circles of a standard newborn screening blotter (Schleicher & Schuell, #903) (*see* **Notes 6** and **7**).
6. Air dry for at least 3 h in a biocontainment hood, when possible.
7. If shipping is required, place each labeled filter in an individual bond envelope containing desiccant (*see* **Note 8**).
8. Seal envelope and enclose in a second, outer bond envelope and ship to a reference laboratory by courier at ambient temperatures (*see* **Note 9**).
9. At the reference laboratory, the DPS can be analyzed immediately or, they can be stored frozen at −70°C and used for "batch-testing" and retrospective analysis (*see* **Note 10**).

3.2. Reagent Preparation

Although different in-house methods exist for the extraction, reverse transcription, and amplification of HIV-1 RNA, the authors opted to use a commercially-available, quality-controlled kit, namely the Roche HIV-1 Monitor assay (*see* **Notes 11** and **12**). The use of a commercial method maximizes reproducibility and renders the technology suitable for large-scale efficacy testing in clinical trials. At the time of analysis (in the research or reference laboratory):

1. Immediately before using, prepare a working lysis reagent by adding a known amount (25 μL) of quantitation standard RNA (QS RNA) to one bottle of lysis reagent (Amplicor HIV-1 Monitor kit, Roche) (*see* **Note 13**). The QS RNA acts as an internal standard to monitor the efficiency of sample preparation, reverse transcription, and amplification. The pink dye confirms the presence QS RNA in the extraction reagent.

2. After determining the number of assays required, prepare the appropriate amount of PCR reaction mix. For 12 quantifications, mix 100 μL of manganese solution with one tube of master mix (Amplicor HIV-1 Monitor kit). Again, the pink dye confirms the addition of manganese.

3.3. RNA Extraction

1. Excise each circle of dried plasma (approx 1.0 cm^2) using clean, acid-depurinated scissors. Cut in three pieces and place in a 1.5-mL screw-cap microfuge tube. Use a different pair of scissors for each patient and each control specimen (*see* **Notes 14** and **15**).
2. Reconstitute the dried plasma by adding 200 μL of sterile, DEPC-treated water to each tube.
3. Dispense 600 μL of working lysis reagent (containing QS RNA) into each tube; cap and incubate for 15 min at 65°C with continuous shaking on an Eppendorf Thermomixer set at 1000 rpm to extract the RNA (*see* **Note 16**).
4. Following incubation, transfer 750 μL of the supernatant to a new tube.
5. Add 750 μL of 100% isopropanol, recap, and vortex briefly (3–5 s) to precipitate the RNA.
6. Centrifuge at approx 16,000*g* for 15 min at room temperature.
7. Aspirate the supernatant, taking great care not to disturb the RNA pellet on the outer shoulder of the tube. Use a fine-tipped, sterile transfer pipet or a pipeting device with disposable tips. It is important to maintain a constant negative pressure during removal of the liquid.
8. Wash the pellet with 1.0 mL of 70% ethanol. Recap and vortex (3–5 s).
9. Recentrifuge at approx 16,000*g* for 5 min at room temperature.
10. Again, carefully aspirate the supernatant without disturbing the pellet.
11. Add 100 μL of specimen diluent (Amplicor HIV-1 Monitor kit), recap, and vortex vigorously for 10 s to resuspend the extract RNA (*see* **Note 17**).
12. Pipet 50 μL to the appropriate PCR tube and amplify by RT-PCR, exactly as specified in the Roche HIV-1 Monitor kit (*see* **Note 18**).

4. Notes

1. Universal precautions are to be used whenever handling blood or other potentially infectious specimens. Essential precautions include the availability of adequate hand washing facilities and work practice controls, as well as the proper use of warning labels and protective equipment such as gloves and lab coats, the routine decontamination of work areas, and the proper disposal of waste material.
2. To reduce the risk of false-positive results and inaccurate quantification in-house and commercial assays that incorporate uracil-*N*-glycosylase (UNG) are routinely used for the prevention of PCR product carryover contamination. Although this approach is highly effective in controlling against small amounts of contamination, it is not a substitute for the extreme care that is required of all PCR-based technologies. Other universal precautions to guard against carryover of PCR

amplicons and cloned sequences include performing sample processing pre-PCR, amplification and detection in separate laboratories or containment hoods, using designated pipetors and plugged tips, cleaning work areas with bleach after each assay, using disposable gloves that are changed frequently, and aliquotting reagents in small volumes suitable for a single assay.

3. To achieve accurate and reproducible quantification, it is important that cells and platelets be effectively removed from the plasma preparation, and that the same specimen processing procedure be used for all comparative studies. If cells are not removed from the preparation, HIV-1 DNA will be amplified in addition to viral RNA. Platelets, if present, may confound quantification by binding small amounts of circulating virus. To remove these components, the Roche Monitor assay recommends a single centrifugation at 800–1600g for 20 min or longer. Other methods have used a two step protocol involving a low-speed centrifugation at 400–800g for 20 min, followed by removal of the plasma and recentrifugation for an additional 20 min at 800g. Despite these differences, it is reassuring that several commercially-developed assays are giving comparable HIV-1 RNA quantification results. In the near future, however, it is likely that methods will become increasingly standardized and that consistent guidelines will be developed to minimize interassay and interlaboratory variability. This is especially important for RT-PCR, where small differences in HIV-1 target RNA, when exponentially amplified, can lead to substantial variations in PCR product yield.

4. Although heparin, acid-citrate-dextrose (ACD), and citrate cell preparation tubes (CCPT) have been successfully used for collection and quantification of HIV-1 RNA in plasma, EDTA is now emerging as the preferred anticoagulant. Heparinized samples require a rather tedious extraction with silica to purify the RNA and prevent heparin inhibition of PCR. Citrate, which is used in solution, dilutes the plasma by an unknown amount (approx 15%) and leads to variable results.

5. Early studies recommended that the plasma be processed within 2–3 h of collection to preserve the integrity of the viral RNA. However, with increased experience, as shown in this chapter, it is becomingly apparent that the HIV-1 virion RNA in plasma is more stable than previously appreciated, presumably a result of the protective presence of the viral coat. As a result, the 2–3 h time period has now been extended to 6 h.

6. All steps in the collection, isolation, and extraction procedure, as well as handling of the filter papers, should be performed using aseptic techniques to prevent degradation of the RNA by nucleases. This includes the use of sterile tubes, pipet tips and reagents, and the wearing of disposable gloves.

7. The authors have routinely used Schleicher & Schuell #903 paper, originally designed for neonatal metabolic screening, as an absorbent matrix and noninfectious transport system *(22,23,25–29)*. This collection device consists of a blotter containing five 1-cm^2 circles for specimen collection and sturdy paper overlay that covers the absorbent blotter and dried sample. A 50-μL aliquot of plasma saturates the circle and may extend slightly beyond. In future studies, it may be

possible to use blotters that have been preimpregnated with 2 *M* guanidine thio-cyanate *(35)* or other preservatives, to reduce the risk of microbial contamination.

8. The plasma spots should be thoroughly dried at room temperature before cover-ing them with the attached paper overlay and sealing them in high-quality, sturdy envelopes, preferably ones that are air-permeable and water-resistant. In regions of excessive humidity, it may be prudent to air-dry in the presence of desiccant. The plastic seal-a-bags used in some early studies are to be avoided since they release undesirable chemicals and cause heat buildup, leading to specimen degradation.

9. When double-packaged using two extra strong bond envelopes, as recommended by the Centers for Disease Control (Atlanta, GA) *(30)*, filter specimens can be safely shipped and transported by mail or courier.

10. Real-time analysis may be required to determine eligibility for a clinical trial, or to alter therapy, whereas batch-testing of serially collected samples may be more appropriate for evaluating therapeutic efficacy in large-scale, blinded trials.

11. HIV-1 RNA quantification is still technically challenging, requiring skilled tech-nologists, stringent quality controls, and standardized reagents and protocols. At present, quantification assays are best performed in a controlled setting using commercial technology. Three assays which show significant promise in this regard are the branched DNA assay from Chiron *(20,21)*, the Amplicor RT-PCR assay from Roche *(17–19)*, and the NASBA amplification system developed by Organon-Teknika. Although each assay has its strengths and limitations, the re-sults appear to be closely related. RT-PCR was selected for this study, since it is currently the most sensitive assay, is readily available, and requires the least amount of specimen, although a small volume assay with improved sensitivity is currently under development at Chiron. A disadvantage of RT-PCR is that it requires a high level of technical skill to avoid cross-contamination of amplifica-tion reactions. In addition, since RT-PCR is based on the exponential amplifica-tion of HIV-1 RNA target sequences, small changes in sample processing can alter the input RNA copy number and lead to significant variation in the final PCR signal. With respect to PCR, there has also been some concern that a single set of primers may not recognize all HIV-1 subtypes equally. This would lead to nonuniform, differential amplification across HIV-1 subtypes. Strict quality con-trol and judicious selection of primers are needed to avoid these potential pitfalls.

12. Of particular note for filter paper methods is the potential of the NASBA assay. A major advantage of NASBA is its ability to selectively amplify RNA is the presence of DNA. The ability to quantify HIV-1 RNA from whole blood, rather than plasma, would simplify field trials by eliminating the need for on-site sepa-ration and isolation of plasma.

13. To compensate for the smaller plasma volume of DPS specimens (50 μL instead of the 200 μL routinely used for fresh or cryopreserved plasma) and to maintain the same relative ratio of QS RNA to specimen RNA, the amount of QS RNA used to prepare the working lysis reagent has been reduced from 100 μL to 25 μL.

14. To depurinate and prevent cross-contamination between specimens, scissors are routinely washed in 0.25 *N* HCl for 10 min, followed by a thorough rinsing in sterile water.

15. In addition to clinical specimens, it is recommended that at least one negative and three positive controls are included in each DPS RT-PCR assay. Controls are prepared by applying measured aliquots (50 μL) of pooled plasma (from uninfected individuals, and infected individuals with known low-intermediate and high-HIV-1 RNA copy numbers) to replicate sets of Schleicher and Schuell #903 filter paper. After air drying in a laminar flow hood, individual filters can be enveloped and stored at –70°C for use as reference standards.

16. DPS are heated at 65°C to ensure that the RNA is efficiently eluted from the filter, and to eliminate any RNA secondary structure.

17. Again, the amount of specimen diluent has been reduced (from 400 to 100 μL) to compensate for the smaller volume of dried plasma specimens. When adjusted in this manner, the RNA input into the PCR reaction is identical to that used in conventional "fresh plasma" assays.

18. The Amplicor HIV Monitor test involves RNA extraction in guanidine thiocyanate, precipitation with isopropanol, and RT-PCR amplification of a 142 base pair HIV-1 *gag* sequence using biotinylated primers, and a single thermostable enzyme (rTth DNA polymerase) that has both reverse transcriptase and DNA polymerase activities. Serial dilutions of the biotinylated PCR product are hybridized to individual wells a microwell plate coated with HIV-specific and QS-specific oligonucleotide probes and quantified in an avidin-horseradish peroxidase colorimetric reaction. The input HIV-1 RNA copy number is then calculated from the known copy number of the QS RNA standard (Amplicor HIV Monitor package insert [Roche]).

19. Since preparation of this chapter, acurate quantification of HIV-1 RNA from dried plasma and dried blood spots (DBS) has been achieved using NASBA/Nuclisense technology *(38)*. As with the Amplicor method, there is a strong correlation between viral RNA levels in liquid plasma, dried plasma, and dried whole blood. In patients with primary HIV-1 infection, the testing of DPS/DBS allows accurate measurement of viral RNA during the intital spike of viremia, and in the subsequent period of suppressed viral replication. In the pediatric setting, testing of DBS is facilitating natural history and perinatal intervention studies in both developed and developing countries (*39,40*; manuscripts in preparation).

References

1. Piatak, M., Saag, M. S., Yang, L. C., Clark, S. J, Lappes, L. C., Luk, K. C., et al. (1993) High levels of HIV-1 in plasma during all stages of infection determined by competitive PCR. *Science* **259**, 1749–1754.
2. Coombs, R., Collier, A. C., Allain, J. P., Nikora, B., Leuther, M., Gjerset, G. F., et al. (1989) Plasma viremia in human immunodeficiency virus infection. *N. Engl. J. Med.* **321**, 1626–1631.

3. Schnittman, S. M., Greenhouse, J. J., Lane, H. C., Pierce, P. F., and Fauci, A. S. (1991) Frequent detection of HIV-1-specific mRNAs in infected individuals suggests ongoing active viral expression in all stages of disease. *AIDS Res. Hum. Retrovir.* **7**, 361–367.

4. Merzouki, A., Mo, T., Vellani, N., Pattullo, A., Estable, M., O'Shaughnessy, M., et al. (1994) Accurate and differential quantitation of HIV-1 tat, rev and nef mRNAs by competitive PCR. *J. Virol. Methods* **50**, 115–128.

5. Michael, N. L., Mo, T., Merzouki, A., O'Shaughnessy, M., Oster, C., Burke, D. S., et al. (1995) Human immunodeficiency virus type 1 cellular RNA load and splicing patterns predict disease progression in a longitudinally studied cohort. *J. Virol.* **69**, 1868,1677.

6. Saksela, K., Stevens, C. E., Rubinstein, P., Taylor, P. E., and Baltimore, D. (1995) HIV-1 messenger RNA in peripheral blood mononuclear cells as an early marker of risk for progression to AIDS. *Ann. Intern. Med.* **123**, 641–648.

7. Furtado, M. R., Kingsley, L. A., and Wolinsky, S. M. (1995) Changes in the viral mRNA expression pattern correlated with a rapid rate of CD4+ T-cell number decline in human immunodeficiency virus type 1-infected individuals. *J. Virol.* **69**, 2092–2100.

8. Ho, D. D., Neumann, A. U., Perelson, A. S., Chen, W., Leonard, J. M., and Markowitz, M. (1995) Rapid turnover of plasma virions and CD4 lymphocytes in HIV-1 infection. *Nature* **373**, 123–126.

9. Wei, X., Ghosh, S. K., Taylor, M. E., et al. Viral dynamics in human immunodeficiency virus type 1 infection. *Nature* (1995) **373**, 117–122.

10. Perelson, A. S., Neumann, A. U., Markowitz, M., Leonard, J. M., Ho, D. D. (1996) HIV-1 dynamics in vivo: virion clearance rate, infected cell life-span, and viral generation time. *Science* **271**, 1582–1586.

11. Mellors, J. W., Kingsley, L. A., Rinaldo, C. R., Todd, J. A., Hoo, B. S., Kokka, R. P., et al. (1995) Quantitation of HIV-1 RNA in plasma predicts outcome after seroconversion. *Ann. Intern. Med.* **122**, 573–579.

12. Ioannidis, J. P. A., Capelleri, J. C., Lau, J., Sacks, H. S., and Skolnik, P. R. (1996) Predictive value of viral load measurements in asymptomatic untreated HIV-1 infection: a mathematical model. *AIDS* **0**, 255–262.

13. Katzenstein, D. A. and Holodniy, M. (1995) HIV viral load quantification, HIV resistance and antiretroviral therapy. *AIDS Clin. Rev.* **96**, 277–303.

14. Kappes, J. C., Saag, M. S., Shaw, G. M., Hahn, B. H., Chopra, P., Chen, S., et al. (1995) Assessment of antiretroviral therapy by plasma viral load testing: standard and ICD HIV-1 p24 antigen and viral RNA (QC-PCR) assays compared. *J. Acquir. Immune Defic. Synd. Hum. Retrovirol.* **10**, 139–149.

15. Vella, S. (1994) HIV therapy advances. Update on a proteinase inhibitor. *AIDS* **8(Suppl 3)**, S25-S29.

16. Kitchen, V. S., Skinner, C., Ariyoshi, K., Lane, E. A., Duncan, I. B., Burckhardt, J., et al. (1995) Safety and activity of saquinavir in HIV infection. *Lancet* **345**, 936,937.

17. Mulder, J., McKinney, N., Christopherson, C., Sninksy, J., Greenfield, L., and Kwok, S. (1994) Rapid and simple PCR assay for quantitation of human immuno-

deficiency virus type 1 RNA in plasma: Application to acute retroviral infection. *J. Clin. Microbiol.* **32,** 292–300.

18. Katzenstein, D. A., Winters, M., Bubp, J., Israelski, D., Winger, E., and Merigan, T. C. (1994) Quantitation of human immunodeficiency virus by culture and polymerase chain reaction in response to didanosine after long-term therapy with zidovudine. *J. Infect. Dis.* **169,** 416–419.

19. Winters, M. A., Tan, L. B., Katzenstein, D. A., and Merigan, T. C. (1993) Biological variation and quality control of plasma human immunodeficiency virus type 1 RNA quantitation by reverse transcriptase polymerase chain reaction. *J. Clin. Microbiol.* **31,** 2960–2966.

20. Cao, Y., Ho, D. D., Todd, J., Kokka, R., Urdea, M., et al. (1995) Clinical evaluation of bDNA signal amplification for quantifying HIV type 1 in human plasma. *AIDS Res. Hum. Retrovir.* 353–361.

21. Pachl, C., Todd, J. A., Kern, D. G., Sheridan, P., Fong, S-J., Stempien, M., et al. (1995) Rapid and precise quantification of HIV-1 RNA in plasma using a branched DNA signal amplification assay. *J. Acquir. Immune Defic. Synd. and Hum. Retrovirol.* **8,** 446–454.

22. Cassol, S., Salas, T., Arella, M., Neumann, P., Schechter, M. T., and O'Shaughnessy, M. (1991)Use of dried blood spot specimens in the detection of human immuno-deficiency virus type 1 by the polymerase chain reaction. *J. Clin. Microbiol.* **29,** 667–671.

23. Cassol, S. A., Lapointe, N., Salas, T., Hankins, C., Arella, M., Fauvel, M., et al. (1992) Diagnosis of vertical HIV-1 transmission using the polymerase chain reaction and dried blood spot specimens. *J. Acquir. Immune Defic. Synd.* **5,** 113–119.

24. Comeau, A. M., Harris, J., McIntosh, K., Weiblen, J., Hoff, R., Grady, G. F., and the AIDS Programme of Boston City Hospital and Children's Hospital. (1992) Polymerase chain reaction in detecting HIV infection among seropositive infants: relation to clinical status and age and to results of other assay. *J. Acquir. Immune Defic. Synd.* **5,** 271–278.

25. Cassol, S., Butcher, A., Kinard, S., Spadoro, J., Sy, T., Lapointe, N., et al. (1994) Rapid screening for the early detection of mother-to-child transmission of HIV-1. *J. Clin. Microbiol.* **32,** 2641–2645.

26. Cassol, S. A., Read, S., Weniger, B. G., Gomez, P., Lapointe, N., Ou, C-Y., et al. (1996) Dried blood spots collected on filter paper: an international resource for the diagnosis and genetic characterization of human immunodeficiency virus type 1. *Mem. Inst. Oswald Cruz,* Rio de Janeiro, **91,** 351–358.

27. Cassol, S., Weniger, B. G., Babu, P. G., Salminen, M. O., Zheng, X., Htoon, M. T., et al. (1996) Detection of HIV-1 env sutypes A, B, C, and E in Asia using dried blood spots: a new surveillance tool for molecular epidemiology. *AIDS Res. Hum. Retrovir.* **12,** 1435–1441.

28. Cassol, S. Amplicor HIV Monitor Assay, version 3, no. 13–93-87374–001 (April 3, 1996). Roche Molecular Systems, Somerville, New Jersey.

29. Cassol, S., Salas, T., Gill, M. J., Montpetit, M., Rudnik, J., Sy, C. T., et al. (1992) Stability of dried blood spot specimens for detection of human immunodeficiency virus DNA by polymerase chain reaction. *J. Clin. Microbiol.* **30,** 3039–3042.

30. Knudsen, R. C., Slazyk, W. E., Richmond, J. Y, and Hannon, W. H. Guidelines for the Shipment of Dried Blood Spot Specimens. Document No. 101011, 13 October 1993. Office of Health and Safety. Centers for Disease control and Prevention. FAX Information Service (40 4. 332–4564), Atlanta, Georgia.

31. Nyambi, P. N., Fransen, K., De Beenhouwer, H., et al. (1994). Detection of human immunodeficiency virus type 1 (HIV-1) in heel prick specimens from children born to HIV-1-seropositive mothers. *J. Clin. Microbiol.* **32,** 2858–2860.

32. National Institutes of Health. (1994). Biosafety, specimen handling and codes, storage and shipment of specimens, in *ACTG Virology Manual for HIV Laboratories.* Division of AIDS, National Institutes of Allergy and Infectious Diseases, Publication NIH-94–3828, pp. LAB-14.

33. Kwok, S. (1990) Procedures to minimize PCR-product carry-over, in *PCR Protocols: A Guide to Methods and Application* (Innis, M. A., Gelfand, S. H., Sninsky, J. J., and White, T. J., eds.) Academic, San Diego, CA, pp. 142–145.

34. National Institutes of Health (1994) Quantitative plasma culture assay, in *ACTG Virology Manual for HIV Laboratories.* Division of AIDS, National Institutes of Allergy and Infectious Diseases, Publication NIH-94–3828, pp. PLA-1.

35. Harvey, M. A., King, T. H., and Burghoff, R. (1996). Impregnated 903 blood collection paper. A tool for DNA preparation from dried blood spots for PCR amplification. A Technical Bulletin from the Research and Development Department, Schleicher and Schuell, Inc., Keene, N. H. 03431; Fax (603) 357–3627.

36. Chin, J. (1990) Current and future dimensions of the HIV and AIDS epidemic in women and children. *Lancet* **336,** 221–224.

37. World Health Organization, Global Programme on AIDS. Current and future dimensions of the HIV/AIDS pandemic. A capsule summary. WHO/GPA/RES/SFI/91. 4: 1–15. World Health Organization, Geneva.

38. Cassol, S., Gill, J. M., Pilon, R., Cormier, M., Voigt, R. F., Willoughby, B., Forbes, J. (1997) Quantification of human immunodeficiency virus type 1 RNA from dried plasma spots collected on filter papaer. *J. Clin. Microbiol.* **35,** 2795–2801.

39. Comeau, A. M., Su, Z., Gerstel, J., Pan, D., Hillyer, G. V., Tuomala, R., et al. (1998) Use of microsample dried blood spot RNA assays for diagnosis of pediatric HIV in the first week of life. Fifth Conference on Retroviruses and Opportunistic Infections, Chicago, February 1–5.

40. Cassol, S., Pilon, R., Janes, M., Hillyer, G. V., Tuomala, R., LaRussa, P., et al. (1998) Dried blood spots (DBS) for monitoring HIV-1 RNA load in neonates and infants. Fifth Conference on Retroviruses and Opportunistic Infections, Chicago, February 1–5.

17

Quantitation of HIV-1 RNA in Genital Secretions

Bruce L. Gilliam

1. Introduction

The continuing spread of the HIV-1 epidemic worldwide has stimulated efforts to develop vaccines and decrease transmission of HIV-1 as noted in **Chapter 8**. Key to this effort is the characterization of the qualities of HIV-1 in genital secretions. Seminal cell and seminal plasma culture have been used to isolate HIV-1 from semen but have low recovery rates of 9–50% *(1–11)*. Culture of vaginal cells have also had low recovery rates of 0–30% *(12–14)*. In an attempt to overcome this problem, HIV-1 has been evaluated in genital secretions using polymerase chain reaction (PCR) techniques. Compared to culture techniques, PCR techniques, both DNA and RNA, have had a higher recovery rate of HIV-1 from genital secretions *(2,3,7,9–11,13–25)*.

The need to determine the infectivity of a given individual has led to the pursuit of quantitative methods for the evaluation of HIV-1 in genital secretions. Quantitative culture yields definitively infectious virus but, as discussed above and in **Chapter 8**, has the limitation of relatively low recovery rates. Quantitative PCR techniques have improved recovery of HIV-1 and allowed more accurate quantification of virus. In addition, PCR is less labor-intensive than culture and can be done on frozen specimens without significant loss of sensitivity. Multiple studies have used quantitative PCR techniques to determine HIV-1 RNA levels in semen and cervicovaginal secretions *(2,3,9–11,14–16,18,21–24)* and a correlation between HIV-1 RNA levels in semen and quantitative seminal cell culture results has been demonstrated *(3,9,11)*.

This chapter provides an overview of the different techniques that may be used to quantitate HIV-1 RNA in genital secretions and the difficulties encountered with these techniques.

From: *Methods in Molecular Medicine, Vol. 17: HIV Protocols*
Edited by: N. L. Michael and J. H. Kim © Humana Press Inc., Totowa, NJ

2. Materials
2.1. Specimen Collection
2.1.1. Semen

1. Sterile specimen container with screw-on lid.
2. Sterile phosphate-buffered saline (PBS), Hank's buffered saline solution (HBSS), or viral transport medium (VTM). Viral transport medium can be easily prepared using the following formula and stored at 4°C for up to 6 mo. The final concentrations of the components is 200 U/mL of nystatin, 1000 U/mL of penicillin, and 1000 µg/mL of streptomycin (*see* **Note 1**).
   (a) 1 mL of penicillin/streptomycin.
   (b) 2 mL of nystatin suspension (10,000 U/mL) (Gibco-BRL, Grand Island, NY).
   (c) RPMI 1640 to bring to 100 mL.
3. Sterile 15-mL Falcon conical tube (PGC, Gaithersburg, MD).
4. Centrifuge.
5. Sterile cryovials.

2.1.2. Cervicovaginal Secretions

1. Sterile speculum.
2. Sterile PBS or viral transport medium (VTM).
3. Sterile plastic transfer pipet—6 mL (Fisher, Pittsburgh, PA), and/or sterile luer lock syringe—10 mL (*see* **Note 2**).
4. Dacron swab (Baxter/VWR Scientific, Westchester, PA).
5. Sno-strips (Akorn, Inc., Abita Springs, LA).
6. Sterile 15-mL Falcon conical tube (PGC, Gaithersburg, MD).
7. Hemoccult single slides (SmithKline Diagnostics, San Jose, CA) or similar test for occult blood.
8. Centrifuge.
9. Sterile cryovials.

2.2. Quantitative HIV-1 RNA Techniques

There are currently three commercially available HIV-1 RNA assays: Organon-Teknika NucliSens HIV-1 QT or NASBA, Roche Amplicor HIV-1 Monitor, and Chiron Quantiplex. It is important to note that the each of these assays has advantages and disadvantages (*see* **Table 1**). When evaluating a commercial or in-house assay for use in the determination of HIV-1 RNA in semen, it is important to take into consideration several factors. Semen usually is limited in volume and is more difficult to obtain than other specimens. Therefore, the amount of sample required to run an assay is important. Likewise, it has been shown that seminal plasma causes inhibition of PCR assays *(3,9,24)*. This is especially important in the quantitative assays. The Organon Teknika Nuclisens (NASBA) assay uses the Boom silica isolation procedure *(26)* to circum-

Table 1.
Advantages and Disadvantages
of Three Commercially Available HIV-1 RNA Assays

	Advantages	Disadvantages
Chiron Quantiplex bDNA	• Most reproducible (lowest coefficient of variation) • Can detect HIV-1 subtypes A–H • No inhibition of assay by mucosal and nonplasma specimens	• High sample input volume • Lower limit of detection (500–10,000 copies/mL)
Roche Amplicor Monitor	• Lower limit of detection (400 copies/mL—can decrease to 50 copies/mL with larger input volume)	• Difficulty detecting some non-subtype-B strains • Inhibition of assay by mucosal and other nonplasma specimens
Organon Teknika	• No inhibition of assay by mucosal and nonplasma specimens • Lower limit of detection (400–1000 copies/mL—with larger input volume can decrease to 40 copies/mL)	• Difficulty detecting some non subtype-B strains

vent this problem and has been shown to be able to detect RNA in semen without inhibition *(3,10,11,24)*. In research settings, this isolation procedure has also been used in combination with the Roche assay to decrease the effects of inhibitors *(3,9)* (*see* **Note 20**). The amount of inhibition that occurs in the Chapter 13 assay when detecting RNA in semen has not been clearly defined. The Chiron assay does not rely on PCR techniques to detect RNA and, therefore, is not affected by inhibition. However, the sample volume (2.0- to 1.0-mL samples in duplicate) required for the assay has precluded investigators from using this assay for RNA detection in genital secretions. Although seminal plasma has been shown to inhibit PCR assays, this effect has not been demonstrated in cervicovaginal secretions *(13,21–23)*.

As studies of HIV-1 are extended worldwide, it is important to remember that not all of the assays detect different HIV-1 subtypes equally *(27–30)*. Therefore, when choosing an assay, one must take into consideration the predominant subtypes in the area being studied. Both Roche and Organon Teknika are developing primers to better detect and quantitate non-subtype-B HIV-1 strains. The Chiron assay appears to be able to detect and quantitate HIV-1 subtypes A–H without difficulty *(27,29,30)*.

2.2.1. Quantitative HIV-1 RNA Assay

1. Any of the following assays can be used:
   Organon Teknika NucliSens HIV-1 QT (or NASBA).
   Roche Amplicor HIV-1 Monitor (*see* **Note 3**).
   Chiron Quantiplex.
   In-house assay such as the one described in Chapter 13.
2. Equipment required varies with which assay is chosen. Check package insert for equipment list for the desired assay.

3. Methods
3.1. Specimen Collection
3.1.1. Semen

See protocol for semen collection in **Subheading 3.1.** of Chapter 8. Note that when collecting semen for PCR only, the use of viral transport medium (VTM) is not necessary.

3.1.2. Cervicovaginal Secretions

The optimal method of collection of female genital secretions, including which secretions to collect and in what order, is still a matter of much debate. This section presents methods for the collection of cervicovaginal secretions. However, it is important to understand that the use of these methods for the collection of cervical and vaginal secretions for RNA quantitation, excepting cervicovaginal lavage with which there is some experience, have not been well validated and have scant published data to support or discount their use.

The methods listed below, which could be used for the separate collection of cervical and vaginal secretions, are not well validated for RNA quantitation in genital secretions but have been derived from the experience of various groups, some collecting similar specimens for different assays (*14,31,32;* Chapter 36). The order in which the specimens are collected has a large impact on the yield of RNA for each specimen type. Therefore, the order of collection from the cervical and vaginal compartments must be kept uniform. The cervicovaginal lavage could be done in addition to or instead of the vaginal swab (or wick).

3.1.2.1. CERVICOVAGINAL LAVAGE

The protocol described in **Subheading 3.1.2.** of Chapter 36 may be used for the collection of cervicovaginal lavage; however, it was optimized for the collection of mucosal secretions for antibody analysis. A modified version of this protocol is for the collection of cervicovaginal secretions for RNA quantitation is as follows:

1. The subject is asked to refrain from penetrative sexual intercourse or vaginal douching within 72 h prior to collection of secretions. Collection of cervicovaginal secretions should be postponed if the patient has not refrained from these activities or is currently menstruating (*see* **Note 4**).
2. The subject is placed in the lithotomy position with feet placed in the stirrups.
3. A sterile speculum, moistened and warmed with warm water (but not lubricant), is gently inserted into the vaginal vault.
4. Using a sterile plastic transfer pipet (or sterile syringe), 3–10 mL of sterile saline is flushed over and around the os and cervix (*see* **Notes 2** and **5**).
5. Using the same apparatus, the lavage is collected from the posterior vaginal fornix (*see* **Note 6**).
6. Place the lavage in a 15-mL Falcon conical tube.
7. Transport specimen to the laboratory on wet ice within 4 h of collection.

3.1.2.2. CERVICAL SECRETIONS COLLECTION

1. Wipe the surface of the cervix with a large cotton swab to remove cervical mucus.
2. If using dacron swabs, place the swab in the cervical os and rotate three to five times. Then place the swab in a sterile container with 0.5–1.0 mL PBS or VTM (*see* **Note 7**).
3. If using cervical wicks (Sno-strips), grasp two strips with exam forceps and apply to the cervical os until secretions wick up to the shoulder of the strips. Place the strips into a collection container. Collect a second pair of strips in the same manner and place in the same collection vial (*see* **Note 8**).
4. Transport specimen to the laboratory on wet ice within 4 h of collection.

3.1.2.3. VAGINAL SECRETIONS COLLECTION

1. Using a dacron swab, wipe each section of the vaginal wall. Wipe from the interior of the vagina towards the introitus (*see* **Note 9**).
2. Place in sterile container with 0.5–1.0 mL of sterile PBS or VTM.
3. Transport specimen to the laboratory on wet ice within 4 h of collection.

3.2. Specimen Processing

3.2.1. Semen

1. Allow liquefaction of semen to occur prior to processing. This usually takes 20–45 min.
2. Measure semen volume and place semen in 15-mL conical tube using a pipet (*see* **Note 10**).
3. Dilute 1 : 1 with sterile PBS, HBSS, or, if culture is desired, VTM containing antibiotics and nystatin (*see* **Note 11**).
4. Semen is centrifuged at 600g for 15 min (*see* **Note 12**).
5. Seminal plasma is carefully pipeted off and aliquoted into cryovials (*see* **Notes 13–15**).
6. Seminal plasma is frozen at −70°C until analysis.

3.2.2. Cervicovaginal Secretions

3.2.2.1. CERVICOVAGINAL LAVAGE

1. Note the volume, color, and the presence of gross blood in the specimen and record.
2. Lavage is centrifuged at 600*g* for 15 min.
3. The supernatant is carefully pipeted off and aliquoted into cryovials (*see* **Notes 14** and **16**).
4. Prior to freezing, test the supernatant for the presence of occult blood by placing 10 µL of the supernatant on a Hemoccult card or similar test system.
5. The lavage is frozen at –70°C until analysis.

3.2.2.2. CERVICAL SECRETIONS—DACRON SWAB

1. Vortex the vial containing the cervical swab.
2. Remove the swab from the vial pressing the swab against the wall of the vial to remove as much fluid as possible. Rotating the swab 360° while pressing against the vial wall is most efficient. Discard swab.
3. Centrifuge at 600*g* for 15 min.
4. Carefully aspirate the supernatant and aliquot into cryovials (*see* **Notes 14** and **16**).
5. Prior to freezing, test the supernatant for the presence of occult blood by placing 10 µL of the supernatant on a Hemoccult card or similar test system.
6. Freeze at –70°C until analysis.

3.2.2.3. CERVICAL SECRETIONS—WICKS

1. Freeze wicks in sterile container at –70°C.
2. Prior to analysis, place the frozen wicks into lysis buffer of chosen assay for elution of RNA (*see* **Notes 17** and **18**).
3. Rock or shake wicks in lysis buffer for 2 h to elute RNA (*see* **Note 18**).
4. Remove wicks from lysis buffer with RNAase-free forceps and discard.
5. Proceed with assay as described in package insert.

3.2.2.4. VAGINAL SECRETIONS

For vaginal swabs, follow instructions for cervical swabs as described above. Likewise, if vaginal wicks were collected, follow the instructions for cervial wicks described above (*see* **Note 9**).

3.3. Quantitative HIV-1 RNA Assays

Any of the three commercially available assays may be chosen as discussed in **Subheading 2.2.** If either the Organon Teknika (Nuclisens or NASBA) assays or the Chiron Quantiplex assay is chosen, follow the protocol as described on the package insert for male or female genital secretions (*see* **Note 19**). Likewise, the protocol described in Chapter 13 can be followed if you wish to produce your own reagents and perform quality control.

The Roche Amplicor HIV Monitor assay may be used as described on the package insert for the detection of RNA in female genital secretions. However, as noted in **Subheading 2.2.**, this assay and other PCR assays are subject to inhibition by inhibitors found in seminal plasma. When using the Roche assay to quantitate HIV-1 RNA in seminal plasma, it has often used in combination with the Boom isolation procedure *(26)* to avoid inhibition *(3,9)*. This procedure is described below and could be used in combination with any PCR assay (*see* **Note 20**). It is important to note that the Quantitation Standard RNA must be added to the lysis reagent prior to the Boom isolation procedure. In addition, much care must be taken in quality control of the silica when performing the Boom procedure in your lab.

Boom Isolation Procedure (*see* **Notes 20** and **21**)
1. Prepare Silica Reagent (*see* **Notes 20** and **22**).
   (a) Add 60 g of silicon dioxide to a 500-mL glass cylinder and bring volume to 500 mL with distilled water. Leave at room temperature overnight.
   (b) Aspirate supernatant by suction and bring volume back up to 500 mL with distilled water. Resuspend silica with vigorous mixing and leave at room temperature for 5 h.
   (c) Aspirate supernatant by suction and adjust silica solution to pH of 2 with concentrated hydrochloric acid (approximately 400 µL).
   (d) Aliquot silica into glass containers and autoclave for 15 min.
   (e) Store silica in the dark at room temperature.
2. Place 900 µL of lysis buffer with QS RNA in a 2.0-mL tube (*see* **Note 23**).
3. Vortex silica vigorously to resuspend in solution.
4. Add 40 µL of the freshly mixed silica solution to each of the tubes containing lysis buffer.
5. Resuspend the silica in each tube by vortexing.
6. Add 200 µL of seminal plasma and vortex the solution vigorously for 5–10 s to thoroughly mix.
7. Incubate tubes at room temperature for 10 min.
8. Resuspend the silica with vigorous vortexing for 5–10 s.
9. Centrifuge the tubes at 10,000g for 15 s.
10. Aspirate the supernatant with a disposable transfer pipet (preferably with a fine tip), using care not to disturb the silica pellet, and discard.
11. Wash procedure:
    (a) Wash the silica pellet with 1 mL of wash buffer and vortex until the pellet is completely resuspended. Use a fresh disposable 1000-µL pipet tip for each tube.
    (b) Centrifuge at 10,000g for 15 s.
    (c) Aspirate the supernatant with a disposable pipet tip (preferably with a fine tip), using care not to disturb the silica pellet, and discard.
    (d) Repeat this procedure four times with the wash reagents and in the order listed below:

(1)Wash buffer

(2)70% Ethanol

(3)70% Ethanol

(4) Acetone (reagent grade > 99% pure)

12. Following the acetone wash, carefully remove any residual acetone with a 100-μL pipet. Make sure to use a new pipet tip for each tube.

13. Place the open tubes in a heating block at 56°C for 10–15 min to dry the silica pellets (*see* **Note 24**). It is a good idea to cover the tubes with tissue to prevent contamination.

14. Add 400 μL of sample diluent to each tube after pellet is dry.

15. Resuspend the pellet by vortexing.

16. Incubate the tube at 56°C for 10 min to elute the RNA.

17. Vortex the tubes for 5 s.

18. Centrifuge the tubes at 10,000*g* for 2 min.

19. Take 50 μL of the supernatant which contains the RNA and place in PCR tubes for amplification (*see* **Note 25**).

20. Follow the Roche package insert or the procedure for your PCR assay from this point on.

4. Notes

1. VTM is not essential, but, if performing culture, it may decrease bacterial and fungal contamination. It has not been shown to inhibit PCR reactions.

2. To perform the wash, one can use a sterile plastic transfer pipet or a sterile syringe. At low volumes such as 3 mL, the transfer pipet works well. However, with volumes of 10 mL, the sterile syringe works better. To facilitate the lavage and its collection, a sterile transfer pipet can be cut below the bulb and fitted onto a 10-mL luer lock syringe. This makes it easier to collect the lavage from the posterior vaginal fornix.

3. If one chooses to do the Boom isolation procedure *(26)* in combination with the Roche assay (*see* **Note 20**) for detection of RNA in seminal plasma, the following materials will be required in addition to those listed in the Roche package insert:

    Dry-heating block

    pH meter

    1000-μL micropipet

    Thin tip-transfer pipettes

    Silicon dioxide (Sigma Chemical Co., St. Louis, MO—*see* **Note 19**)

    DEPC distilled water

    Concentrated hydrochloric acid

    Acetone (reagent grade > 99% pure)

4. This time limitation is based on the length of time that semen has been documented to persist in the vagina following vaginal intercourse. Douches are prohibited because they may alter the characteristics of the cervicovaginal secretions and, therefore, may affect the RNA recovery and quantitation.

5. The amount of sterile saline used for the lavage is a matter of debate. It is important in a given study to utilize the same volume to avoid confounding. The larger the volume, the more dilution occurs. Generally, most studies use between 5 and 10 mL of saline.

6. Some advocate flushing this aspirate of instilled PBS over the vaginal wall and reaspirating it from the posterior vaginal fornix prior to placing the specimen in the 15-mL conical tube (*see* **Subheading 3.1.2.** of Chapter 36).

7. Both dacron swabs and Sno-strips have been used to collect cervical secretions. No comparisons have been performed between these two techniques and there is little published data to support one method over the other.

8. Rarely, there is bleeding with insertion of the Sno-strips into the cervical os. If this occurs with the first pair of strips, a second pair is not collected and cervicovaginal lavage is not performed until the bleeding has stopped.

9. Dacron swabs of the vaginal wall have been shown to have lower yield than swabs of the cervical os when evaluating HIV-1 DNA *(20)*. There is little published data on the use of swabs for evaluation of vaginal HIV-1 RNA; however, the preliminary data of some suggest that this may be a useful method for the collection of vaginal RNA. In theory , wicks could also be used to collect vaginal secretions. However, there is little data regarding the utility of wicks (i.e., filter paper or Sno-strips) for the collection of vaginal secretions. In addition, collection of a good specimen is dependent on the natural moisture of the vaginal mucosa which can be affected by many environmental and cultural factors.

10. At this point, it can be very useful to count the number of white blood cells (WBC) in the semen, as inflammation in the male genital tract has been associated with increased shedding of HIV-1 *(8,33)*. This has been done using a variation of the Endtz test *(34,35)* as summarized below.

Endtz Test

1. Prepare a stock solution of benzidine by dissolving 125 mg of benzidine (Sigma Chemical Co., St. Louis, MO) in 50 mL of 96% ethanol. Add 50 mL of distilled water and store in a brown bottle at room temperature. This solution usually is good for approx 1 yr.

2. Prepare a working solution by adding 5 μL of 30% H_2O_2 to 4 mL of the benzidine stock solution. It is generally recommended to prepare this solution fresh when needed.

3. Add 20 μL of the working solution to 20 μL of liquefied semen and let sit for 5 min at room temperature.

4. Add 20 μL of PBS to the semen/benzidine solution and vortex briefly.

5. Place 10 μL of this mixture in a hemocytometer and count the peroxidase positive (brown staining) cells in the four large squares of the hemocytometer (alternatively, one can count five small squares in the central grid).

6. The number of peroxidase-positive cells/ejaculate is the number of brown cells counted multiplied by 10,000. Inflammation is considered to be present when there are $\geq 1 \times 10^6$ peroxidase-positive cells/mL of semen *(8,35)*.

11. Seminal plasma has also been separated from seminal cells without dilution **(33)**, although it may be more difficult if the specimen is viscous (*see* **Note 13** in Chapter 8 and **Note 12** of this chapter). This offers the advantage that the specimen is not being diluted. Seminal cell culture may still be done if the semen is not diluted. In that case, following the initial centifugation, the seminal cells would be washed twice with HBSS and then cultured as described in Chapter 8.

12. Some advocate spinning the seminal plasma again at high speed following separation from the cells to clarify the plasma of cellular debris. This can be done at 10,000*g* for 5 min.

13. Seminal plasma can, at times, be quite viscous. It can be difficult at times to aliquot the seminal plasma. In andrology labs, incompletely liquefied viscous semen has been passed through a 19-gage needle to decrease viscosity; however, introducing needles into a retrovirology lab presents risks to the lab personnel and using this method could shear DNA that is present. An alternative is to try passing the semen through a micropipet tip, which removes the risk of needle sticks.

14. Aliquots of any size can be made, however, a reasonable size is 250–500 µL. This size aliquot allows multiple aliquots for analysis even in an ejaculate of small volume. Also, this eliminates the multiple freeze–thaw cycles often encountered if larger aliquots are used. This also pertains to cervicovaginal secretions specimens.

15. If seminal plasma culture is desired, seminal plasma would then be processed as described in **Subheading 3.4.** of Chapter 8.

16. If desired, the vaginal cells may be washed and cultured (or frozen) using the method described for seminal cell culture in Chapter 8.

17. The number of wicks utilized for analysis can be varied. In general, at least two wicks should be used for analysis. As one would expect, yield will improve if all four wicks are used in the analysis.

18. It appears that performance is improved if the wicks are thawed in the lysis buffer *(31)*. Care must be taken to touch the wicks with only RNAase-free gloves or forceps. The volume of lysis buffer used should be adequate to cover wicks while rocking or shaking to facilitate elution. This volume could vary from 1 to 9 mL. The Organon Teknika Nuclisens or NASBA assay, with which the author has the most experience, can be ordered with 9-mL lysis buffer tubes, ideal for larger sample input volumes or situations such as this. This procedure has been used effectively to quantitate HIV-1 RNA in dried blood spots *(31)*. Alternatively, the procedure described in Chapter 16 for the quantitation of RNA in dried plasma spots using the Roche assay can be utilized for the cervical wicks. The amount of QS RNA used in preparation of the working lysis reagent and the reduction in the amount of specimen diluent described to compensate for the smaller volume of the DPS specimens would need to be adjusted depending on the number of wicks being analyzed.

19. If using the NASBA assay, it is generally better to dilute the calibrators to increase the sensitivity at the low end of the assay. This is important in genital secretions given that many specimens have RNA levels at the lower end of the assay's dynamic range. Follow the package insert directions to dilute the calibrators.

20. It is important to note that Organon Teknika has patented the Boom isolation procedure *(26)* and, therefore, all patent laws should be observed when using this

procedure. In addition, Organon Teknika has plans to market their isolation materials separately from their Nuclisens and NASBA assays, obviating the need for preparing the silica reagent and performing quality control. Any questions regarding Organon Teknika's patents should be directed to legal services at Organon Teknika (1-800-682-2666).

21. This procedure *(26)* has been used successfully in combination with the Roche assay to detect HIV-1 RNA in semen *(9)* and the methods described are adapted from these protocols.

22. The importance of using high quality silica with a small variance in the size of the silica beads to avoid shearing of the RNA should be emphasized. You may use any silica that meets these standards. Sigma is one of the companies through which silicon dioxide is commercially available.

23. The lysis buffer with QS RNA is prepared as directed on the Roche package insert or as would be for an in-house PCR assay.

24. When dry, the pellets will fragment easily when the tube is gently tapped.

25. At this point, the samples may be frozen at −20°C or, preferably at −70°C. If the samples are frozen prior to the amplification step, the samples must be thawed. After they are thawed, follow steps 15–19 of the Boom isolation procedure.

References

1. Vernazza, P. L., Eron, J. J., and Fiscus, S. A. (1996) Sensitive Method for the detection of infectious HIV in semen of seropositive individuals. *J. Virol. Methods* **56**, 33–40.

2. Van Voorhis, B., Martinez, A., Mayer, K., and Anderson, D. J. (1991) Detection of human immunodeficiency virus type 1 in semen from seropositive men using culture and polymerase chain reaction deoxyribonucleic acid amplification techniques. *Fertil. Steril.* **55**, 588–594.

3. Dyer, J., Gilliam, B. L., Eron, Jr., J. J., Grosso, L., Cohen, M. S., and Fiscus, S. (1996) Quantitation of human immunodeficiency virus type 1 RNA in cell-free seminal plasma: comparison of NASBA and amplicor reverse transcription PCR amplification. *J. Virol. Methods* **60**, 161–170.

4. Vernazza, P. L., Eron, Jr., J. J., Cohen, M. S., van der Horst, C. M., Troiani, L., and Fiscus, S. A. (1994) Detection and biologic characterization of infectious HIV-1 in semen of seropositive men. *AIDS* **8**, 1325–1329.

5. Krieger, J. N., Coombs, R. W., Collier, A. C., Koehler, J. K., Ross, S. O., Chaloupka, K., Murphy, V. L., and Corey, L. (1991) Fertility parameters in men infected with human immunodeficiency virus. *J. Infect. Dis,* **164**, 464–469.

6. Krieger, J. N., Coombs, R. W., Collier, A. C., Ross, S. O., Speck, C., and Corey, L. (1995) Seminal shedding of human immunodeficiency virus type 1 and human cytomegalovirus: Evidence for different immunologic controls. *J. Infect. Dis.* **171**, 1018–1022.

7. Krieger, J. N., Coombs, R. W., Collier, A. C., Ho, D., Ross, S. O., Zeh, J. E., and Corey, L. (1995) Intermittent shedding of human immunodeficiency virus in semen: implications for sexual transmission. *J. Urol.* **154**, 1035–1040.

8. Anderson, D. J., O'Brien, T. R., Politch, J. A., Martinez, A., Seage, III, G. R., Padian, N., Horsburgh, Jr., R., and Mayer, K. H. (1992) Effects of disease stage and zidovudine therapy on the detection of human immunodeficiency virus type 1 in semen. *JAMA* **267,** 2769–2774.

9. Coombs, R. W., Speck, C. E., Hughes, J. P., Lee, W., Sampoleo, R., Ross, S. O. et al. (1998) Association between cultivable virus in semen, syncytium-inducing phenotype, and short-term variation of HIV-1 RNA levels in semen and blood. *J. Infect. Dis.* **177,** 320–330.

10. Gilliam, B. L., Dyer, J. R., Fiscus, S. A, Marcus, C., Zhou, S., Wathen, L., Freimuth, W. W., Cohen, M. S., and Eron, Jr., J. J. (1997) Effects of reverse transcriptase inhibitor therapy on the HIV-1 viral burden in semen. *J. Acquir. Immun. Defic. Syndr. Hum. Retrovirol.* **15,** 54–60.

11. Vernazza, P. L., Gilliam, B. L., Dyer, J., Fiscus, S. A., Eron, J. J., Frank, A. C., and Cohen, M. S. (1997) Quantitation of HIV in semen: Correlation with antiviral treatment and immune status. *AIDS* **11,** 987–993.

12. Henin, Y., Mandelbrot, L., Henrion, R., Pradinaud, R., Coulaud, J. P., and Montagnier, L. (1993) Virus excretion in the cervicovaginal secretions of pregnant and nonpregnant HIV-infected women. *J. Acquir. Immune. Def. Syndr.* **6,** 72–75.

13. Nielson, K., Boyer, P., Dillon, M., Wafer, D., Wei, L. S., Garratty, E., Dickover, R. E., and Bryson, Y. J. (1996) Presence of human immunodeficiency virus type 1 and HIV-1-specific antibodies in cervicovaginal secretions of infected mothers and in the gastric aspirates of their infants. *J. Infect. Dis.* **173,** 1001–1004.

14. Goulston, C., Stevens, E., Gallo, D., Mullins, J. I., Hanson, C. V., and Katzenstein, D. (1996) Human immunodeficiency virus plasma and genital secretions during the menstrual cycle. *J. Infect. Dis.* **174,** 858–861.

15. Hamed, K. A., Winters, M. A., Holodniy, M., Katzenstein, D. A., and Merigan, T. C. (1993) Detection of human immunodeficiency virus type 1 in semen: effects of disease stage and nucleoside therapy. *J. Infect. Dis.* **167,** 798–802.

16. Mermin, J. H., Holodniy, M., Katzenstein, D. A., and Merigan, T. C. (1991) Detection of human immunodeficiency virus DNA and RNA in semen by the polymerase chain reaction. *J. Infect. Dis.* **164,** 769–772.

17. Tindall, B., Evans, L., Cunningham, P., McQueen, P., et al. (1992) Identification of HIV-1 in semen following primary HIV-1 infection. *AIDS* **6(9),** 949–952.

18. Liuzzi, G., Bagnarelli, P., Chirianni, A., Clementi, M., Nappa, S., Tullio Cataldo, P., et al. (1995) Quantitation of HIV genome copy number in semen and saliva. *AIDS* **9,** 651–653.

19. Clemetson, D. B. A., Moss, G. B., Willerford, D. M., Hensel, M., Emonyi, W., Holmes, K. K., et al. (1993) Detection of HIV DNA in cervical and vaginal secretions: prevalence and correlates among women in Nairobi, Kenya. *JAMA* **269,** 2860–2864.

20. John, G. C., Nduati, R. W., Mbori-Ngacha, D., Overbaugh, J., Welch, M., Richardson, B. A., Ndinya-Achola, J., Bwayo, J., Krieger, J., Onyango, F., and Kreiss, J. K. (1997) Genital shedding of human immunodeficiency virus

type 1 DNA during pregnancy: Association with immunosuppression, abnormal cervical or vaginal discharge, and severe vitamin A deficiency. *J. Infect. Dis.* **175,** 57–62.

21. Rasheed, S., Li, Z., Xu, D., and Kovacs, A. (1996) Presence of cell-free human immunodeficiency virus in cervicovaginal secretions in independent of viral load in the blood of human immunodeficiency virus-infected women. *Am. J. Obstet. Gynecol.* **175,** 122–129.

22. Lennox, J., Ellerbrock, T. V., Palmore, M., Hart, C., Schnell, C., Bush, T., Evans-Strickfaden, T., and Conley, L. (1997) Effect of antiretroviral therapy on vaginal HIV RNA level. Fourth Conference on Retroviruses and Opportunistic Infections, Washington, DC, Abstract 727.

23. Hart, C., Palmore, M., Wright, T., Lennox, J., Evans-Strickfaden, T., Bush, T., Schnell, C., Conley, L., and Ellerbrock, T. V. (1997) Correlation of cell-free and cell-associated HIV RNA levels in plasma and vaginal secretions. Fourth Conference on Retroviruses and Opportunistic Infections, Washington, DC, Abstract 25.

24. Gupta, P., Mellors, J., Kingsley, L., Riddler, S., Singh, M. K., Schreiber, S., Cronin, M., and Rinaldo, C. R. (1997) High viral load in semen of human immunodeficiency virus type-1 infected men at all stages of disease and its reduction by therapy with protease and nonnucleoside reverse transcriptase inhibitors. *J. Virol.* **71,** 6271–6275.

25. Xu, C., Politch, J. A., Tucker, L., Mayer, K. H., Seage, G. R., and Anderson, D. J. (1997) Factors associated with increased levels of human immunodeficiency virus type 1 DNA in semen. *J. Infect. Dis.* **176,** 941–947.

26. Boom, R., Sol, C. J., Salimans, M. M., Jansen, C. L., Wertheim-van Dillen, P. M., and van der Noordaa, J. (1990) Rapid and simple method for purification of nucleic acids. *J. Clin. Microbiol.* **28,** 495–503.

27. Coste, J., Montes, B., Reynes, J., Peeters, M., Segarra, C., Vendrell, J. P., Delaporte, E., and Segondy, M. (1996) Comparative evaluation of three assays for the quantitation of human immunodeficiency virus type 1 RNA in plasma. *J. Med. Virol.* **50,** 293–302.

28. De Wolf, F., Von Briessen, H., Holmes, H., Bakker, M., Cornelissen, C., and Goudsmit, J. (1996) HIV-1 subtype specific differences in plasma RNA levels related to rate and amount of virus produced in PBMC culture. XI International Conference on AIDS, Vancouver, Abstract Tu.A.155.

29. Dunne, A. L. and Crowe, S. M. (1996) Comparison of branched chain DNA and RT-PCR for quantifying six different HIV-1 subtypes in plasma. XI International Conference on AIDS, Vancouver, Abstract LB.A.6005.

30. Rouzioux, C., Burgard, M., Chaix, M. L., Manigart, O., Ivanoff, S., Doussin, A., Ngo, N., Tachet, A., Blanche, S., and Mayaux, M. J. (1997) Quantification of "non B" subtype HIV-1 RNA: Underestimation is frequent for all "non B" subtypes with monitor and NASBA QT tests. Fourth Conference on Retroviruses and Opportunistic Infections, Washington, DC, Abstract 285.

31. Grosso, L., Schock, J., Shepard, R., Brambilla, D., Cronin, M., and Fiscus, S. (1997) Quantitation of plasma HIV-1 RNA from blood dried on filter paper.

Fourth Conference on Retroviruses and Opportunistic Infections, Washington, DC, Abstract 620.

32. Artenstein, A. W., VanCott, T. C., Sitz, K. V., Robb, M. L., Wagner, K. F., Veit, S. C. D., Rogers, A. F., Garner, R. P., Byron, J. W., Burnett, P. R., and Birx, D. L. (1997) Mucosal immune responses in four distinct compartments of women infected with human immunodeficiency virus type 1: A comparison by site and correlation with clinical information. *J. Infect. Dis.* **175,** 265–271.

33. Cohen, M. S., Hoffman, I. F., Royce, R. A., Kazembe, P., Dyer, J. R., Daly, C. C., Zimba, D., Vernazza, P. L., Maida, M., Fiscus, S. A., Eron, Jr., J. J., and the AIDSCAP Malawi Research Group. (1997) Reduction of concentration of HIV-1 in semen after treatment of urethritis: implications for prevention of sexual transmission of HIV-1. *Lancet* **349,** 1868–1873.

34. Endtz, A. W. (1974) A rapid staining method for differentiating granulocytes from "germinal cells" in papanicolaou-stained semen. *Acta. Cytol.* **18,** 2–7.

35. Politch, J. A., Wolff, H., Hill, J. A., and Anderson, D. J. (1993) Comparison of methods to enumerate white blood cells in semen. *Fertil. Steril.* **60,** 372–375.

18

Detection of Nucleic Acids in Cells and Tissues by *In Situ* Polymerase Chain Reaction

Omar Bagasra, Lisa E. Bobroski, Mohammad Amjad, Matthew Memoli, and Maureen V. Abbey

1. Introduction

The solution-based polymerase chain reaction (PCR) method for amplification of defined gene sequences has proved a valuable tool not only for basic
researchers but also for clinical scientists. Using even a minute amount of DNA
or RNA and choosing a thermostable enzyme from a large variety of sources,
one can enlarge the amount of the gene of interest, which can be analyzed and
sequenced. Therefore, genes, or segments of gene sequences present only in a
small sample of cells or small fraction of mixed cellular populations can be
examined. One of the major drawbacks of the solution-based PCR technique is
that the procedure does not allow for the association of amplified signals of a
specific gene segment with the histological cell type(s) *(1–2)*. For example, it
would be advantageous to determine what types of cells in the peripheral blood
circulation or in pathological specimens carry HIV-1 gene sequences, a vector
used for gene therapy, an aberrant gene in a leukemia patient, or to determine
the percentage of leukemia cells present following antitumor therapy.

The ability to identify individual cells in a tissue section that express specific genes of interest or carry them in a latent form, provides a great advantage
in determining various aspects of normal (as opposed to pathological) conditions. For example, this technique could be used in determination of viral or
tumor burden, before and after therapy in lymphomas or leukemias, in which
specific aberrant gene translocations are associated with certain types of
malignancy *(3)*. In case of HIV-1 infection or other viral infections, one can
determine the effects of therapy or putative antiviral vaccination by evaluating

From: *Methods in Molecular Medicine, Vol. 17: HIV Protocols*
Edited by: N. L. Michael and J. H. Kim © Humana Press Inc., Totowa, NJ

the number of cells still infected with viral agent, post-chemotherapy or vaccination *(4–7)*. Similarly, one can potentially determine the preneoplastic lesions by examining tumor suppressor genes (i.e., p53 mutations associated with certain tumors or oncogenes or other aberrant gene sequences which are known to be associated with certain types of tumors) *(3)*. In the area of diagnostic pathology, determination of the origin of metastatic tumors is a perplexing problem. By utilizing the proper primers for genes that are expressed by certain histological cell types, one can potentially determine the origin of metastatic tumors by performing reverse transcriptase-initiated *in situ* PCR *(3)*.

The author's laboratories have been using *in situ* PCR techniques for several years, and they have developed simple, sensitive protocols for both RNA and DNA *in situ* PCR that proved reproducible in multiple double-blinded studies *(4–6,8–14)*. By use of multiple labeled probes, one can detect various signals in a single cell *(2,14)*. Additionally, under special circumstances, one can perform immunohistochemistry, RNA and DNA amplification at a single-cell level ("triple labeling") *(2,14)*.

To date, the authors have successfully amplified and detected HIVs, SIVs, HPVs, HBVs, CMV, EBV, HHV-6, HHV-8, HSV, p53 and its mutations, mRNA for surfactant Protein A, estrogen receptors, and inducible nitrous oxide synthesis (iNOS)-gene sequences associated with multiple sclerosis by DNA and RNA (RT *in situ* PCR). Tissue types have included peripheral blood mononuclear cells (PBMC), lymph nodes, spleen, skin, breast, lungs, placenta, spermatozoa, cytological specimens, Kaposi's sarcoma, and cultured cells prepared by formalin-fixation or frozen sections. This technique has also been successfully applied to brain tissue of HIV-1 seropositive patients *(1–6,8–21)*. In the following pages, the authors present a detailed protocol currently being utilized in their laboratory. For more details, see the specific publications cited at the end of the chapter (especially **ref. *1***).

2. Materials

2. 1. Slides

Heavy, Teflon-coated glass slides with 3-, 10-, 12-, or 14-mm diameter wells for cell suspensions, or single oval wells for tissue sections are available from Cel-line Associates of New Field, NJ (1-800-662-0973), or Erie Scientific of Portsmouth, NH (1-800-258-0834). These specific slide designs are particularly useful, since the Teflon coating serves to form distinct wells, each of which serves as a small reaction "chamber" when the coverslip is attached. Furthermore, the Teflon coating helps to keep the nail polish from entering the reaction chamber, and multiple wells allow for both a positive and a negative control on the same slide.

2.2. Coplin Jars and Glass Staining Dishes

Suitable vessels for simultaneously washing, fixing, and staining 4–20 glass slides are available from several vendors, including Fisher Scientific.

2.3. Paraformaldehyde Solution

1. Add 12 g paraformaldehyde (Merck ultra pure Art No. 4005) to 600 mL 1X phosphate-buffered saline (PBS).
2. Heat at 65°C for 10 min.
3. When the solution starts to clear, add 4 drops 10 N NaOH and stir.
4. Adjust to neutral pH and cool to room temperature.
5. Filter on Whatman number 1.

2.4. Standard Buffers

1. 10X PBS stock solution pH 7.2 to 7.4: Dissolve 20.5 g $NaH_2PO_4 \cdot H_2O$ and 179.9 g $Na_2HPO_4 \cdot 7H_2O$ (or 95.5 g Na_2HPO_4) in about 4 L double-distilled water. Adjust to the required pH (7.2–7.4). Add 701.3 g NaCl and make up to a total volume of 8 L.
2. 1X PBS: Dilute the stock 10X PBS at 1:10 ratio (i.e., 100 mL 10X PBS and 900 mL of water for 1 L). Final concentration of buffer should be 0.01 M phosphate and 0.15 M NaCl.
3. Hydrogen peroxide (H_2O) in PBS: Dilute stock in 30% hydrogen peroxide (H_2O_2) at a 1:100 ratio in 1X PBS for a final concentration of 0.3% H_2O_2.
4. 20X SSC: Dissolve 175.3 g of NaCl and 88.2 g of sodium citrate in 800 mL of water. Adjust the pH to 7.0 with a few drops of 10 N solution of NaOH. Adjust the volume to 1 L with water. Sterilize by autoclaving.
5. 2X SSC: Add 100 mL of 20X SSC to 900 mL of water.

2.5. Proteinase K Solution

Dissolve powder from Sigma (St. Louis, MO) in water to obtain 1 mg/mL concentration. Aliquot and store at –20°C. Working solution (6.7 µg/mL): Dilute 1 mL of stock (1 mg/mL) into 150 mL of 1X PBS.

2.7. Streptavidin Peroxidase

Dissolve powder from Sigma in PBS to make a stock of 1 mg/mL. Just before use, dilute stock solution in sterile PBS at a 1:30 ratio.

2.8. Color Solution

1. Dissolve one 3-amino-9-ethyl-carbazole (AEC) (Sigma) tablet in 2.5 mL of N,N dimethyl formamide. Store at 4°C in the dark.
2. Working Solution: 5 mL of 50 mM sodium acetate buffer, pH 5.0, 250 µL AEC solution, 25 µL 30% H_2O_2. Make fresh before each use, keeping solution in the dark.
3. 50 mM sodium acetate buffer pH 5.0: Add 74 mL of 0.2 N acetic acid (11.55 mL glacial acid/L) and 176 mL of 0.2 M sodium acetate (27.2 g sodium acetate trihydrate in 1 L) to 1 L of deionized water and mix.

2.9. In Situ *Hybridization Buffer*

1. Formamide, denatured salmon sperm DNA (ssDNA), and 50X Denhardt's solution are available through many vendors including Boehringer-Mannheim, Sigma, and Promega (Madison, WI).
2. *In situ* hybridization buffer: 2.5 mL formamide, 0.5 mL 10 mg/mL ssDNA, 0.5 mL 20X SSC, 1 mL 50X Denhardt's solution, 0.05 mL 10% SDS, 0.45 mL distilled water.
3. Heat denature ssDNA at 94°C for 10 minutes before adding to the solution.

3. Methods
3.1. Peparation of Glass Slides

Before one can perform *in situ* reactions by this protocol, the proper sort of glass slide with Teflon appliqué must be obtained. The glass surface must then be treated with the proper sort of silicon compound. Both of these factors are very important, for the following reasons. First, one should always use glass slides that are partially covered by a Teflon coating. Not only does the glass withstand well the stress of repeated heat-denaturation, but it also presents the right chemical surface—silicon oxide—that is needed for proper silanization. Furthermore, slides with special Teflon coatings that form individual "wells" are useful because vapor-tight reaction chambers can be formed on the surface of the slides when cover slips are adhered with coatings of nail polish around the periphery. These reaction chambers are necessary because within them, proper tonicity and ion concentrations can be maintained in aqueous solutions during thermal cycling—conditions that are vital for proper DNA amplification. The Teflon coating serves a dual purpose in this regard. First, the Teflon helps keep the two glass surfaces slightly separated, allowing for reaction chambers about 20 µm in height to form between. Second, the Teflon border helps keep the nail polish from entering the reaction chambers when the polish is being applied. This is important, since any leakage of nail polish into a reaction chamber can compromise the results in that chamber. Even if one is using an advanced thermal cycler with humidification, use of the Teflon-coated slides is still recommended, since the hydrophobicity of the Teflon combined with the pressure applied by a coverslip helps spread small volumes of reaction cocktail over the entire sample region without forcing much fluid out the periphery.

In order to prepare glass slides properly, follow this procedure:

1. Prepare the following 2% 3-aminopropyltriethoxysilane (AES) solution just prior to use: 5 mL AES (Sigma) and 250 mL acetone. 250 mL of AES solution is sufficient to treat 200 glass slides.
3. Put solution into a Coplin jar or a glass staining dish and dip glass slides in 2% AES for 60 s. Allow to dry for 1–2 h at room temperature or overnight.

4. Dip slides five times into a fresh vessel containing 1000 mL of distilled water.
5. Repeat **step 3** three to four times, changing the water each time.
6. Air dry in laminar-flow hood from a few hours to overnight, then store slides in a sealed container at room temperature. Try to use slides within 15 d of silanization.

3.2. Preparation of Tissue

3.2.1. Cell Suspensions

To use peripheral blood leukocytes, first isolate cells on a Ficoll-Hypaque density gradient (*see* Chapter 1). Tissue culture cells or other single-cell suspensions can also be used. Prepare all cell suspensions with the following procedure:

1. Wash twice cells with 1X PBS.
2. Resuspend cells in PBS at 2×10^6 cells/mL.
3. Add at least 10 μL of cell suspension to each well of the slide using a P20 micropipet, spreading across surface of the slides.
4. Air dry slide in a laminar-flow hood.

3.2.2. Adherent Cultured Cells

There are several types of slides which are designed to support in situ PCR after they are attached on the glass slides. We favor Falcon CultureSlides. The cells are grown on this type of slide. If certain primary cell cultures require attachment factors or growth media, they could be used in conjunction with this cell culture system. After appropriate confluence is achieved (usually >60%), cells are gently washed with 1X PBS, heat-fixed, and fixed overnight with 2% paraformaldehyde.

3.2.3. Paraffin-Fixed Tissue

Routinely-fixed paraffin tissue sections can be amplified quite successfully. This permits the evaluation of individual cells in the tissue for the presence of a specific RNA or DNA sequence. For this purpose, tissue sections are placed on specially designed slides that have single wells (*see* **Subheading 2.1.** for more details). In the author's laboratory, they routinely use placental tissues, central nervous system (CNS) tissues, cardiac tissues, etc., that are cut to 5–6-μm thickness (*see* **Note 1**).

1. Place tissue section upon the glass surface of the slide.
2. Incubate the slides in an oven held at 60–80°C (depending on the type of paraffin used to embed the tissue) for 1 h to melt the paraffin.
3. Dip the slides in electron microscopy (EM) grade xylene solution for 5 min, then in EM grade 100% ethanol for 5 min (EM grade reagents are benzene-free).
4. Repeat these washes two or three times, in order to completely rid the tissue of paraffin.
5. Dry the slides in an oven at 80°C for 1 h.

3.2.4. Frozen Sections

It is possible to use frozen sections for *in situ* amplification. However, the morphology of the tissue following the amplification process is generally not as good as with paraffin sections. The cryogenic freezing of the tissue, combined with the lack of paraffin substrate during sectioning, compromises the integrity of the tissue (*see* **Note 2**). Usually, thicker slices must be made, and the tissue "chatters" in the microtome. Definitive diagnoses are made from paraffin sections. This rule of thumb extends to the amplification procedure as well. To use frozen sections perform the following procedure:

1. Use as thin a slice as possible (down to 4–6 μm).
2. Apply section to slide.
3. Dehydrate for 10 min in 100% methanol (*see* **Note 3**).
4. Air dry in a laminar-flow hood.
5. Proceed with heat treatment described below.

3.3. In Situ *Amplification:* Low Abundance of DNA and RNA Targets

For all sample types, the following steps comprise the basic preparatory work which must be done before any amplification–hybridization procedure. The flowchart is depicted in **Fig. 1**.

3.3.1. Heat Treatment

Place the slides with adhered tissue or cells on a heat block at 105°C for 0.5–2 min to stabilize the cells or tissue on the glass surface of the slide (*see* **Note 4**).

3.3.2. Fixation and Washes

1. Place the slides in a solution of 2% paraformaldehyde (PFA) in PBS, pH 7.4, for 2 h at room temperature. Use of the recommended Coplin jars or staining dishes facilitates these steps.
2. Wash the slides once with 3X PBS for 10 min, agitating periodically with an up and down motion.
3. Wash the slides with 1X PBS for 10 min, agitating periodically with an up and down motion.
4. Repeat once with fresh 1X PBS.
5. At this point, slides with adherent tissue could be stored at –80°C until use. If this is desired, first dehydrate slides with 100% ethanol.
6. If biotinylated probes or peroxidase-based color development are to be used, the samples should be further treated with a 0.3% solution of hydrogen peroxide in PBS in order to inactivate any endogenous peroxidase activity. Incubate the slides overnight either at 37°C or at room temperature. Then wash the slides once with 1X PBS. If other probes are to be used, proceed directly to the following proteinase K digestion.

Typical *In-Situ* Protocol

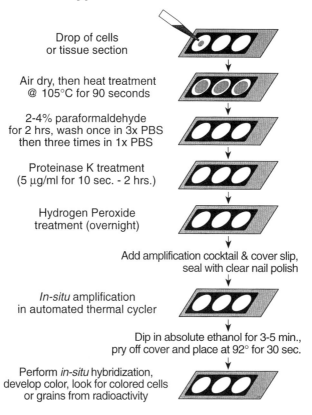

Drop of cells
or tissue section

Air dry, then heat treatment
@ 105°C for 90 seconds

2-4% paraformaldehyde
for 2 hrs, wash once in 3x PBS
then three times in 1x PBS

Proteinase K treatment
(5 µg/ml for 10 sec. - 2 hrs.)

Hydrogen Peroxide
treatment (overnight)

Add amplification cocktail & cover slip,
seal with clear nail polish

In-situ amplification
in automated thermal cycler

Dip in absolute ethanol for 3-5 min.,
pry off cover and place at 92° for 30 sec.

Perform *in-situ* hybridization,
develop color, look for colored cells
or grains from radioactivity

Fig. 1. Overview of *in situ* PCR protocol. Please refer to text for details and modifications.

3.3.3. Proteinase K Treatment

1. Treat samples with 6 µg/mL proteinase K in 1X PBS for 5–60 min at room temperature or at 55°C (*see* **Note 5**).
2. After 5 min, look at the cells under the microscope at 400X. If the majority of the cells of interest exhibit uniform-appearing, small, round, "salt-and pepper" dots on the cytoplasmic membrane, then stop the treatment immediately with **step 3**. Otherwise, continue treatment for another 5 min and re-examine.
3. After proper digestion, heat slides on a block at 95°C for 2 min to inactive the proteinase K.
4. Rinse slides in 1X PBS for 10 s.
5. Rinse slides in distilled water for 10 s.
6. Air dry.

3.3.4. Reverse Transcription Variation: DNase Treatment

If DNA sequences are to be amplified, skip to **Subheading 3.3.6.** If RNA sequences are to be amplified, two options are available. The first and more elegant method is to use primer pairs that flank RNA splice junctions within the gene of interest, because these particular sequences will be more closely opposed in the mRNA. By using this type of primer selection, one can omit the following DNase step and proceed directly to reverse transcription. The second approach is to treat the cells or tissue with a DNase solution following the proteinase K digestion. This step destroys all of the endogenous DNA in the cells so that only RNA survives to provide signals for amplification (*see* **Note 6**). Obviously, this treatment will obviate the ability to amplify DNA sequences from treated tissues.

1. Prepare a RNase-free, DNase solution: 40 mM Tris-HCl, pH 7.4, 6 mM MgCl$_2$, 2 mM CaCl$_2$, 100 U/µL final volume of DNase (use RNase-free DNase, such as 1000 U/µL RQ1 DNase, cat # 776785 from Boehringer) (*see* **Note 7**).
2. Add 10–15 µL of solution to each well.
3. Incubate the slides at 37°C in a humidified chamber for 1 h (*see* **Note 8**).
4. After incubation, rinse the slides with a similar solution that was prepared without the DNase I.
5. Wash the slides twice with DEPC-treated water.

3.3.5. Reverse Transcriptase Reaction

Next, DNA copies complementary to the targeted RNA sequence are prepared using the enzyme reverse transcriptase (RT) so that these complementary DNA (cDNA) sequences can be amplified by the PCR. First, either a gene-specific primer or oligo-dT is hybridized to the mRNA. Second, these short RNA:DNA heteroduplexes are extended with RT (*see* **Note 9**). The RT is then heat-inactivated, and the PCR is performed. The length of the amplicon must be kept small (*see* **Note 10**) and the oligonucleotide primers chosen carefully (*see* **Note 11**) to optimize the RT-PCR.

A specific master mix tailored for the RT enzyme chosen (*see* **Note 12**) is prepared in sterile 1.5-mL microfuge tubes held on ice. If using AMV (avian myoblastosis virus) or MMLV (Moloney murine leukemia virus) RT enzyme: 4.0 µL 5X reaction buffer (250 mM Tris-HCl, pH 8.3, 375 mM KCl, 15 mM MgCl$_2$), 8 µL 2.5 mM dNTPs, 0.5 µL RNasin (40 U/µL), 1.0 µL 20 µM antisense primer, 6.0 µL sterile water, 0.5 µL (10 U) AMV RT for a total volume of 20.0 µL. If using Superscript II enzyme (Gibco-BRL, Gaithersburg, MD) (an engineered form of Moloney murine leukemia virus RT lacking RNase H activity): 4.0 µL 5X reaction buffer (as supplied with enzyme), 8 µL 2.5 mM dNTPs, 0.5 µL RNasin (40 U/µL), 1.0 µL 20 µM antisense primer, 2.0 µL 0.1 M dithiothreitol, 4.0 µL sterile water, and 0.5 µL Superscript II enzyme (100 U) for a total volume of 20.0 µL.

Table 1
Master Mix for DNA PCR

Ingredients	Volume
25 μ*M* forward primer (i.e., SK 38 for HIV-1)	5.0 μL
25 μ*M* reverse primer (i.e., SK 39 for HIV-1)	5.0 μL
10 m*M* each dNTP	2.5 μL
Taq DNA polymerase (Ampli-Taq 5 U/μL)[a]	1.0 μL
10X PCR buffer	10.0 μL
Water	76.5 μL
Total volume	100.0 μL

[a]Other thermostable polymerase enzymes have also been used quite successfully.

Once the master mixes are prepared, perform the following:

1. Add 10–15 μL of the appropriate master mix to each well.
2. Carefully place the coverslip on top of the slide.
3. Incubate slides at 42°C or 37°C for 1 h in a humidified atmosphere.
4. Incubate slides at 92° C for two min to inactivate the RT enzyme.
5. Remove the coverslip and wash the slide twice with distilled water.
6. Proceed with the amplification procedure, which is the same for both DNA and RNA based protocols.

3.3.6. DNA Amplification

1. Prepare an amplification cocktail containing the following: 1.25 μ*M* of each primer, 200 μ*M* (each) dNTP, 10 m*M* Tris-HCl, pH 8.3, 50 m*M* KCl, 1.5 m*M* MgCl$_2$, 0.001% gelatin, and 0.05 U/μL *Taq* DNA polymerase. A convenient recipe that we use in our laboratory is given in **Table 1**.
2. Layer 10–15 μL of amplification solution onto each well with a P20 micropipet so that the whole surface of the well is covered with the solution. Be careful: do not touch the surface of the slide with the tip of the pipet.
3. Add a glass coverslip (22 × 60 mm) and carefully seal the edge of the coverslip to the slide with 2 coats of clear nail polish (*see* **Note 13**). If using tissue sections, use a second slide instead of a coverslip (*see* **Note 14**).
4. Allow nail polish to completely dry (not sticky to the touch) (*see* **Note 15**).
5. Place slides in a thermocycling instrument (*see* **Note 16**).
6. Run 30 cycles of the following amplification protocol: 94°C, 30 s; optimal annealing temperature (*see* **Note 17**), 1 min; 72°C, 1 min. It is likely that these times/temperatures will require optimization for the specific thermocycler and specific digonucleotides being used. A "hot start" technique may be considered (*see* **Note 18**).
7. Dip slides in 100% EtOH for at least 5 min in order to dissolve the nail polish.

8. Pry off the coverslip using a razor or other fine blade. The coverslip generally pops off easily.
9. Scratch off any remaining nail polish on the outer edges of the slide so that fresh coverslips will lay evenly in the subsequent hybridization/detection steps.
10. Place slides on a heat block at 92°C for 1 min. This treatment helps immobilize the intracellular signals.
11. Wash slides with 2X SSC at room temperature for 5 min.
12. The amplification protocol is now complete and one can proceed to the labeling/hybridization procedures.

3.3.7. Direct Incorporation of Nonradioactive, Labeled Nucleotides

Several nonradioactive labeled nucleotides are available from various sources (i.e., dCTP-Biotin, digoxin 11-dUTP). These nucleotides can be used to directly label amplification products, so the proper secondary agents and chromogens can then be used to detect the directly labeled *in situ* amplification products (*see* below). However, in the author's opinion, the greatest specificity is only achieved by conducting amplification followed by subsequent *in situ* hybridization. In the direct labeling protocols, nonspecific incorporation can be significant, and even if this incorporation is minor, it still leads to false-positive signals similar to nonspecific bands in gel electrophoresis following solution-based DNA or RT amplification. Therefore, the authors strongly discourage the direct incorporation of labeled nucleotides as part of an *in situ* amplification protocol.

The only exceptions to this recommendation is when one is screening a large number of primer pairs for optimization of a specific assay. To perform such screenings, add the following to the amplification cocktail detailed in **Subheading 3.3.6.**: 4.3 μ*M* labeled nucleotide (either 14-biotin dCTP or 14-biotin dATP or 11-digoxigenin dUTP) along with cold nucleotide to achieve a 0.14 m*M* final concentration. Also, if one has worked out the perfect annealing system, either using Robocycler or equivalent system, then direct incorporation can be used without fear of nonspecific labeling, which was discussed elsewhere in detail *(16)*.

3.3.8. Multiple Signals and Multiple Labels in Individual Cells

DNA, mRNA, and protein can all be detected simultaneously in individual cells *(2,14)*. Proteins can be labeled by rhodamine-labeled antibodies. Then, both RNA and DNA *in situ* amplification is performed with the cells. If primers for spliced mRNA are used and if these primers fail to amplify sequences from genomic DNA (if the intron is sufficiently large), then both DNA and cDNA amplification can be carried out simultaneously. In this case, the RT step must be performed without the DNase I pretreatment. Subsequently, products can be labeled with different kinds of probes, resulting in different colors of signal. For example, proteins can have a rhodamine-labeled probe, mRNA can show a fluorescein isothiocyanate (FITC) signal (FITC-conjugated probe, >20 different fluorochromes are available) and DNA can have been labeled with a biotin-peroxidase probe or a fluorochrome with different color emission. Each will show a different signal within an individual cell *(2,14)*.

3.4. In Situ *Hybridization*

The in situ hybridization (ISH) technique has been successfully applied in both the research and clinical settings. However one single easy to use universal procedure has not been developed. Therefore, specific needs of the diagnostic or research goals must be considered in choosing a suitable protocol. In comparing ISH with other methods one has to realize what is being detected. For example, the immunocytochemical method localizes protein within a cell or on cell surface and therefore identifies gene expression. However, these assays cannot yield useful information on post-translational processing of the gene product or differentiate between the uptake and storage of the protein and the site of synthesis of the protein. In addition, needs several hundred copies of the proteins are needed to be able to identify an expression signal. Also, most of the protein are destroyed by formalin fixation methods making it difficult to identify the protein in most of the pathological specimens. In mRNA extraction methods that utilize the isolation of nucleic acids from cells (filter hybridization assays), there can be a dilution of the target sequence by the RNA from cells with little or no target. These methods provide no distribution information. They provide only an average measurement of the nucleic acid target present in the mixed cell population. Therefore, ISH is a very powerful technique when the target is focally distributed within a single cell or certain histological cell types with in a tissue. Consequently, ISH has greater sensitivity than filter assays if the gene expression is taking place in a small subpopulation of cells. The major limitation of ISH is relative insensitivity, as compared to *in situ* PCR. By utilizing ISH, one can detect as low as 20 copies of mRNA. However, success of that degree of sensitivity is limited to only few highly specialized laboratories and to few specific genes. More realistically, detection of >100 copies/cell would be an attainable goal for a laboratory not specialized in ISH. In order to detect a single copy of gene integrated, or to detect very low levels of gene expression (few copies of mRNA), the gene sequences can be amplified *in situ* by DNA or RNA (RT)-*in situ* PCR and then utilize ISH to detect the amplicons.

Analyzing gene expression by ISH after RT can provide information on the site of mRNA synthesis which provides information about the cellular origin of protein synthesis and demonstrates in the amounts of synthesis (level of gene expression). This permits an understanding of the cell types involved in the production of certain proteins in gene regulation and in identification of

Table 2
In Situ Hybridization Master Mix

Ingredients	Volume
Probe (biotinylated, or digoxigenin)	2 µL
Deionized formamide	50 µL
20X SSC^a	10 µL
50X Denhardts solution	20 µL
10 mg/mL ssDNA^a	10 µL
10% SDS	1 µL
H_2O	7 µL
Total volume	100 µL

^{a}The salmon sperm should be denatured at 94°C for 10 min before it is added to the hybridization buffer. Two percent bovine serum albumin (BSA) can be added if nonspecific binding is observed. Add 7 µL of 30% BSA solution and eliminate the water accordingly.

cell types infected by various infectious agents. In combination with immuno-histochemistry, differential expression of a gene in different cell types or different stages of development can be analyzed at the microscopic levels.

3.4.1. Choice of Probes for ISH

Many ISH protocols employ [^{3}H]- or [^{35}S]-labeled nucleic acid probes followed by autoradiographic detection. Although this method can be very sensitive and 3H-labeled probes generate well resolved autoradiographic signals, it is time consuming and technically difficult. Other high radiation emitting isotopes can be used, but they give nonspecific background.

Nonisotopic methods for ISH offer the advantages of probe stability, sensitivity, spatial resolution, and great time saving. The nonisotopic adaptations are generally simpler and faster than autoradiography, and the sensitivity of nonradioactive methods has increased over the years as the parameters influencing the hybridization efficiency and signal specificity have become more optimized. Factors contributing to increased use of nonisotopic methods include faster color development time, chemically stable probes with no special disposal requirements, and different labeling and detection systems that can be used to facilitate the analysis of several probes simultaneously.

3.4.2. ISH Procedure

1. Prepare a solution containing: 20–50 pM/mL of the appropriate probe, 50% deionized formamide, 2X SSC buffer, 10X Denhardt's solution, 0.1% sonicated salmon sperm DNA, and 0.1% SDS. A convenient recipe is given in **Table 2**.

2. Add 10 μL of hybridization mixture to each well, and add coverslips.
3. Heat slides on a block at 95°C for 5 min to denature the double-stranded DNA.
4. Incubate slides at 48°C for 2–4 h in a humidified atmosphere (*see* **Note 19**).

3.4.3. Posthybridization Protocol
for Peroxidase-Based Color Development

1. Wash slides in 1X PBS twice for 5 min each time.
2. Add 10–15 μL of streptavidin-peroxidase complex (1 mg/mL stock diluted 1:30 in 1X PBS, pH 7.2).
3. Gently apply the coverslips.
4. Incubate slides at 37°C for 1 h.
5. Remove coverslip, wash slides with 1X PBS twice for 5 min each time.
6. Mix chromogen: 5 mL 50 mM acetate buffer, 25 mL 30% H_2O_2, 250 mL AEC.
7. Add to each well 100 μL of AEC in the presence of 0.03% hydrogen peroxide in 50 mM acetate buffer, pH 5.0.
8. Incubate slides in the dark at 37°C for 10 min to develop the color.
9. Observe slides under a microscope. If color is not strong enough, develop for another 10 min.
10. Rinse slides with tap water and allow to dry.
11. Add 1 drop of 50% glycerol in PBS, and apply the coverslips.
12. Analyze with optical microscope. Positive cells will be stained a brownish red.

3.5. Validation and Controls

The validity of *in situ* amplification–hybridization should be examined in every run. Attention is especially necessary in laboratories using the technique for the first time because occasional technical pitfalls lie on the path to mastery. In an experienced laboratory, it is still necessary to continuously validate the procedure and to confirm the efficiency of amplification. To do this, the authors routinely run two or three sets of experiments in multiwelled slides simultaneously in order to validate both amplification and the subsequent hybridization/detection steps.

In the author's lab, we frequently work with HIV. A common validation procedure mixes HIV-1 infected cells with HIV-1 uninfected cells in a known proportion (i.e. 1:10, 1:100, etc.) and is used to confirm that the detection results are appropriately proportionate. To examine the efficiency of amplification, a cell line that carries a single copy or two copies of cloned HIV-1 virus *(1,2,4–6,8–11,15–19)* is used to ensure that proper amplification and hybridization has 0occurred.

In all amplification procedures, the authors use one slide as a control for nonspecific binding of the probe. Here they hybridize the amplified cells with an unrelated probe. The authors use HLA-DQα and β-actin probes and primers with PBMC and other tissue sections as positive controls, to check various parameters of our system.

In case one is using tissue sections, a cell suspension lacking the gene of interest can be used as a control. These cells can be added on top of the tissue section and then retrieved after the amplification procedure. The cell suspension can then be analyzed with the specific probe to see if the signal from the tissue leaked out and entered the cells floating above. The authors suggest that researchers carefully design and employ appropriate positive and negative controls for their specific experiments. In the case of RT-*in situ* amplification, β-actin, β-globulin, HLA-DQα, and other endogenous-abundant RNAs can be used as the positive markers. Of course, one should always have a RT-negative control for RT *in situ* amplification, as well as DNase and non-DNase controls. Control reactions lacking *Taq* DNA polymerase both with and without primers should always be included.

4. Notes

1. Other laboratories prefer to use sections up to 10-μm thickness, but in the author's experience, amplification is often less successful with thicker sections, and multiple cell layers can often lead to difficult interpretation as a result of superimposition of cells. However, if tissues that contain particularly large cells are used (such as ovarian follicles), then thicker sections may be appropriate.
2. It is very important to use tissues that were frozen in liquid nitrogen or were placed on dry-ice immediately after they were harvested before autolysis began to take place. If tissues are slowly frozen by simply placing them at −70°C, ice crystals will form inside the tissues with resulting morphologic distortion.
3. If surface antigens are lipoprotein and denature in methanol, use 2% paraformaldehyde or other reagent.
4. This step is absolutely critical, and one may need to experiment with different periods in order to optimize the heat treatment for specific tissues. The author's laboratory routinely uses 90 s for DNA target sequences, and 30–45 s for RNA sequences.
5. The time and temperature of incubation should be optimized carefully for each cell line or tissue-section type. With too little digestion, the cytoplasmic and nuclear membranes will not be sufficiently permeable to primers and enzyme, and amplification will be inconsistent. With too much digestion, the membranes will either deteriorate during repeated denaturation or worse, signals will leak out. In the first case, cells will not contain the signal and high background will result. In the latter case, many cells will show pericytoplasmic staining or "rim staining" representing the leaked signals going into the cells not containing the signals. Attention to detail here can often mean the difference between success and failure, and this procedure should be practiced rigorously with extra sections before continuing on to the amplification steps.
   In the author's laboratory, proper digestion parameters vary considerably with

tissue type. Typically, lymphocytes will require 5–10 min at 25°C or room temperature, CNS tissue will require 12–18 min at room temperature, and paraffin-fixed tissue will require between 15–30 min at room temperature. However, these periods can vary widely and the appearance of the "salt and pepper dots" is the important factor. Unfortunately, the appearance of the "salt and pepper dots" is less prominent in paraffin sections.

The critical importance of these dots should not be underestimated, since an extra 2–3 min of treatment after the appearance of dots will result in leakage of signals. An alternate to observation of "dots" method is to select a constant time and treat slides with varying amounts of proteinase K. For example, treat slides for 15 min in 1–6 µg/mL of proteinase K.

6. All reagents for RT *in situ* amplification should be prepared with RNase-free water. In addition, the silanized glass slides and all glassware should be RNase-free, which the authors insure by baking the glassware overnight in an oven before use in the RT-amplification procedure.

7. Some cells (e.g., pancreas) are particularly rich in ribonuclease. In this circumstance, add the following ribonuclease inhibitor to the DNase I solution: 1000 U/mL placental ribonuclease inhibitor (e.g., RNasin) plus 1 mM DTT. Also, some investigators prefer to use a long incubation period with a lower concentration of DNase (1 U/mL for 18 h).

8. If liver tissue is being used, this incubation should be extended an additional hour.

9. In the author's laboratory, the authors use antisense downstream primers for their gene of interest, since they already know the sequence of most genes they study. However, oligo (dT) primers can alternatively be used to convert all mRNA populations into cDNA and then perform the *in situ* amplification for a specific cDNA. This technique is also useful when performing simultaneous amplification of several different gene transcripts. For example, if one is attempting to detect the expression of various cytokines, an oligo (dT) primer can be used to prime reverse transcription of all of the mRNA in a cell or tissue section into cDNA. Then, more than one type of cytokine can be amplified, and detection of the various types with different probes which develop into different colors can occur.

10. In all RT reactions, it is advantageous to reverse transcribe only relatively small fragments of mRNA (<1.5 kilobases). Larger fragments may not completely reverse transcribe as a result of the presence of secondary structures. Furthermore, the RT enzymes are not very efficient in transcribing large mRNA fragments. However, this size restriction does not apply to DNA amplification reactions since the thermostable DNA-dependent DNA polymerases are more processive than RT enzymes. In *in situ* DNA reactions, the authors routinely amplify genes up to 300 base pairs.

11. The length for both sense and antisense primers should be 14–22 base pairs. At the 3' ends, primers should contain a GC-type base pairs (e.g., GG, CC, GC, or CG) to facilitate complementary strand formation. The preferred GC content of the primers is from 45–55%. Try to design primers so that they do not form intra-

or interstrand base pairs. Furthermore, the 3' ends should not be complementary to each other, or else they will form primer dimers.

12. Avian myoblastosis virus reverse transcriptase and MMLV reverse transcriptase give comparable results in our laboratory. However, it is important to read the manufacturer's descriptions of the RT enzyme and to make certain that the proper buffer is used. An alternative RT enzyme is available which lacks RNase H activity (degradation of single stranded RNA in an RNA:DNA heteroduplex) and, thus, is more processive. It is called Superscript II and is available from Gibco-BRL. It is suitable for reverse transcription of long mRNAs. It is also suitable for routine RT amplification, and in the author's laboratory, it has proven to be more efficient than the two enzymes described above.

13. Be certain to carefully paint the polish around the entire periphery of the coverslip or the edges of the dual slide, because the polish must completely seal the coverslip-slide assembly in order to form a small reaction "chamber" that can contain the water vapor during thermal cycling. For effective sealing, do not use colored polish or any other nail polish which is especially "runn." The author's laboratory prefers to use Wet & Wild Clear nail polish. Proper sealing is very important, because this keeps reaction concentrations consistent through the thermal cycling procedure, and concentrations are critical to proper amplification. However, be certain to apply the nail polish very carefully so that none of the polish gets into the actual chamber where the cells or tissues reside. If any nail polish does enter the chamber, discard that slide, since the results will be questionable. Please bear in mind that the painting of nail polish is truly a learned skill; therefore, it is strongly recommended that researchers practice this procedure several times with mock slides before attempting an experiment.

14. In the case of thick tissue sections, it is best to use another identical blank slide for the cover instead of a coverslip. Apply the amplification cocktail to the appropriate well of the blank slide, place an inverted tissue-containing slide atop the blank slide, and seal the edges as described. Invert the slide once again so that the tissue-containing slide is on the bottom. This technique can be modified to accommodate a hot start (*see* **Note 18**).

15. An alternate to nail polish is to utilize a "self seal," which , when mixed directly into the amplification cocktail, seals the slides at it edges, limiting the evaporation of the "cocktail". The authors have utilized this "self seal" in thier laboratory extensively, and it has given excellent results. This is available from M.J. Research.

16. Various types of thermocycler will work in this application; however, some instruments work much better than others. In the author's laboratory, two types are used: a standard, block-type thermocycler that normally holds sixty 0.5-mL tubes, but which can be adapted with aluminum foil, paper towels and a weight to hold 4–6 slides. They also use dedicated thermocyclers that are specifically designed to hold 12 or 16 slides. It is understood that other investigators have used stirred-air, oven-type thermocyclers quite successfully. However, these systems are prone to cracking glass slides during cycling. Thermocyclers dedicated

to glass slides are now available from several vendors, including Barnstead Thermolyne (Iowa), Coy Corporation (Minnesota), Hybaid (England), Perkin Elmer (California), and MJ Research (Massachusetts). The author's laboratory has used an MJ Research PTC-100-16MS, PTC-100-16MS, and DNA-Engine Twin-Tower 16x2 quite successfully. Recently, this company has combined the slide and tubes into a single block, allowing the simultaneous confirmation of *in situ* amplification in a tube. Furthermore, there are newer designs of thermal cyclers which incorporate humidification chambers. However, the authors do not yet have sufficient experience with this technology to verify whether they eliminate the need for sealing the slides with nail polish during thermal cycling. Nonetheless, the humidified instruments are especially useful in the reverse transcription and hybridization steps, where a humidified incubator is otherwise needed.

The authors suggest that the manufacturer's instructions on the use of a thermocycler be followed bearing in mind the following points. First, glass does not easily make good thermal contact with the surface on which it rests. Therefore, a weight to press down the slides and/or a thin layer of mineral oil to fill in the interstices will help thermal conduction. If using mineral oil, make certain that the oil is well smeared over the glass surface so that the slide is not merely floating on air bubbles beneath it. Second, the top surfaces of slides lose heat quite rapidly through radiation and convection. Therefore, use a thermocycler which envelopes the slide in an enclosed chamber (as in some dedicated instruments), or insulate the tops of the slides in some manner. Insulation is particularly critical when using a weight on top of the slides, for the weight can serve as an unwanted heat sink if it is in direct contact with the slides. Third, good thermal uniformity is imperative for good results. Poor uniformity or irregular thermal change can result in cracked slides, uneven amplification, or completely failed reactions. If adapting a thermocycler that normally holds plastic tubes, use a layer of aluminum foil to spread out the heat.

17. Annealing temperatures for reverse transcription and for DNA amplification can be chosen according to the following formula: Tm of the primers $= 81.5°C + 16.6$ (Log M) $+ 0.41$ (G + C%) $- 500/n$, where n = length of primers, M = molarity of the salt in the buffer, usually 0.047 M for DNA reactions and 0.070 M for RT reactions. If using AMV RT, the value will be lower according to the following formula: Tm of the primers $= 62.3°C + 0.41$ (G + C%) $- 500/n$. A simpler version could be used for primers of 18 bases or below: $Tm = 4°C$ (# of GC pairs) $+ 2°C$ (# of AT pairs). Usually, primer annealing is optimal at 2°C above its Tm. However, this formula provides only an approximate temperature for annealing, since base-stacking, near-neighbor effect, and buffering capacity may play a significant role for a particular primer. Optimization of the annealing temperature should be carried out first with solution-based reactions. It is important to know the optimal temperature before attempting to conduct *in situ* amplification, since *in situ* reactions are simply not as robust a solution-based ones. The authors hypothesize that this is due to the fact that primers do not have easy access to DNA templates inside cells and tissues, since numerous membranes, folds, and

other small structures can keep primers from binding homologous sites as readily as they do in solution-based reactions.

There are two additional ways to determine the real annealing temperatures. First, utilize a thermocycler designed with a temperature gradient block for the rapid empirical determination of annealing temperatures (Robocycler, Stratagene, La Jolla, CA). Second, use Touchdown PCR *(14)*.

18. There is much debate as to whether a hot start helps to improve the specificity and sensitivity of amplification reactions. In the author's laboratory, they find that hot start adds no advantage in this regard. Rather, it adds only technical difficulty to the practice of the *in situ* technique. However, a variation of the hot start which uses anti-*Taq* DNA polymerase antibody in the PCR master mix (containing the DNA polymerase) may resolve this problem. The anti-*Taq* antibody keeps the polymerase "blocked" until the first cycle of 92°C when the antibody becomes denatured and the DNA polymerase becomes active. This modification essentially serves the same function as the hot start procedure but without its difficulties.

19. The optimal hybridization temperature must be calculated for each probe, as described in **Note 17**.

References

1. Bagasra, O., Seshamma, T., Hansen, J., and Pomerantz, R. (1995) In situ polymerase chain reaction and hybridization to detect low abundance nucleic acid targets, in *Current Protocols in Molecular Biology* (Ausubel et al., eds.), Sec 14.8.1.
2. Bagasra, O., Lavi, U., Bobroski, L., Khalili, K., Pestaner, J. P., and Pomerantz, R. J. (1996) Cellular reservoirs of HIV-1 in the central nervous system of infected-individuals: identification by the combination of in situ PCR and immunohistochemistry. *AIDS* **10**, 573–585.
3. Pestaner, J. P., Bibbo, M., Bobroski, L., Seshamma, T., and Bagasra, O. (1994) Potential of in situ polymerase chain reaction in diagnostic cytology. *Acta Cytologia* **38**, 676–680.
4. Bagasra, O., Hauptman, S. P., Lischner, H.W., Sachs, M., and Pomerantz, R. J. (1992) Detection of HIV-1 provirus in mononuclear cells by in situ PCR. *New Engl. J. Med.* **326**, 1385–1391.
5. Bagasra, O., Seshamma, T., Oakes, J., and Pomerantz, R. J. (1993) Frequency of cells positive for HIV-1 sequences assessed by *in situ* polymerase chain reaction. *AIDS* **7**, 82–86.
6. Bagasra, O., Seshamma, T., Oakes, J., and Pomerantz, R. J. (1993) High percentages of CD4-positive lymphocytes harbor the HIV-1 provirus in the blood of certain infected individuals. *AIDS* **7**, 1419–1425.
7. Nuovo, G. J. (1994) *PCR In Situ Hybridization Protocols and Applications*, 2nd. ed. Raven, New York.
8. Bagasra, O., Seshamma, T., and Pomerantz, R. J. (1993) Polymerase chain reaction in situ: intracellular amplification and detection of HIV-1 proviral DNA and other specific genes. *J. Immunol. Meth.* **158**, 131–145.
9. Bagasra, O. and Pomerantz, R. J. (1993) HIV-1 provirus is demonstrated in

peripheral blood monocytes in vivo: a study utilizing an in situ PCR. *AIDS Res. Hum. Retrovir.* **9**, 69–76.

10. Bagasra, O., Farzadegan, H., Seshamma, T., Oakes, J., Saah, A., and Pomerantz, R. J. (1994) Human immunodeficiency virus type 1 infection of sperm in vivo. *AIDS* **8**, 1669–1674.

11. Bagasra, O., Michaels, F., Mu, Y., Bobroski, L., Spitsin, S. V., Fu, Z. F., and Koprowski, H. (1995) Activation of the inducible form of nitric oxide synthetase in the brains of patients with multiple sclerosis. *Proc Natl. Acad. Sci. USA* **92**, 12041–12045.

12. Lattime, E. C., Mastrangelo, M. J., Bagasra, O., and Berd, D. (1995) Expression of cytokine mRNA in human melanoma tissue. *Cancer Immunol. Immunother.* **41**, 151–156.

13. Mehta, A., Maggioncalda, J., Bagasra, O., Thikkavarapu, S., Saikumari, P., Nigel, F. W., and Block, T. (1995) In situ PCR and RNA hybridization detection of herpes simplex virus sequences in trigeminal ganglia of latently infected mice. *Virology* **206**, 633–640.

14. Pereira, R. F., Halford, K. W. O'Hara, M. D., Leeper, D. B., Sokolov, B. P., Pollard, M. D., Bagasra, O., and Prockop, D. J. (1995) Cultured stromal cells from marrow serve as stem cells for bone, lung and cartilage in irradiated mice. *Proc. Natl. Acad. Sci. USA* **92**, 4857–4861.

15. Bagasra, O. (1990) Polymerase chain reaction in situ. *Amplifications* (March 1990), Editorial note, 20–21.

16. Bagasra, O. and Pomerantz, R. J. (1994) In situ polymerase chain reaction and HIV-1, in *Clinics of North America* (Pomerantz, R. J., ed.), W. B. Saunders, Philadelphia, pp. 351–366.

17. Bagasra, O., Hui, Z., Bobroski, L., Seshamma, T., Saikumari, P., and Pomerantz, R. J. (1995) One step amplification of HIV-1 mRNA and DNA at a single cell level by in situ polymerase chain reaction. *Cell Vision* **2**, 425–440.

18. Bagasra, O. and Pomerantz, R. J. (1995) Detection of HIV-1 in the brain tissue of individuals who died from AIDS, in *PCR in Neuroscience* (Gobinda Sarkar, ed.), Academic, pp. 339–357.

19. Bagasra, O., Seshamma, T., Pastanar, J. P., and Pomerantz, R. (1995) Detection of HIV-1 Gene sequences in the brain tissues by in situ polymerase chain reaction, in *Technical Advances in AIDS Research in the Nervous System* (Majors, E., ed.), Plenum, NY, pp. 251–266.

20. Qureshi, M. N., Barr, C. E., Seshamma, T., Pomerantz, R. J., and Bagasra, O. (1994) Localization of HIV-1 proviral DNA in oral mucosal epithelial cells. *J. Infect. Dis.* **171**, 190–193.

21. Winslow, B. J., Pomerantz, R. J., Bagasra, O., and Trono, D. (1993) HIV-1 latency due to the site of proviral integration. *Virology* **196**, 849–854.

19

Determination of the Promoter Activity of HIV-1 Using the Chloramphenicol Acetyltransferase Reporter Gene Assay

Loretta Tse and Nelson L. Michael

1. Introduction

RNA transcripts are produced from the 5' long terminal repeat (LTR) of human immunodeficiency virus type-1 (HIV-1) under the complex control of viral regulatory sequences *(1–7)*. The LTR from a prototypical, laboratory-adapted HIV-1 (HXB2) can be divided into modulatory, core promoter, and transactivating regions (**Fig. 1**). The modulatory regions include elements with limited homology to AP-1 enhancer sequences at positions -347 to -329 relative to the cap site *(8)*, two NF-AT sites at positions -292 to -255 *(9)*, a USF site at positions -159 to -173 *(10–12)*, a TCF-1α site at positions -139 to -124 *(13)*, and two NF-kB enhancer elements at positions -104 to -81 *(14)*. The core positive strand promoter is composed of three Sp1 binding sites located at positions -78 through -47 and a TATA box at positions -28 to -24 *(15,16)*. A 59-base pair region which confers transcriptional transactivating potential to the core promoter elements by the viral Tat protein is located within the R region of the LTR at positions +1 to +59 *(17,18)*. This transactivating region (TAR) folds into alternate RNA stem-loop structures that are found in the 5' termini of all viral transcripts. The TAR element mediates a substantial increase in transcriptional initiation and elongation through interactions with the viral Tat protein and other cellular factors *(3,19–22)*. The HIV-1 LTR possesses a variable structure in natural infection *(23,24)* and Much of our understanding of the HIV-1 enhancer/promoter has been gained from the use of artificial reporter system constructions. These plasmids contain portions of the HIV-1 enhancer/

From: *Methods in Molecular Medicine, Vol. 17: HIV Protocols*
Edited by: N. L. Michael and J. H. Kim © Humana Press Inc., Totowa, NJ

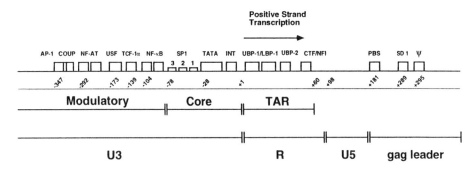

Fig. 1. LTR/gag leader region of HIV-1. A schematic drawing of the LTR/gag leader region of HIV-1 is shown. The positions of cis-acting regulatory sequences are given on the heavy line and genomic positions relative to the initiation of positive strand transcription (shown by the arrow) are given on the thinner line below. The functional and structural regions of the HIV-1 LTR are given at the bottom of the figure. The schematic is not drawn to scale. PBS, primer binding site; SD 1, splice donor 1 (major 5' splice donor); y, packaging signal.

promoter cloned 5' to reporter genes whose expression can be detected and quantitated with a high degree of sensitivity and precision after transfection into suitable mammalian target cells. There are a variety of reporter genes available, such as β-galactosidase, firefly luciferase, and chloramphenicol acetyltransferase. Since these reporter genes do not express in the absence of a heterologous promoter, their expression is a direct measure of the promoter activity of the HIV-1 LTR sequences cloned 5' to them. The authors will describe an adaptation of a specific reporter gene assay, first described by Gorman in 1984 *(26)*, that measures expression of the bacterial antimicrobial resistance gene chloramphenicol acetyltransferase (CAT) under the transcriptional control of a heterologous promoter in eukaryotic cells. This CAT reporter gene assay has been adapted to monitor HIV-1 promoter activity in neoplastic human T-cell lines transiently transfected with HIV-1 LTR sequences cloned 5' to the CAT gene (LTR-CAT reporter plasmids). An example of a prototypical LTR-CAT reporter plasmid is shown in **Fig. 2**

Promoter activity is determined by measurement of the CAT activity contained in crude lysates of T-cells 40 h post-transfection with both LTR-CAT reporter and β-galactosidase expression plasmids. CAT activity is normalized to total protein and β-galactosidase activity to control for cell lysis and transfection efficiency variation, respectively. CAT mediates the transfer of acetyl groups from acetyl coenzyme A to chloramphenicol. Thus, the conversion of nonacetylated to acetylated chloramphenicol is used to determine CAT activity.

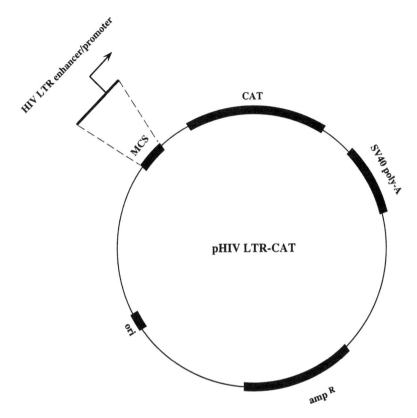

Fig. 2. Basic elements of a LTR-CAT reporter plasmid. A schematic illustration of a generic LTR-CAT reporter construct, which contains an bacterial origin of replication (ori), the ampicillin resistance gene (Amp[R]), a multiple cloning site for enhancer/promoter sequences insertion 5' of the CAT gene, and a SV40 derived poly A signal to ensure proper transcription termination 3' polyadenylation. The start site of transcription directed from HIV LTR enhancer/promoter sequences is shown by the arrow. Note that the relative size of each element is not necessary drawn to scale.

2. Materials
2.1. Plasmid Vector Construction

1. CAT expression plasmids are available in a variety of plasmid vectors that can be readily obtained from colleagues or from commercial sources such as Invitrogen (San Diego, CA), Promega (Madison, WI), and Stratagene (La Jolla, CA). A typical CAT reporter plasmid contains a multiple cloning site 5' to the CAT gene to facilitate insertion of HIV-1 enhancer/promoter sequences and a eukaryotic poly-A signal sequence 3' to the CAT gene to maximize CAT gene expression (*see* **Fig. 2**).

βgal, an expression vector producing β-galactosidase under the control of MV immediate early gene promoter (and with the SV40 poly-A signal aces cloned 3' to the β-galactosidase gene) can be easily constructed from only available plasmids or commercially obtained from the suppliers listed ep 1.

A plasmid to be used to normalize DNA concentrations for each electroporation reaction ("filler plasmid"). This plasmid should not contain a eukaryotic promoter. pBluescript II, pUC19, pBR322, or other, similar plasmids can be used and are readily obtainable from colleagues or from the vendors noted in **Subheading 2.1.1.**

4. All plasmids propagated in *Escherichia coli* cells should contain a selectable marker gene (e.g., ampicillin, tetracycline, kanamycin) to facilitate subcloning.
5. Approximately 500 μg of each of the final constructions can be prepared using the Qiagen Plasmid Maxi Kit (Qiagen, Chatsworth, CA) or by double banding in CsCl-EtBr dye-density gradients.

2.2. Cell Strains

Continuous human T-cell lines, such as SupT1, H9, Jurkat, or A3.01, can be obtained from the NIH AIDS Research and Reference Reagent Program (Rockville, MD) or the American Type Culture Collection (Rockville, MD). SupT1 cells will be used in the assays described in this chapter (*see* **Note 1**).

2.3. Reagents and Equipment for Electroporation

An electroporation system with capacitance extender and sterile, 0.4 cm gap electroporation cuvets can be obtained from Bio-Rad (Emeryville, CA). Sterile 6-well culture plates and pipets are supplied by Costar (Cambridge, MA). All solutions and reagents used for electroporation should be sterilized by passage through a 0.45–μM sterile filter (Costar). Fine-tipped disposable plastic transfer pipets are supplied by PGC Scientific (Gaithersburg, MD).

1. TE: 10 mM Tris-HCl, pH 7.4, 1 mM ethylenediamine tetra-acetic acid (EDTA).
2. RPMI/20% FCS media: RPMI 1640 media (ABI, Columbia, MD), supplemented with 20% heat-inactivated fetal calf serum (Sigma, St. Louis, MO), 100 U/mL penicillin, 100 μg/mL streptomycin, and 2 mM L-glutamine (each from ABI).

2.4. Reagents and Equipment for Human T-cell Line Culture

1. SupT1 cells are maintained in RPMI/10% FCS media: RPMI 1640 media supplemented with 10% heat-inactivated fetal calf serum, 100 U/mL penicillin, 100 μg/mL streptomycin, and 2 mM L-glutamine.
2. Cells are cultured in a humidified tissue culture incubator held at 37°C with a 5% CO_2 atmosphere.
3. Temperature-controlled, table-top centrifuge (e.g., Beckman Model GS6R).
4. Tissue culture flasks and pipets are supplied by Costar.

2.5. Reagents and Equipment for the Preparation of Cell Lysates

1. Standard microfuge.
2. Dry ice–70% ethanol bath.
3. Water bath held at 37°C.
4. 0.25 M Tris-HCl, pH 7.4.
5. Phosphate buffered saline (PBS). PBS may be obtained commercially in sterile bottles. If desired, it may be made using the recipe given in **steps 6–8**.
6. Mix 1.15 g anhydrous Na_2HPO_4, 0.23 g anhydrous NaH_2PO_4, and 9.00 g NaCl with 950 mL distilled water.
7. Adjust pH to between 7.2 and 7.4 with either 1 M HCl or 1 M NaOH and bring total volume to 1000 mL with distilled water.
8. Filter sterilize by passage through a 0.45-μM pore size filter unit.

2.6. Reagents and Equipment for Quantitation of Cell Lysate Total Protein

96-well, flat-bottom microtiter plates (Immulon 1) are supplied by PGC Scientific (Gaithersburg, MD), albumin standards and Coomassie Protein Assay solution are provided by Pierce Chemical Co. (Rockford, IL), and an ELISA plate reader with Soft Max Pro software is supplied by Molecular Devices Corporation (Sunnyvale, CA).

2.7. Reagents and Equipment for the β-Galactosidase Assay

1. β-galactosidase Enzyme Assay System is supplied by Promega.
2. ELISA plate reader (*see* **Subheading 2.6.**).

2.8. Reagents and Equipment for the CAT Assay

1. [^{14}C]-chloramphenicol is supplied by Amersham (Arlington Heights, IL).
2. Acetyl CoA lithium salt is supplied by Pharmacia LKB Biotech (Piscataway, NJ).
3. CAT reaction mix: 0.25 M Tris-HCl, pH 7.4, 0.5 μCi/mL [^{14}C]-chloramphenicol, 0.45 mM acetyl coenzyme A. This mix should be freshly prepared just prior to performing the assay.
4. Microfuge tube compatible, rotary-evaporation system equipped for organic solvent use. The UVS Speed-Vac system by Savant Instruments (Farmingdale, NY) works well for this application.
5. Chromatography tanks and Whatman 3MM paper are supplied by Fisher Scientific (Columbia, MD).
6. Flex-silica gel plates-1B (dimensions 20 × 20 cm), ethyl acetate, chloroform, and methanol are supplied by J.T. Baker (Phillipsburg, NJ).
7. Kodak XAR-5 film is supplied by Standard Medical Imaging (Columbia, MD).
8. Metal autoradiography cassettes are supplied by Sigma.
9. Storage phosphor imaging systems are supplied by Molecular Dynamics.

3. Methods

3.1. Preparation of Plasmid DNAs for Transfection

1. Plasmid DNAs should be resuspended at approx 1 mg/mL concentrations in sterile TE buffer and held at 4°C prior to transfection.

3.2. Preparation of Human T-Cell Lines for Transfection

1. SupT1 cells should be maintained in RPMI/10% FCS media at a density of $1-2 \times 10^6$ cells/mL by biweekly 1:3 passage.
2. SupT1 cells are resuspended at a density of 1×10^6 cells/mL in RPMI/10% FCS media 6–12 h prior to transfection to ensure that the culture is in log-phase growth at the time of transfection.

3.3.Transfection of T-Cell Lines by Electroporation

1. Determine the total number of transfection reactions to be performed and pipet 3.5 mL of RPMI/20% FCS media into that number of wells of 6-well tissue culture plates.
2. 1.5×10^7 SupT1 cells are required for each transfection. Pellet the appropriate number of cells at 300g for 7 min at 4°C in a temperature-controlled, table-top centrifuge. Resuspend the cells in RPMI/20% FCS medium at a density of 5×10^7 cells/mL and hold on ice.
3. For each transfection reaction, pipet 300 μL of SupT1 cell suspension into individual, sterile 1.5-mL microfuge tubes and hold on ice.
4. Pipet 2 μg of the pCMVβgal plasmid into each microfuge tube containing the cell suspension.
5. Pipet a range from 0 (negative control) to 20 μg of LTR-CAT reporter gene plasmid into each microfuge tube (*see* **Note 2**).
6. If other plasmids are to be used in cotransfection studies, pipet them into the appropriate microfuge tubes at this point (*see* **Note 4**).
7. Finally, pipet an appropriate amount of "filler plasmid" into each microfuge tube to bring the total amount of plasmid DNA in each tube up to a uniform amount (typically 20–40 μg).
8. Mix each DNA/cell suspension thoroughly by tapping on each tube (*see* **Note 5**) and hold on ice for 20 min.
9. For each reaction, aspirate and remix the cell/DNA suspension with a sterile, 1.0-mL pipet tip, dispense into a sterile, 0.4-cm gap electroporation cuvet, and immediately place into the electroporation device.
10. Deliver a 240 volt, 960 μF electrical pulse to the cuvet (*see* **Note 4**). A film of denatured cell fragments will appear in the cuvet after the pulse.
11. Immediately place the cuvet on ice and hold for an additional 20 min (*see* **Note 5**).
12. Aspirate the cuvet contents into a media containing well of a 6-well plate using a sterile, disposable, fine-tipped transfer pipet. Then draw approx 1 mL of the media in that well and rinse the cuvet with this media before returning the rinse to the well ("rinse-transfer technique").

13. Place the 6-well plates in the tissue culture incubator for the next 40 h (approx 2 cell generations).

3.4. Preparation of the Cell Lysate

1. For each well of a 6-well plate, aspirate and discard approximately ≥ 2 mL of media using a fine-tipped transfer pipet taking care not to disturb the cells which are settled on the bottom of the well.
2. Using the same pipet, gently resuspend the cells in the residual media (approx 1 mL), transfer to a 1.5-mL microfuge tube, and spin at 6000 rpm for 2 min in a standard microfuge. Aspirate and discard the supernatant fluid. Recentrifuge the tubes for a few seconds to collect residual traces of media and carefully aspirate and discard it to leave a moist cell pellet (*see* **Note 6**).
3. Resuspend the cell pellet in 85 μL of 0.25 *M* Tris-HCl, pH 7.4 by vortexing.
4. Placing the samples in a dry ice–70% ethanol bath for 5 min.
5. Immediately place the samples in a 37°C water bath for 1 min.
6. Repeat the above freeze-thaw cycles three additional times.
7. Microfuge the samples at 12,000 rpm for 5 min at 4°C. Remove the supernatant fluid to new microfuge tubes (*see* **Note 7**).

3.5. Quantitative Protein Determination

1. Pipet 6 μL of each of the albumin standards into wells A1 through A7 of a microtiter plate (the albumin standard concentrations are 1500, 1000, 500, 400, 250, 100, and 75 μg/mL). These standards need to be prepared from the initial concentration of 2 mg/mL supplied by Pierce by dilution into sterile PBS. The standards should be stored at –20°C between uses.
2. Pipet 5 μL of 0.25 *M* Tris-HCl, pH 7.4 into each of two wells for each transfection lysate to be tested.
3. Pipet 1 μL of lysate into each of two wells containing the Tris buffer to achieve a 1:6 dilution.
4. Add 300 μL of Coomassie dye reagent to each well containing diluted lysate or albumin standard.
5. Optical density (OD) is determined on an automated plate reader at 405 nm. Determine the protein concentration of the diluted transfection lysates by interpolation to the albumin standards. To compute the protein concentrations of the undiluted lysates, multiply the diluted protein concentration by 6 (the value of the dilution factor) (*see* **Note 8**).

3.6. β-galactosidase Activity Determination

1. Thaw the system components and will each well.
2. Place the 2X assay buffer on ice.
3. Prepare dilutions of the 1 U/μL β-galactosidase standard stock solution as follows: add 10 μL of the stock to 990 μL of 1X reporter lysis buffer (RLB) and vortex. Add 10 μL of this 1:100 stock dilution to another 990 μL aliquot of RLB to make a 1:10,000 stock dilution. Finally, add 0, 2, 4, 6, 8, 10, 20, 30, 40, and 50 μL

of 1:10,000 stock to the appropriate amounts of 1X RLB to bring the final volume to 50 μL.

4. Mix 17 μL of each transfection lysate with 33 μL of 1X RLB in 1.5 mL microfuge tubes.

5. Pipet each of the β-galactosidase standards and diluted cell lysates (50 μL) into separate wells of a 96-well microtiter plate.

6. Pipet 50 μL of 2X assay buffer into each well containing diluted β-galactosidase standard or transfection lysate and cover the plate.

7. Incubate the plate at 37°C for 0.5–3.0 h or until a faint yellow color has developed. The color intensity of all of the transfection lysates should be within the range of color intensities of the β-galactosidase standards.

8. Stop the color development by adding 150 μL of 1 *M* sodium carbonate to each well and mix by gentle pipeting to avoid bubble formation.

9. Read the plate in an automated plate reader with a 420-nm (or 405-nm) filter. The β-galactosidase activities for each transfection lysate are determined by interpolation of the standard curve.

3.7. Chloramphenicol Acetyltransferase (CAT) Assay

1. For each CAT assay to be performed, pipet the lysate volume necessary to deliver 15 μg of total protein into 1.5-mL microfuge tubes (*see* **Note 9**).

2. Add 100 μL of CAT reaction mix to each microfuge tube and vortex to mix.

3. Incubate reactions at 37°C for 1 h (*see* **Note 10**).

4. Add 1 mL ethyl acetate to each reaction, vortex for 30 s, and spin in a microfuge at 12,000 rpm for 5 min to effect phase separation.

5. Remove 900 μL of the upper (ethyl acetate) layer to new 1.5-mL microfuge tubes (*see* **Note 11**).

6. Evaporate the ethyl acetate in a rotary-vacuum system equipped for organic solvents (*see* **Note 12**).

7. During the evaporation step, prepare a chromatography tank containing 95 mL of chloroform and 5 mL of methanol in a chemical fume hood. Add a piece of Whatman 3MM paper to one (long) side of the tank and allow it to become saturated with solvent.

8. Using a pencil, mark silica thin-layer chromatography (TLC) plates with 12 pencil marks each which are 1.5 cm apart and 1.5 cm from the bottom of the plate. This horizontal line of marks defines the "origin" of the plate.

9. Resuspend the evaporated samples in 10 μL of fresh ethyl acetate, vortex, and immediately spot onto the TLC plate. Allow the plate to dry for 1 min.

10. Clamp the TLC plate to a 20 × 20 cm glass plate and place into the chromatography tank with the "origin" marks closest to, but not immersed in, the solvent.

11. Develop the TLC plate in the tank for 1.5 h.

12. Remove the TLC plates and air dry.

13. The TLC plate is visualized and quantitatively analyzed by either direct autoradiography or storage phosphor imaging technology (*see* **Note 13**). The slowest migrating spot (origin proximal) is nonacetylated [^{14}C]-chloramphenicol. One,

two, or three spots may be seen in each lane with a higher degree of mobility. These spots correspond to mono, di, and triacetylated forms of $[^{14}C]$-chloramphenicol, respectively (*see* **Note 14**).

14. The percent conversion of non-acetylated to acetylated $[^{14}C]$-chloramphenicol forms is the standard description of CAT activity. Percent conversion = 100 × (radioactivity in all acetylated chloramphenicol forms)/(radioactivity in all acetylated chloramphenicol forms) + (radioactivity in nonacetylated-chloramphenicol forms). The CAT assay exhibits a linear response from 0.1–25%. Values outside of this range will necessitate another CAT assay with an appropriate adjustment in the assay conditions (*see* **Note 15**).

3.8. Calculation of Promoter Activity

1. The raw CAT activity calculated in **Subheading 3.7.14.** has been determined from uniform amounts of lysate total protein to control for differential cell lysis. However, DNA transfection efficiency can vary by over tenfold in a series of electroporations. Normalization for transfection efficiency can be accomplished by measurement of β-galactosidase activity expressed from the pCMVβgal plasmid that was cotransfected into the SupT1 cells along with the LTR-CAT reporter plasmid.
2. Determine the geometric mean (or median) value for all of the β-galactosidase activities from the transfection lysates.
3. Calculate the corrected CAT activity according to the following formula:

Corrected CAT activity = (percent conversion) ×
(geo. mean or median β-galactosidase activity)/(β-galactosidase activity).

4. Notes

1. Human T-cell lines, such as SupT1, are highlighted in this protocol as they can be infected by laboratory adapted HIV-1 strains but not by most HIV-1 strains directly obtained from infected patients. Thus, T-cell lines represent more of a "natural" target cell for HIV-1 than other commonly used cell types for LTR-CAT assays such as COS-1 cells. True natural target cells, such as primary human T-cells, can also be used for these experiments, but the level of promoter activity obtained from them is very low.
2. The basal level promoter activity of most LTR-CAT plasmids using the assay conditions described here is best typically optimized in the 2–10 μg range of plasmid input put this needs to be titrated in the expanded range given. Transfections in the absence of LTR-CAT reporter plasmids and with LTR-CAT reporter plasmids lacking HIV-1 enhancer promoter sequences are critical specificity controls.
3. Expression of transcription factors with positive or negative effects upon the basal level promoter activity of the HIV-1 LTR are frequently tested in the LTR-CAT assay. The HIV-1 Tat protein, acting through the TAR element, is the most commonly tested factor. Cotransfection of a wild-type Tat expression vector with a HIV-1 LTR-CAT plasmid will boost basal level promoter activity by approx 100-fold.

4. The optimal voltage for any given cell type varies widely and must be optimized prior to extensive experimentation. Optimal voltages for T-cells range from 180 to 250 V. Capacitance is almost always optimal at 960 μF.

5. Multiple samples can be processed during this 20 min step. At the conclusion of the last electroporation reaction, hold the last sample on ice for the full 20 min. It is acceptable if the other reactions are held for somewhat longer times on ice.

6. These cell pellets can be stored at –20°C for several days at this step, if necessary.

7. Alternatively, the cell lysates can be prepared by sonication. Cell pellets are resuspended in 100 μL of 0.25 M Tris-HCl, pH 7.4, held on ice, and then subjected to six 1–2 s pulses at setting 2 using a sonicator microtip attachment. Cell lysates prepared with either method can be stored at –20°C for many months, although some activity is lost over time. Thus, lysates that are to be directly compared to each other should be prepared on the same day.

8. The optimal lysate dilution to fit the linear range of the albumin standards is typically 1:6 but may have to be empirically determined for any given experiment.

9. The optimal amount of lysate protein to ensure CAT activity within the linear range of the assay must be empirically determined. If basal level promoter activity is compared to Tat-transactivated activity in the same experimental series, the 100-fold difference in CAT activity will require the use of varying amounts of lysate protein to uniformly obtain activities within the linear range of the assay.

10. The length of this incubation can be shortened in order to reduce the CAT activity, but it is more practical to vary the amount of input cell lysate.

11. This extraction preferentially partitions chloramphenicol forms into the organic phase.

12. Ethyl acetate is a highly volatile, toxic solvent. An evaporation system designed to contain such solvents must be employed at this step to minimize exposure of laboratory personnel to this solvent.

13. If access to a storage phosphor imaging system is available, the plate scan be exposed to a storage phosphor screen for 2–16 h, scanned, and the signals quantitated. Otherwise, the plate can be subjected to direct autoradiography overnight at room temperature without an intensifying screen with Kodak XAR-5 film directly applied to the TLC plate. The resulting autoradiograph can then be analyzed by quantitative densitometry. Finally, the autoradiograph could be used as a guide to scrape off the relevant portions of the TLC plate into scintillation vials for [^{14}C] determination by liquid scintillation counting.

14. Nonacetylated chloramphenicol has a lower affinity for the chloroform:methanol solvent system than the acetylated chloramphenicol forms. Thus, higher order chloramphenicol acetylation products migrate with increasing mobility in the solvent system.

15. Newer technology is available to measure CAT activity through differential partitioning of chloramphenicol forms in scintillant fluid systems for the direct determination of chloramphenicol acetylation. Although some investigators have turned to these assay systems, many (including the authors) have not done so owing to the inability of these systems to allow for the visualization of distinct

chloramphenicol forms. There are also commercially available kits to measure CAT protein with ELISA technology, but the authors have found this latter technology to be unreliable.

References

1. Arrigo, S. J., Weitsman, S., Zack, J. A., and Chen, I. S. (1990) Characterization and expression of novel singly spliced RNA species of human immunodeficiency virus type 1. *J. Virol.* **64,** 4585–4588.
2. Cullen, B. R. and Greene, W. C. (1989) Regulatory pathways governing HIV-1 replication. *Cell* **58,** 423–426.
3. Feinberg, M. B., Baltimore, D., and Frankel, A. D. (1991) The role of Tat in the human immunodeficiency virus life cycle indicates a primary effect on transcriptional elongation. *Proc Natl Acad Sci USA* **88,** 4045–4049.
4. Greene, W. C. (1990) Regulation of HIV-1 gene expression. *Annu. Rev. Immunol.* **8,** 453–475.
5. Guatelli, J. C., Gingeras, T. R., and Richman, D. D. (1990) Alternative splice acceptor utilization during human immunodeficiency virus type 1 infection of cultured cells. *J. Virol.* **64,** 4093–4098.
6. Schwartz, S., Felber, B. K., Benko, D. M., Fenyo, E. M., and Pavlakis, G. N. (1990) Cloning and functional analysis of multiply spliced mRNA species of human immunodeficiency virus type 1. *J. Virol.* **64,** 2519–2529.
7. Muesing, M. A., Smith, D. H., Cabradilla, C. D., Benton, C. V., Lasky, L. A., and Capon, D. J. (1985) Nucleic acid structure and expression of the human AIDS/lymphadenopathy retrovirus. *Nature* **313,** 450–458.
8. Franza, B. J., Rauscher, F., Josephs, S. F., and Curran, T. (1988) The Fos complex and Fos-related antigens recognize sequence elements that contain AP-1 binding sites. *Science* **239,** 1150–1153.
9. Siekevitz, M., Josephs, S. F., Dukovich, M., Peffer, N., Wong-Staal, F., and Greene, W. C. (1987) Activation of the HIV-1 LTR by T cell mitogens and the trans-activator protein of HTLV-I. *Science* **238,** 1575–1578; also, Erratum (1988) *Science* **239,** 451.
10. Garcia, J. A., Wu, F. K., Mitsuyasu, R., and Gaynor, R. B. (1987) Interactions of cellular proteins involved in the transcriptional regulation of the human immunodeficiency virus. *Embo. J.* **6,** 3761–3770.
11. Giacca, M., Gutierrez, M. I., Menzo, S., Di, F. F., and Falaschi, A. (1992) A human binding site for transcription factor USF/MLTF mimics the negative regulatory element of human immunodeficiency virus type 1. *Virology* **186,** 133–147.
12. Lu, Y., Stenzel, M., Sodroski, J. G., and Haseltine, W. A. (1989) Effects of long terminal repeat mutations on human immunodeficiency virus type 1 replication. *J. Virol.* **63,** 4115–4119.
13. Waterman, M. L., Fischer, W. H., and Jones, K. A. (1991) A thymus-specific member of the HMG protein family regulates the human T cell receptor C alpha enhancer. *Genes Dev.* **5,** 656–669.

14. Nabel, G. and Baltimore, D. (1987) An inducible transcription factor activates expression of human immunodeficiency virus in T cells. *Nature* **326**, 711–713; also, Erratum (1990) *Nature* **344**, 178.

15. Muesing, M. A., Smith, D. H., and Capon, D. J. (1987) Regulation of mRNA accumulation by a human immunodeficiency virus trans-activator protein. *Cell* **48**, 691–701.

16. Rosen, C. A., Sodroski, J. G., and Haseltine, W. A. (1985) The location of cis-acting regulatory sequences in the human T cell lymphotropic virus type III (HTLV-III/LAV) long terminal repeat. *Cell* **41**, 813–823.

17. Sodroski, J., Patarca, R., Rosen, C., Wong-Staal, F., and Haseltine, W. (1985) Location of the trans-activating region on the genome of human T-cell lymphotropic virus type III. *Science* **229**, 74–77.

18. Arya, S. K., Guo, C., Josephs, S. F., and Wong-Staal, F. (1985) Trans-activator gene of human T-lymphotropic virus type III (HTLV-III). *Science* **229**, 69–73.

19. Kao, S. Y., Calman, A. F., Luciw, P. A., and Peterlin, B. M. (1987) Anti-termination of transcription within the long terminal repeat of HIV-1 by tat gene product. *Nature* **330**, 489–493.

20. Laspia, M. F., Rice, A. P., and Mathews, M. B. (1989) HIV-1 Tat protein increases transcriptional initiation and stabilizes elongation. *Cell* **59**, 283–292.

21. Lu, X., Welsh, T. M., and Peterlin, B. M. (1993) The human immunodeficiency virus type 1 long terminal repeat specifies two different transcription complexes, only one of which is regulated by Tat. *J. Virol.* **67**, 1752–1760.

22. Selby, M. J., Bain, E. S., Luciw, P. A., and Peterlin, B. M. (1989) Structure, sequence, and position of the stem-loop in tar determine transcriptional elongation by tat through the HIV-1 long terminal repeat. *Genes Dev.* **3**, 547–558.

23. Koken, S. E., van, W. J., Goudsmit, J., Berkhout, B., and Geelen, J. L. (1992) Natural variants of the HIV-1 long terminal repeat: analysis of promoters with duplicated DNA regulatory motifs. *Virology* **191**, 968–972.

24. Michael, N. L., d'Arcy, L., Ehrenberg, P. K., and Redfield, R. R. (1994) Naturally occurring genotypes of the human immunodeficiency virus type 1 long terminal repeat display a wide range of basal and Tat-induced transcriptional activities. *J. Virol.* **68**, 3163–3174.

25. Michael, N. L., Vahey, M. T., d'Arcy, L., Ehrenberg, P. K., Mosca, J. D., Rappaport, J., and Redfield, R. R. (1994) Negative-strand RNA transcripts are produced in human immunodeficiency virus type 1-infected cells and patients by a novel promoter downregulated by Tat. *J. Virol.* **68**, 979–987.

26. Gorman, C. M., Moffat, L. F., and Howard, B. H. (1982) Recombinant genomes which express chloramphenicol acetyltransferase in mammalian cells. *Mol. Cell Biol.* **2**, 1044–1051.

20

In Vitro Techniques for Studies of HIV-1 Promoter Activity

Fabio Romerio and David M. Margolis

1. Introduction

A rather unique feature of the human immunodeficiency virus type-1 (HIV-1) is the structural complexity of the regulatory sequences located in the long-terminal repeat (LTR) promoter region and the number of cellular and viral transcription factors known to interact with these sequences and modulate HIV gene expression (*see* **ref.** *1*). The HIV-1 LTR can be schematically divided into four functional regions: (1) the negative regulatory element (NRE) encompassing nuceotides -350 to -190 with respect to the transcription start site; (2) the enhancer (-140 to -81), containing two binding sites for the transcription factor NFκB; (3) the basal promoter (located between -80 and $+1$), including a typical TATAA box and three binding sites for the transcription factor Sp1; and (4) the trans-activation response (TAR) element, a bulged stem-and-loop structure present in the nascent RNA ($+1$ to $+59$) transcript that provides a binding site for Tat activation of HIV-1 transcription. In addition, a novel regulatory DNA element, named IST (Initiator of Short Transcripts), has been shown to be present in the HIV-1 LTR (position -5 to $+26$), encompassing the binding site for transcription factors YY1 and late SV40 transcription factor (LSF, or CP-2, or LBP-1) (*see* **refs.** *2* and *3*). IST directs the RNA polymerase II to synthesize short (59–61 nt), correctly initiated, nonpolyadenylated transcripts that prematurely terminate at the TAR stem–loop structure. The function of these transcripts remains unclear (*see* **ref.** *4*).

Because of the complexity of the HIV-1 regulatory sequences, an accurate assessment of the contribution of specific cis- or trans-acting elements to the HIV-1 transcription is often difficult to obtain from in vivo studies. Cotrans-

From: *Methods in Molecular Medicine, Vol. 17: HIV Protocols*
Edited by: N. L. Michael and J. H. Kim © Humana Press Inc., Totowa, NJ

fection of HIV-1 LTR-driven reporter genes or viral molecular clones, along with vectors expressing specific transcription factors, offers a means to study HIV-1 promoter activity in vivo. Nonetheless, these assays may present several drawbacks, namely difficulties in estimating the effects due to the overexpression of transcription factors or to external factors that might interfere with the system under analysis. In general, any element that may influence the HIV-1 promoter activity and escape experimental control also affects the accuracy and reproducibility of the experiments. Therefore, in vitro techniques are employed as a means to study HIV-1 transcription under rigorously controlled conditions. These methods allow a deeper and more accurate understanding of all the components involved in the regulation of HIV-1 gene expression at the transcriptional level. Additionally, the information obtained from these experiments may be helpful in planning in vivo approaches to study HIV-1 transcriptional regulation.

Here, we describe a two-step procedure for the in vitro study of the HIV-1 promoter. In the first step, the in vitro transcription reaction, a plasmid DNA carrying sequences from the HIV-1 promoter is incubated in the presence of nuclear extract and ribonucleotides. Transcription factors present in nuclear extract (prepared according to the procedure reported in **ref. 5**) retain their ability to assemble functional preinitiation complexes with DNA template and, in the presence of ribonucleotides, synthesize RNA molecules. The use of mutated cis- and/or trans-acting elements as well as the employment of particular reaction conditions allow an accurate and detailed analysis of the promoter. The in vitro transcription reaction is carried out in the presence of a control plasmid to assess the promoter specificity of the observed effects.

In the second step, the synthesized RNA is purified and analyzed by either primer extension or RNase protection, providing an assessment of the rate of promoter activity. The primer extension assay (*see* **Fig. 1**) involves the annealing of a radiolabeled DNA oligonucleotide to the RNA transcript. The RNA : DNA hybrid is incubated in the presence of nucleotides and reverse transcriptase to extend the oligonucleotide from its 3'-OH terminus using RNA molecule as a template. The reverse transcriptase stops when it reaches the 5' end of the template RNA; therefore, all the extension products are of the same length. In the RNase protection assay (*see* **Fig. 1**), a radiolabeled runoff transcipt is synthesized from a bacteriophage promoter located downstream of the eukaryotic promoter; this riboprobe is complementary to the RNA to be analyzed. The RNA synthesized in the in vitro reaction of the HIV-1 promoter and the riboprobe are annealed and incubated in the presence of ribonuclease T1, which digests the single-strand sequences. The extended products from the primer extension assay or the digestion products from the RNase protection assay are subjected to separation on polyacrylamide gel and visualized by autoradiography. Changes in the levels of RNA synthesized in the in vitro

1) *in vitro* transcription reaction

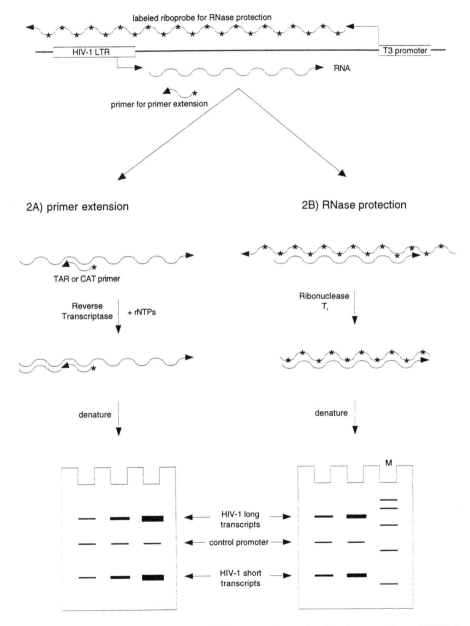

Fig. 1. Schematic representation of the procedures for in vitro studies of HIV-1 promoter activity.

Table 1
Sequence of the Oligonucleotides Used in the Primer Extension Analysis

TAR oligonucleotide: 5'-GTTCCCTAGTTAGCCAGAGAGCTCCCAGGCTC-3'
CAT oligonucleotide: 5'-GATGCCATTGGGATATATCAACGGT-3'

reaction are reflected by a corresponding variation in the intensity of the bands detected by autoradiography.

2. Materials and Reagents
2.1. Nuclear Extract, Plasmids, and Probes

Nuclear extract for in vitro transcription reactions are usually prepared according to the protocol of Dignam *(5)*. We usually prepare the HIV–LTR template and control template DNA for the in vitro transcription reaction and for the preparation of the riboprobe (in diethyl pyrocarbonate [DEPC]-treated water or RNase-free Tris-HCl, EDTA [TE]) by alkaline lysis and polyethylene glycol (PEG)-precipitation procedure (*see* **ref. 6**) or using the Quiagen Plasmid Kit (Chatsworth, CA). HIV–LTR–CAT reporter constructs are convenient templates for these studies, as they are widely available, and constructs containing a wide variety of mutations have been described. The oligonucleotide we generally use for the primer extension assay is complementary to nucleotides +56 to +24 with respect to the transcription start site. The sequence of this oligonucleotide is reported in **Table 1**: this probe allows the simultaneous detection of both long and short transcripts originating at the HIV-1 LTR. We also include the CAT reporter gene cloned downstream of the HIV-1 LTR sequences. Performing the primer extension with a mixture of these two probes and an oligonucleotide specific for the control plasmid transcripts in the presence of an internal control that allows standardization of transcriptional activity between reactions.

2.2. Reagents and Buffers

As a general rule, all the reagents, buffers and disposable supplies used for these procedures should be RNase-free: they can be directly purchased or sterilized by autoclave or filtration. We use ribonucleotides, RNase inhibitor, 50 mM MgCl$_2$, 100 mM DTT, avian myeloblastosis virus (AMV) reverse transcriptase, 5× AMV reaction buffer, T3 RNA polymerase, and 5× T3 reaction buffer from Promega (Madison, WI). Polynucleotide kinase (PNK) and 10× PNK buffer are available from New England Biolabs (Beverly, MA). We obtain deoxynucleotides from Perkin Elmer; proteinase K, pheno/chloroform/ isoamyl alcohol (25 : 24 : 1), yeast tRNA, Quick Spin Columns, and RNase-free DNase1 from Boehringer Mannheim (Indianapolis, IN); radiolabeled nucleotides [γ-^{32}P] adenosine triphospahte (ATP) (10 mCi/mL; 6000 Ci/mmol) and [α-^{32}P]CTP (20 mCi/mL; 800 Ci/mmole) from Amersham (Arlingtom Heights, IL). RNase T1 can be obtained from GIBCO (Gaithersburg, MD) and formamide (Molecular Biology Grade) from Sigma (St. Louis, MO). The composition of the nuclear extract buffer is as follows: 20 mM HEPES pH 7.9, 100 mM KCl, 0.2 mM EDTA, 0.5 mM DTT, 20% glycerol. The transcription reaction stop buffer contains 0.3 M Tris-HCl, pH 7.4, 0.3 M sodium acetate, 0.5% sodium dodecyl sulfate (SDS), 2 mM EDTA, and 3 µg/mL tRNA. The 10× hybridization buffer is 0.4 M piperazine-N,N'-bis[2-ethanesulfonic acid] (PIPES), pH 6.4, 10 mM EDTA, 4 M NaCl. The RNase digestion buffer contains 10 mM Tris-HCl, pH 7.5, 0.3 M NaCl, and 5 mM EDTA. The sequencing gel loading buffer contains 95% formamide, 20 mM EDTA, 0.025% bromphenol (BPB), and 0.025% xylenecyanol (XC). The RNA loading buffer is 80% formamide, 1mM EDTA, 0.025% BPB, and 0.025% XC.

3. Methods

3.1. In Vitro Transcription Reaction

1. The in vitro transcription reaction produces RNA to be analyzed; 200 ng of LTR-driven plasmid and control promoter-driven plasmid (such as β-globin or Adenovirus Major Late promoter) are mixed with 50 µg of nuclear extract in a reaction containing 1.6 mM rNTPs, 20 U of RNase inhibitor (Promega,Madison,WI), and 3 mM MgCl$_2$.

2. The final volume is brought to 25 µL with nuclear extract buffer, and the reaction is incubated at 30°C for 1 h. The reaction can be supplemented with purified or semipurified column fractions containing activators, repressors, or control transcription factors if desired. The reaction is stopped by adding 175 µL of stop buffer and 10 µL of 20 mg/mL proteinase K.

3. After 30 min at 55°C, the reaction is extracted twice with phenol/chloroform/isoamyl alcohol and the RNA is precipitated with 10 µg of tRNA and 500 µL of ethanol by incubating the tubes in a dry ice/ethanol bath for 15 min and by centrifugation at 4°C for 30 min at 10,000g.

4. The amount of LTR-driven and control promoter-driven plasmids should be optimized on a case-by-case basis. The linearization of the plasmid template is not necessary; in our laboratory, we usually employ supercoiled plasmid. The volume of nuclear extract depends on the protein concentration; however, the Dignam protocol for nuclear extract preparation is standardized so that the final concentration is usually between 6 and 8 mg/mL.

3.2. Primer Extension

1. The primers used to detect transcripts are labeled by phosphorylation at the 5' terminus: 50–100 ng of oligonucleotide are mixed with 1µL of 10× PNK buffer, 4µL of [γ-^{32}P]ATP and 1 µL of 10 U/µL T4 Polynucleotides kinase in a 10-µL reaction and incubated at 37°C for 30–60 min.

2. The labeled probe is separated from the unincorporated nucleotides by gel filtration over a Quick Spin Column according to the instructions of the manufacturer.
3. The RNA recovered form the in vitro transcription reaction is mixed with 5×10^4 cpm of labeled primer in a 20-µL reaction containing 2 µL of 10× hybridization buffer and 0.4 µL of 10% SDS: the RNA and the primer are annealed by incubating the mixture overnight at 37°C.
4. The next day, 10 µg of tRNA, 9 µL of 9 M ammonium acetate, and 190 µL of water are added and the RNA is precipitated to 200 µL in isopropanol at room temperature for 15 min.
5. The RNA is pelleted by centrifugation at 4°C for 30 min at 15,000 rpm, washed with 70% ethanol, and resuspended in 10 µL of a mixture containing 10 mM DTT, 2 U/µL (1 µL) of RNase inhibitor, 1× AMV buffer, 1 mM dNTPs, and 0.1 U/µL AMV reverse transcriptase.
6. After 1 h at 42°C, the reaction is stopped by adding 20 µL of sequencing gel loading buffer. The samples (2000–5000 cpm) are heated at 85°C for 5 min, chilled on ice and run on a 8–12% denaturing polyacrylamide gel for 2–2.5 h at 200 V.
7. At the end of the run, the gel is transferred to film and autoradiography is performed for 16–24 h at –70°C with one intensifying screen.
8. It is a good practice to purify the oligonucleotides to be labeled over a 12–16% denaturing polyacrylamide gel; this reduces the chances of obtaining nonspecific priming and spurious bands (*see* **ref. 7**). The addition of formamide to the hybridization mix provides more stringent conditions for annealing; the optimal concentration of formamide must be determined empirically. In reactions requiring the employment of two or more primers, it is important to use 5×10^4 cpm per each probe in order to obtain signals detectable with relatively short exposures.

3.3. RNase Protection

1. The first step of this assay is the in vitro synthesis of the radiolabeled riboprobe; this is performed by incubating 0.25–0.5 µg of linearized and gel-purified plasmid template with 1 µL of 5× T3 RNA Pol buffer, 10 µL of 24 mM 3 rNTPs (ATP, GTP, and TTP), 2 µL of 100 mM DTT, 5 µL of [α-^{32}P]CTP, 20 U of RNase inhibitor, and 10 U of T3 RNA polymerase in a 20-µL reaction for 30–60 min at 37°C with 50 µg of proteinase K and 20 µL of 10% SDS.
2. 500,000 cpm of labeled RNA is added to 10–40 µg of total RNA, dried in vacuo, and resuspended in 3 µL of 10X hybridization buffer, 3 µL of water, and 24 µL of formamide and then heated to 85°C for 20 min with occasional stirring to dissolve the nucleic acids.
3. Anneal 8-12 h between 45°C and 55°C. Optimum annealing temperatures will vary for each driver–tracer combination and will need to be titrated.
4. Cool reaction to room temperature and add 300 µL of RNase digestion buffer. Add concentrated RNase T1 and RNase A to final concentrations of 2 and 40 µg/mL, respectively, and incubate at 22°C for 1 h.

5. Add 20 μL of 10% SDS and 10 μL of freshly prepared 10 mg/μL Proteinase K and digest at 37°C for 30 min.
6. After phenol/chloroform and chloroform extraction, RNA is ethanol precipitated with 10 μg of tRNA, resuspended in RNA loading buffer and run on a 6% denaturing polyacrylamide gel at 30 V/cm. The gel is then exposed at −70°C.

4. Notes

1. The accuracy and reliability of the assays described depend on the inclusion of appropriate controls. As mentioned before, a control promoter, whose activity remains unaffected by the addition of the factors to be tested, should be included in the in vitro transcription reaction. A control promoter that has widely been used is that derived from the Adenovirus Major Late promoter (*see* **ref. 3**). Specific probes should be designed for the analysis of the control RNA.
2. The sensitivity of these assays allows quantitative analysis of the results; this can be performed by scanning the autoradiograms with a densitometer and by analyzing the acquired image with an appropriate software (Image 1.59 for Apple Macintosh; National Institutes of Health, Bethesda, MD).

References

1. Haseltine, W. A. and Wong-Staal, F. (1991) *Genetic Structure and Regulation of HIV,* Raven, New York.
2. Margolis, D. M., Somasundaran, M., and Green, M. R. (1994) Human transcription factor YY1 represses human immunodeficiency virus type 1 transcription and virion production. *J. Virol.* **68,** 905–910.
3. Kato, H., Horikoshi, M., and Roeder, R. G. (1991) Repression of HIV-1 transcription by a cellular protein. *Science* **251,** 1476–1479.
4. Sheldon, M., Ratnasabapathy, R., and Hernandez, N. (1993) Characterization of the inducer of short transcripts, a human immunodeficieny virus type 1 transcriptional element that activates the transcription of short RNAs. *Mole. Cell. Biol.* **13,** 1251–1263.
5. Dignam, D. J. (1990) Preparation of extracts from higher eukaryotes. *Meth. Enzymol.* **182,** 194–203.
6. Sambrook, J., Fritsch, E. F., and Maniatis, T. (eds.) (1989) *Molecular Cloning: A Laboratory Manual,* 2nd ed., Cold Spring Harbor Laboratory Press, Cold Spring Harbor, NY.
7. Ausubel, F. M., Brent, R., Kingston, R. E. Moore, D. D., Seidman, J. G., Smith, J. A., and Struhl, K. (1995) *Current Protocols in Molecular Biology,* Wiley, New York.

21

Detection of Polymorphisms in the HIV-1 Coreceptor CCR5 Using Single-Strand Conformation Polymorphism

Maureen P. Martin and Mary Carrington

1. Introduction

The *CCR5* gene encodes a cell-surface chemokine receptor molecule, which serves as a coreceptor for macrophage-tropic strains of HIV-1 *(1–3)*. Mutations in this gene may alter expression or function of the protein product, thereby altering chemokine binding or HIV-1 infection of cells on which the receptor is normally expressed. Indeed, it was recently shown that individuals homozygous for a mutant allele (*CCR5-Δ32*) characterized by a 32-bp deletion in the coding region of the *CCR5* gene, are relatively resistant to HIV-1 infection *(4–6)*. This allele causes a frame shift at amino acid 185, and homozygous individuals fail to express detectable cell-surface CCR5 molecules. It is possible that other as-yet unidentified variants play a role in HIV-1 infectivity and outcome. Several additional mutations, most of which are single-base substitutions, have been identified in the coding region of the *CCR5* gene using the single-strand conformation polymorphism (SSCP) technique *(7)*.

SSCP analysis following amplification of DNA by the polymerase chain reaction (PCR) is a rapid and sensitive screening method for detecting sequence variation, including single-base substitutions, over relatively short fragments of DNA *(8,9)*. It has been utilized successfully in detecting mutations in a number of genes, including *CFTR (10,11)* and *p53 (12)*, as well as detection of polymorphisms in HLA class II genes *(13)*.

The method involves PCR amplification of DNA, followed by heat denaturation and resolution of the amplified product by polyacrylamide gel electrophoresis. Under nondenaturing gel conditions, single-stranded DNA has a unique conformation (secondary structure) that is in part determined by

From: *Methods in Molecular Medicine, Vol. 17: HIV Protocols*
Edited by: N. L. Michael and J. H. Kim © Humana Press Inc., Totowa, NJ

intrastrand molecular interactions, and therefore by its nucleotide sequence. Changes in the latter are detected as a shift in electrophoretic mobility owing to the alteration in the folded structure. Theoretically, DNA amplified from an individual homozygous at a given region exhibits two bands on electrophoresis corresponding to each of the single DNA strands, whereas in a heterozygote four bands are seen. Occasionally, additional bands are observed because some DNA sequences can have more than one stable conformation, but these tend to be lighter in intensity (**Fig. 1**). Homoduplex bands are also present, and heteroduplex bands can be observed in heterozygotes because it is difficult to inhibit reannealing of the DNA completely. However, these duplex patterns can be useful in distinguishing heterozygous from homozygous samples.

A simple protocol for SSCP that has been used to detect polymorphisms in the *CCR5* gene as well as other chemokine receptor genes is described herein. It involves PCR amplification of portions of the gene with radioactively labeled dNTP, denaturation of the amplified sample, gel electrophoresis, and interpretation of the banding patterns observed. The entire procedure can be performed in a day, and thus serves as an efficient and accurate means for screening large numbers of samples. Overall, the method is able to detect 90–100% of polymorphisms in a given gene if the conditions are optimized *(9,11)*. Modifications for optimization of the technique are described in the **Subheading 4.**

2. Materials

2.1. Polymerase Chain Reaction (PCR)

1. DNA isolated from tissue or cells using standard protocols, at a concentration of 50–100 ng/μL.
2. Oligonucleotide primers (10 μ*M*) complementary to the 5'- and 3'-ends of the region to be amplified. Ideally the size of the PCR product for SSCP should be between 200 and 400-bp (*see* **Note 1**).
3. α^{32}P-dCTP (3000 Ci/mmol). Obtain fresh, and use within 2 wk (the half-life of ^{32}P is about 14 d).
4. Deoxynucleotide stock solution (2 m*M* each dATP, dTTP, and dGTP plus 1 m*M* dCTP). The concentration of dCTP in the deoxynucleotide stock solution is decreased by 50% in order to ensure adequate incorporation of labeled dCTP.
5. 10X PCR buffer (100 m*M* Tris-HCl, pH 8.3, 500 m*M* KCl).
6. 25 m*M* MgCl$_2$.
7. *Taq* DNA polymerase (5 U/μL) (*see* **Note 2**).

2.2. Preparation of PCR Product for Electrophoresis

1. Ninety-six-well plates for dilution of samples. These should be heat-resistant, since the samples will be heat denatured at 95°C.
2. Denaturing dye solution (10 m*M* NaOH, 95% formamide, 0.05% bromphenol blue, and 0.05% xylene cyanol).

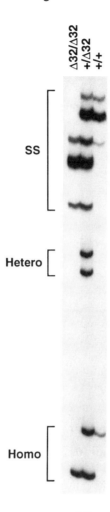

Fig. 1. SSCP analysis of the *CCR5* gene following PCR amplification. Electrophoresis was performed on a 5% acrylamide gel at 4°C for 4.5 h +/+ = homozygous wild-type; Δ32/Δ32 = homozygous deletion mutation; +/Δ32 = heterozygous wild type and deletion mutation. SS denotes the single-strand conformations (note the presence of extra bands representing alternative conformers). Heteroduplex bands (hetero) are present in the heterozygous sample. A single homoduplex band (homo) is seen in the homozygotes, whereas two bands are present in the heterozygote.

3. Heating block or oven for heat denaturation of samples.
4. Ice for rapid cooling of denatured samples.

2.3. Nondenaturing Gel Electrophoresis

1. Glass plates (20 × 40 cm) for casting gels.

2. 0.04-cm spacers and combs.
3. 30% Acrylamide/*bis*-acrylamide (37.5:1) solution.
4. 10X Tris-borate-EDTA (TBE) buffer (0.89 M Tris, 0.89 M boric acid, 0.02 M disodium EDTA, pH 8.3).
5. 10% Ammonium persulfate: This should be made fresh weekly.
6. *N,N,N',N'*-Tetramethylethylenediamine (TEMED).
7. Sequencing gel apparatus and high-voltage power supply.
8. Whatman filter paper.
9. Vacuum gel dryer.
10. X-ray film and film developer (automatic or manual).

3. Methods
3.1. PCR

1. Prepare the PCR reaction in a total volume of 20 μL containing: 2 μL 50–100 ng/μL DNA, 2 μL of each primer (final concentration 1 μM), 2 μL dNTP stock solution, 2 μL 10X PCR buffer (final concentration 1X), 1.6 μL $MgCl_2$ (final concentration 2 mM), 0.05–0.1 μL a^{32}P-dCTP (3000 Ci/mmol) (*see* **Note 3**), and 0.1 μL *Taq* polymerase.
2. Amplify in a programmable thermal cycler using the following parameters: 3 min at 94°C, 30 cycles of 30 s at 94°C, 30 s at 55°C, and 1 min at 72°C, with a final 5-min extension step at 72°C.
3. Store samples at –20°C if electrophoresis cannot be performed immediately. Ideally, the samples should be run as soon as possible after PCR to avoid radioactive decay and consequent loss of signal.

3.2. Preparation of PCR Product for Electrophoresis

1. Mix 3 μL of PCR product with 10 μL denaturing dye solution in a 96-well plate.
2. Immediately before loading the gel, heat the samples at 95°C for 3 min and place on ice. Rapid cooling minimizes the formation of duplex DNA.

3.3. Nondenaturing Gel Electrophoresis

1. Prepare the gel mix by combining 52 mL distilled deionized H_2O, 15 mL 30% acrylamide/*bis*-acrylamide (final concentration 5%), 7.5 mL 10X TBE (final concentration 1X), 450 μL 10% ammonium persulfate, and 45 μL TEMED (75 mL final volume). It may be necessary to change the concentration of the gel, use a different gel matrix, or alter conditions such as temperature or time to identify all alleles.
2. Immediately pour a 20 × 40 × 0.04 cm gel (*see* **Note 4**) using the above mix, taking care to avoid air bubbles, and allow to polymerize for at least 1 h. TEMED will cause the gel to polymerize, so it is essential to pour the gel soon after adding it to the mix.
3. Assemble the gel on the sequencing gel apparatus, and load the upper and lower chambers with 1X TBE running buffer. Remove the comb, and rinse the wells with electrophoresis buffer (1X TBE).

4. Load 3.5 μL of each sample mix. Control samples of known alleles should also be included on each gel.
5. Run the gel at 50 W constant power for 4.5 h at 4°C. Constant cooling of the gel is critical for good band separation. Alternatively, the gel may be run overnight at room temperature (10 W) (*see* **Notes 5** and **6**).
6. After electrophoresis, carefully pry the glass plates apart, lay Whatman paper directly onto the gel, slowly lift the gel from the plate, cover the gel with plastic film, and dry on a vacuum gel dryer for 30 min. Expose to X-ray film overnight.
7. Develop film. If the gel is over- or underexposed, the duration of exposure can be appropriately altered.

3.4. Interpretation of Results

Compare the banding patterns of the unknown samples with the control samples. All unique banding patterns should be sequenced and run on future gels as controls. **Figure 1** illustrates an SSCP gel in which an amplified portion of the *CCR5* gene was analyzed. Lane one represents DNA from an individual homozygous for the deletion allele ($\Delta32/\Delta32$), whereas lane 3 represents homozygosity for the wild type allele. DNA from a heterozygous individual ($+/\Delta32$, lane 2) has bands representing both wild-type and deletion alleles. In addition, heteroduplex bands, which have a faster mobility, are noted in the second lane below the bands representing the single-stranded DNA. Homoduplexes have the fastest mobility and these bands are present below the heteroduplex bands (*see* **Notes 7–10**).

4. Notes

1. The ideal product size for SSCP analysis is 200–400 bp, but larger fragments can also be analyzed if the fragment is first digested with appropriate restriction enzymes.
2. The use of Amplitaq Gold™ (Perkin-Elmer Corp., Norwalk, CT) which is a modified *Taq* polymerase is useful in improving the efficiency and specificity of the PCR. The enzyme does not become enzymatically active until it is exposed to a high temperature (95°C for 8–12 min), thus conferring a hot start to the PCR.
3. An alternative to the use of radiolabled dNTP in the PCR, is to label the primers with γ^{32}P-dATP. This can, in some cases, increase the specific activity of the PCR product *(14)*.
4. The gel plates should be free of irregularities, such as warping, because this will cause the gel to run unevenly, thereby distorting the banding patterns and making interpretation of the results difficult.
5. The temperature of the gel is an important variable and the best separation is obtained at 4°C. Care should be taken to maintain constant cooling of the gel. Therefore, if electrophoresis is performed in a cold room, the door should be kept closed as much as possible to ensure that the temperature is maintained at 4°C. In addition, if there are leaks in the gel rig with resultant loss of buffer, the gel will overheat, and band separation will be affected.

6. If the power supply is interrupted by a power outage, for example, and power is then reapplied, separation of bands will be suboptimal.

7. The concentration of acrylamide and the percentage of crosslinking (defined as the ratio of *bis*-acrylamide/acrylamide X 100), both exert an effect on the pore size of the gel and can influence separation patterns *(9)*. In some cases, it may be necessary to change these variables in order to identify all mutations.

8. For some base changes, the addition of 2–10% glycerol may significantly alter the mobility of the strands and may therefore be useful for efficient strand separation. It has been suggested that glycerol may act as a weak denaturant, thus partially opening the folded single-stranded DNA *(14)*. Addition of other neutral compounds, such as urea, formamide, dimethylsulfoxide (DMSO), 1-butanol, glucose, or sucrose, at a concentration of 5–10% may also improve resolution of some polymorphisms by their effect on the secondary structure *(9)*.

9. Commercially available gel matrices, such as Long Ranger™ (FMC BioProducts, Rockland, ME), may also improve strand separation.

10. Samples loaded at the ends of the gel usually have curved bands because of inefficient cooling, so in some cases, it may be necessary to rerun these samples in the center of the gel.

References

1. Alkhatib, G., Combadiere, C., Broder, C. C., Feng, Y., Kennedy, P. E., Murphy, P. M., and Berger, E. A. (1996) CC CKR5: A RANTES, MIP-1a, MIP-1b receptor as a fusion cofactor for macrophage-tropic HIV-1. *Science* **272,** 1955–1962.

2. Deng, H., Liu, R., Ellmeier, W., Choe, S., Unutmaz, D., Burkhart, M., Di Marzio, P., Marmon, A., Sutton, R., and Hill, C. M. (1996) Identification of a major co-receptor for primary isolates of HIV-1. *Nature* **381,** 661–666.

3. Dragic, T., Litwin, V., Allaway, G. P., Martin, S. R., Huang, Y., Nagashima, K. A., Cayanan, C., Maddon, P. J., Koup, R. A., Moore, J. P., and Paxton, W. A. (1996) HIV-1 entry into CD4$^+$ cells is mediated by the chemokine receptor CC-CKR5. *Nature* **381,** 667–673.

4. Dean, M., Carrington, M., Winkler, C., Huttley, G. A., Smith, M. W., Allikmets, R., Goedert, J. J., Buchbinder, S.P., Vittinghoff, E., Gomperts, E., et al. (1996) Genetic restriction of HIV-1 infection and progression to AIDS by a deletion allele of the CKR5 structural gene. *Science* **273,** 1856–1862.

5. Samson, M., Libert, F., Doranz, B. J., Rucker, J., Liesnard, C., Farber, C.-M., Saragosti, S., Lapouméroulie, C., Cognaux, J., Forceille, C., et al. (1996) Resistance to HIV-1 infection in Caucasian individuals bearing mutant alleles of the CCR-5 chemokine receptor gene. *Nature* **382,** 722–725.

6. Liu, R., Paxton, W. A., Choe, S., Ceradini, D., Martin, S. R., Horuk, R., MacDonald, M., Stuhlmann, H., Koup, R. A., and Landau, N. R. (1996) Homozygous defect in HIV-1 coreceptor accounts for resistance of some multiply-exposed individuals to HIV-1 infection. *Cell* **86,** 367–377.

7. Carrington, M., Kissner, T., Gerrard, B., Ivanov, S., O'Brien, S. J., and Dean, M. (1997) Novel alleles of the chemokine receptor gene CCR5. *Am. J. Hum. Genet.* **61,** 1261–1267.

8. Orita, M., Suzuki, Y., Sekiya, T., and Hayashi, K. (1989) Rapid and sensitive detection of point mutations and DNA polymorphisms using the polymerase chain reaction. *Genomics* **5,** 874–879.

9. Glavac, D. and Dean, M. (1993) Optimization of the single-strand conformation polymorphism (SSCP) technique for detection of point mutations. *Hum. Mutation* **2,** 404–414.

10. Dean, M., White, M. B., Amos, J., Gerrard, B., Stewart, C., Khaw, K., and Leppert, M. (1990) Multiple mutations in highly conserved residues are found in mildly affected cystic fibrosis patients. *Cell* **61,** 863–870.

11. Ravnik-Glavac, M., Glavac, D., and Dean, M. (1994) Sensitivity of single-strand conformation polymorphism and heteroduplex method for mutation detection in the cystic fibrosis gene. *Hum Mol Genet* **3,** 801–807.

12. Mashiyama, S., Murakami, Y., Yoshimoto, T., and Sekiya, T. (1991) Detection of p53 gene mutations in human brain tumors by single-strand conformation polymorphism analysis of polymerase chain reaction products. *Oncogene* **6,** 1313–1318.

13. Carrington, M., Miller, T., White, M., Gerrard, B., Stewart, C., Dean, M., and Mann, D. (1992) Typing of HLA-DQA1 and DQB1 using DNA single-strand conformation polymorphism. *Hum Immunol* **33,** 208–212.

14. Hayashi, K. (1991) PCR-SSCP: a simple and sensitive method for detection of mutations in the genomic DNA. *PCR Methods Appl* **1,** 34–38.

22

Sequence-Specific Priming as a Rapid Screen for Known Mutations

Mary Carrington

1. Introduction

Mutations in a large number of genes have now been identified that ultimately alter the expression or function of the corresponding protein, thereby inducing a particular disease state. These mutations may be found frequently in the disease population, but may also be present to some extent in normal individuals. On the other hand, alterations of the prototypic or wild type allele, again affecting protein expression or function, can result in some level of protection against certain diseases. The latter situation is well-exemplified by an allele of the *CCR5* chemokine receptor gene, *CCR5Δ32*, which does not encode a functional protein on cell surfaces (*see 1* for review). Since CCR5 behaves as a coreceptor with CD4 for macrophage-tropic strains of HIV-1, homozygotes for the *CCR5Δ32* allele are highly, though not completely, protected against HIV-1 infection. Similarly, a single base change in the *CCR2* gene, *CCR2-64I*, is associated with delayed progression to AIDS after HIV-1 infection *(2)*.

Identification of novel alleles of genes can be accomplished by a number of techniques with varying levels of efficiency. Once a variant of interest has been identified, it is necessary to employ a method that allows rapid and accurate screening of large numbers of samples for that variant in order to determine its effect on a particular disease. One such method, termed sequence-specific priming technique (SSP), is commonly used for allelic differentiation of the highly polymorphic genes of the major histocompatibility complex (e.g., *3–5*). Test primers are designed to recognize only a specific allele (or specific set of alleles) by placing the complementary allele-specific base at the 3'-end of either the forward or reverse primer. Additional control primers complementary to regions conserved in all samples being tested must

From: *Methods in Molecular Medicine, Vol. 17: HIV Protocols*
Edited by: N. L. Michael and J. H. Kim   © Humana Press Inc., Totowa, NJ

be included in each amplification reaction to provide evidence that the DNA could in fact be amplified. Obviously, the control primers must amplify a region that is either sufficiently longer or shorter than that from the test primers. Thus, each amplification is a multiplex, or combination of two amplifications of a single sample in a single tube. The control primers need not recognize sequences in the same general area as that recognized by the test primers. For example, test primers for the *CCR2-64I* mutation may be multiplexed with control primers for a conserved region of the *HLA-A* gene. PCR reactions are run through an agarose gel, the gel is stained, and the presence or absence of amplified product is observed. A lane of the gel should have a single band of known size (product of control primers) if that sample is negative for the test allele, but two bands (one representing product from control primers and one from test primers) if that sample is positive for the test allele.

2. Materials

2.1. Primers

Primers may be obtained from a number of commercial sources. The primers arrive from the company dry and can be resuspended in approx 1 mL distilled water as stock primers and their optical density measured to determine their concentration. Primers that have been diluted to a working concentration can be briefly stored at 4°C, but stock primers should be kept at –70°C for long-term storage.

2.2. Polymerase Chain Reaction (PCR)

1. DNA (100 ng/µL).
2. Oligonucleotide primers (each at 10 µM).
3. Deoxynucleotide stock solution containing 2 mM of each dATP, dTTP, dGTP, and dCTP).
4. 10X PCR buffer containing 100 mM Tris-HCl, pH 8.3, and 500 mM KCl.
5. MgCl$_2$ (25 mM).
6. *Taq* polymerase.

2.3. Gel Electrophoresis

1. Horizontal gel electrophoresis apparatus and power supply. For screening large numbers of samples, it is useful to have an apparatus that holds a wide gel template in which two combs can be inserted (one beneath the other) such that 100 samples can be analyzed on a single gel.
2. 1.5% Electrophoresis-grade agarose in 1X TAE buffer (10X TAE = 0.4 *M* Tris and 0.01 *M* EDTA titrated to pH 7.8 with glacial acetic acid) and 0.5 µg/mL ethidium bromide. Ethidium bromide is a mutagen and should be handled with gloves when in solution and with both gloves and face mask when weighing the powder form.

3. Orange G loading buffer (0.5% Orange G, 20% Ficoll, and 100 m*M* EDTA).
4. UV light box with Polaroid camera attachment.

3. Methods
3.1. Primer Design

The specificity of the test primers for the corresponding allele is of critical importance in this technique (*see* **Note 1**). Generally, specific amplification can be achieved using either a specific forward primer with a generic reverse primer or vice versa, and therefore, this technique is useful in screening samples for a known point substitution. For example, given the following alleles, which differ by a single base substitution, a primer (let us assume it is a forward primer) specific for allele 2 can be designed.

Allele 1 3' . . . ggt atc tcg aag gtt ctg aca at<u>A</u> cct tga . . . 5'
Allele 2 3' . . . ggt atc tcg aag gtt ctg aca at<u>C</u> cct tga . . . 5'
Primer 2A 5'tag agc ttc caa gac tgt ta<u>G</u> 3'

Since this forward primer is specific for allele 2, allele 1 should not amplify, even though the reverse primer recognizes both allele 1 and allele 2 (*see* **Note 2**).

3.2. PCR

1. The recipe for a single sample amplification is given below (*see* **Note 3**). However, a PCR cocktail containing all ingredients except for the DNA can be prepared and distributed into tubes containing individual DNA samples.

10X PCR buffer	1.5 μL
dNTP mix	1.5 μL
MgCl$_2$	1.2 μL
Forward test primer	1.5 μL
Reverse test primer	1.5 μL
Forward control primer	1.5 μL
Reverse control primer	1.5 μL
Taq	0.1 μL
DNA	0.4 μL
dH$_2$O	4.3 μL
Total	15 μL

2. The DNA is amplified in a programmable thermal cycler using the following parameters: 3 min at 94°C, follwed by 30 cycles of 30 s at 94°C, 30 s at 55°C, and 1 min at 72°C, with a final 5-min extension step at 72°C.
3. Samples may be stored at −20°C if necessary.

3.3. Gel Electrophoresis

1. Prepare the agarose gel by mixing 1.5% agarose in 1X TAE. For example, for the Centipede Wide-format Electrophoresis System (Model # D-3, Owl Scientific, Woburn, MA), add 9 g of agarose to 600 mL 1X TAE, and heat to a boil until the

agarose is in solution. Cool for 20 min to about 60°C (determine temperature with a thermometer), add 15 mL ethidium bromide to the solution, and gently mix. Pour into gel template, and allow this to solidify for 30 min. If the agarose is too hot, the template will warp.

2. Pour 1 L 1X TAE into the electrophoresis chamber, which will ultimately cover the top of the agarose gel.
3. Add 3 µL Orange G loading buffer to each sample and load 12–15 µL into the wells of the gel.
4. Apply 50–60 V to the gel for 1.5 h. For smaller gels, both parameters can be reduced.
5. Place gel over a UV light source (using protective eye wear), and photograph the gel for a permanent record.

4. Notes

1. If any product is observed using the specific primer in amplification of negative control samples, it may be necessary to alter the amplification conditions, such as temperature or buffer composition (particularly $MgCl_2$). Additionally, the introduction of an additional site of noncomplementarity between the test primer and the negative control DNA, which necessarily introduces a single site of noncomplementarity between the test primer and the corresponding allele, may also eliminate nonspecific amplification. Let us assume that primer 2A given in the **Subheading 3.** erroneously amplifies allele 1 to some degree. Primer 2B shown below would be a second option for specific amplification of allele 2.

   Allele 1 3' . . . ggt atc tcg aag gtt ctg a<u>C</u>a at<u>A</u> cct tga . . . 5'
   Allele 2 3' . . . ggt atc tcg aag gtt ctg a<u>C</u>a at<u>C</u> cct tga . . . 5'
   Primer 2B 5'tag agc ttc caa gac t<u>A</u>t ta<u>G</u> 3'

   This strategy provides increased specificity of the primer in spite of a single mismatch between the primer and the corresponding allele, provided this mismatch is located 4–6 bases from the 3'-end of the primer.
2. An alternative to using four primers (two test and two control) is the use of three primers where two forward primers, for example, recognizing neighboring sequences (100–200 bp apart) are designed such that one primer is specific for the test allele, but the other is generic (i.e., recognizes all known alleles). A single generic reverse primer is then designed that will amplify with both the test and control forward primers. In this situation, it is generally best to place the forward test primer closer to the reverse primer and the forward control primer further away. The test allele in positive samples tends to amplify more vigorously than the control in this configuration.
3. The small volume in the amplification reaction (15 µL) is used in order to conserve reagents. Therefore, the material evaporates readily if the tubes remain at room temperature for long periods of time (e.g., overnight), and this results in little or no visible product on the gels, even after reconstitution with buffer. Also, condensation on the sides of the tubes of the amplified material may be observed after amplification, and it is then necessary to spin the tubes very briefly in a centrifuge.

References

1. D'Souza, M. P. (1996) Chemokines and HIV-1 second receptors. *Nat. Genet.* **2,** 1293–1300.
2. Smith, M. W., Dean, M., Carrington, M., et al. (1997) Contrasting genetic influence of *CCR2* and *CCR5* variants on HIV-1 infection and disease progression. *Science* **277,** 959–965.
3. Powis, S. H., Tonks, S., Mockridge, I., et al. (1993) Alleles and haplotypes of the MHC-encoded ABC transporters *TAP1* and *TAP2*. *Immunogenet.* **37,** 373–380.
4. Krausa, P., Bodmer, J. G., and Browning, M.J. (1993) Defining the common subtypes of HLA-A9, A10, A28, and A19 by use of ARMS/PCR. *Tissue Antigens* **42,** 91–99.
5. Bunce, M., O'Neill, C. M., Barnardo, M. C. N. M., et al. (1995) Phototyping: comprehensive DNA typing for HLA-A, B, C, DRB1, DRB3, DRB4, DRB5 & DQB1 by PCR with 144 primer mixes utilizing sequence-specific primers (PCR-SSP). *Tissue Antigens* **46,** 355–367.

23

Quantitation of HIV-1 Entry Cofactor Expression

James L. Riley and Richard G. Carroll

1. Introduction

Infection of CD4+ T-lymphocytes by HIV-1 is initiated by binding of the virus to the CD4 receptor on the lymphocyte surface, followed by fusion of the virus with the cell membrane *(1)*. However, expression of CD4 on certain non-human cells does not render them permissive for HIV-1 entry, suggesting that an additional entry cofactor is required *(2,3)*. The identity of this cofactor remained elusive until Berger and colleagues reported that the α-chemokine receptor fusin/CXCR4 functions as the entry cofactor for T-cell line-tropic isolates of HIV-1 *(4)*. Subsequent progress in the field has been rapid. To date, three β-chemokine receptors (CCR2b, CCR3, and CCR5) have also been identified as HIV-1 entry cofactors *(5)*.

It has been shown that in CD4+ T cells, HIV-1 entry cofactor expression is regulated by the method of cell activation *(6)*. Therefore, susceptibility or resistance to infection may be determined by how a cell is activated. Furthermore, chemokine receptors are a potential target for therapies or vaccines, as individuals homozygous for a defective CCR5 allele are resistant to infection and heterozygotes may have a slower course of disease progression *(5)*.

The method presented here provides a highly reproducible way to measure the levels of mRNA encoding these receptors in cells. Since it is an RT-PCR based assay, it is much faster and more sensitive than a Northern blot. Furthermore, the low levels of expression of some chemokine receptor transcripts present formidable obstacles to detection by Northern blotting. The use of limited PCR cycles and liquid hybridization permits semiquantitative analysis of transcript levels. Rather than relying on a standard curve containing known quantities of RNA, which is laborious and requires intensive quality control to

From: *Methods in Molecular Medicine, Vol. 17: HIV Protocols*
Edited by: N. L. Michael and J. H. Kim © Humana Press Inc., Totowa, NJ

ensure reproducibility, this assay uses twofold dilutions of the reverse transcriptase (RT) product to demonstrate a linear response to template input.

The importance of being within the linear response range of the assay can not be overstated. Valid comparisons between samples can only be made in the linear range of the PCR reaction. To make each PCR reaction fall in the linear response range, the initial cDNA template is diluted depending on the receptor transcript being assayed. For example, CXCR4 is highly expressed, so the RT product is diluted 300-fold, whereas CCR5 is poorly expressed and only a 1:3 dilution is made. There are two advantages of dilution of cDNA input versus altering the number of PCR cycles: first, multiple chemokine receptors can be analyzed in the same thermocycler and second, relative differences between chemokine receptor transcripts can be assessed.

A disadvantage of this protocol is that absolute numbers generated from analysis are relative to that one experiment and cannot be used to compare two separate experiments. In order to compare separate experiments, the data must be normalized to the expression of a housekeeping gene such as GADPH. This also suffers from drawbacks in time course experiments, as GADPH transcript expression is enhanced by cell activation.

This method can be broken down into four sections: RNA preparation, cDNA preparation, PCR reaction, and liquid hybridization.

2. Materials

2.1. RNA Isolation

In order do this assay, high-quality RNA is required. RNase-free conditions must be maintained throughout the isolation. These include using dedicated, RNase-free reagents, dedicated micropipetors with aerosol-resistant tips, and, if possible, a dedicated RNA preparation area.

1. RNA STAT-60 (cat. no. CS-111, Tel-Test, Friendswood, TX).
2. Chloroform (cat. no. 36, 692-7, Sigma, St. Louis, MO).
3. Isopropanol (cat. no. 9084-01, J. T. Baker, Philipsburg, NJ).
4. Ethanol (cat. no. 64-17-5, Warner Graham, Cockeysville, MD).
5. RNase-free DNase I (cat no. 776785, Boehringer Mannheim, Indianapolis, IN).
6. Phenol/chloroform/isoamyl alcohol (cat. no. 101001, Boehringer Mannheim).
7. DEPC dH$_2$0 cat. no. (351-068-130, Quality Biological, Gaithersburg, MD).
8. 3 M Sodium acetate, pH 5.2 (cat no. 351-035-060, Quality Biological).
9. Screw-top microcentrifuge tubes (cat. no. 72.692.005, Sarstedt, Newton, NC).

2.2. RT-PCR Reaction

1. StrataScript RT-PCR Kit (cat. no. 200420, Stratagene, LaJolla, CA).

2.3. PCR Reaction

1. Ampli-Taq DNA polymerase 5 U/µL (cat. no. 0145, Perkin Elmer Cetus, Philipsburg, NJ).

2. 10X PCR buffer (cat. no. N808-0129, Perkin Elmer).
3. 200 mM dNTPs (cat. no. 1 227 049, Boehringer Mannheim) made up in ddH$_2$0 and aliquoted into 300-μL stocks stored at –20°C.
4. GeneAmp PCR reaction tubes (cat. no. N801-0180, Perkin Elmer Cetus).
5. Primers (*see* **Table 2** for sequence) 20 mM and aliquoted into 150-μL stocks.
6. Mineral oil (cat. no. 186-2302, Perkin Elmer Cetus),

2.4. Liquid Hybridization

1. Hoefer Minigel System (cat. nos. SE 275, SE 2119-2 1.0-mm, SE 211A-10 1.0-mm, SE 250). This system is ideal because multiple gels can be poured simultaneously, run times are fast, and loading and cleanup are easy. Other systems can be used, but if the gels are more than 1.0 mm thick, they may have to be dried down before exposure to film or the PhosphorImager.
2. 40% solution of Acrylamide/bis-acrylamide 19:1 (cat. no. A 2917, Sigma).
3. 10% ammonium persulfate, freshly made (cat. no. 15523-012, Gibco-BRL, Gaithersburg, MD).
4. TEMED (cat. no. 5524UB, Gibco-BRL).
5. [γ-^{32}P]ATP 6000 Ci/mmol (cat. no. NEG-002Z, DuPont NEN, Boston, MA).
6. T4 Polynucleotide kinase (cat. no. 201L, New England Biolabs, Beverly, MA).
7. 10X TBE (cat. no. 351-001-130, Quality Biological)
8. Oligo hybridization buffer: 66.7 mM NaCl, 45 mM ethylene diamine tetra-acetic acid (EDTA), pH 8.0.
9. 5X DNA loading solution (cat. no. 351-028-030, Quality Biological).

3. Methods
3.1. Preparation of Total RNA from Cells

This section is adapted from the RNA STAT-60 protocol provided by the manufacturer. The end product of this step is purified cellular RNA free from DNA.

1. Spin the cells down in a polypropylene tube in a Beckman table top centrifuge for 7 min at 600g. Remove the supernatant. Do not wash the cells. By flicking, break up the pellet, and add 1 mL of RNA STAT per 1 × 10^7 cells. Gently pipet the RNA STAT solution up and down several times to ensure all of the cells come in contact with the RNA STAT. Transfer the RNA mixture to screw-top microcentrifuge tubes in 1 mL aliquots. Thus, for 3 × 10^7 cells, three microcentrifuge tubes are needed. In order to prevent the RNA from degrading during preparation, process the tubes in batches of 12.
2. Allow the mixture to sit at room temperature for 5 min. Note that at this point the samples can be stored at –70°C for at least a month. Add 0.3 mL of CHCl$_3$ and shake vigorously for 15 s. Do not vortex. Allow the samples to sit for 3 min and spin at full speed in a 4°C microcentrifuge for 15 min.
3. Carefully transfer the upper phase to a new tube, and add 0.5 mL of isopropanol. Store the samples at room temperature for 10 min, and spin at full speed in a 4°C microcentrifuge for 10 min. Carefully remove the supernatant. A white pellet should be visible at this point.

4. Add 0.7 mL of 75% EtOH made with DEPC dH$_2$0 to each sample, mix, and spin at full speed in a 4°C microcentrifuge for 5 min. Carefully remove all of the supernatant. After most of the supernatant is removed, a 1 min spin and the use of a thin gel loading tip is useful to remove the remaining supernatant.

5. Air dry for a few minutes and resuspend the pellets in 0.13 mL of DEPC water. At this point, if multiple tubes were used for the same sample, they may be recombined; keep the total volume for each sample at 0.13 mL in order to reduce the number of tubes for subsequent steps. The pellets resuspend with little effort; if they do not, high levels of genomic DNA may be present.

6. Add 15 µL of virtually any restriction enzyme buffer (the authors use NEB #2) and 5 µL RNase-free DNase I. Place at 37°C for 30 min. Add 150 µL of phenol:chloroform:isoamyl alcohol (25:24:1) to each sample, vortex, and spin at full speed in a 4°C microcentrifuge for 10 min.

7. Transfer the top phase to a new tube and add 15 µL of 3 *M* sodium acetate and 375 µL of 100% EtOH. Store at –70°C for at least 30 min, and spin at full speed in a 4°C microcentrifuge for 15 min. Remove the supernatant, and wash with 75% EtOH as above. Resuspend the pellet in 25 µL per 1 × 10^7 initial cells. Remove 2 µL of sample to perform spectrophotometric determination of RNA concentration.

3.2 Making cDNA from RNA

This protocol is adapted from the manufacturer's procedure (Stratagene) and will make cDNA from the RNA. A duplicate of each sample is created that will not receive RT enzyme. This is a critical control for subsequent PCR reactions, because it demonstrates that all the observed signal is derived from input RNA rather than contaminating genomic DNA.

1. In a clean area free of any plasmid DNA (a dedicated biosafety hood is ideal) mix 5 µg of RNA with DEPC water to a volume of 38 µL in a 2-mL screw-top tube. For each RNA sample, make two cDNA reactions. RT will be added to only one of these. Add 3 µL of the random primers supplied in the kit, mix, and denature at 65°C for 5 min. Allow the reaction to cool to room temperature for 10 min.

2. Make two Master Mixes. All reagents are in the kit. Add the RNase block inhibitor immediately prior to use. Multiply the 1X value by the number of samples +1 to get the volume needed to make each mix. To avoid confusion, it is advisable to separate the tubes based on whether they receive RT or not (*see* **Table 1**).

3. Add 9 µL of each Master Mix to the proper samples. Mix and place samples at 37°C for 1 h. Transfer samples to 90°C for 5 min and then place on ice.

3.3. Chemokine Receptor PCR of cDNA Samples

Standard PCR precautions should be employed to minimize the risk of contamination. These include the use of a dedicated biohazard hood and dedicated PCR reagents, as well as the use of aerosol-resistant pipet tips during all manipulations.

Table 1
RT Master Mix

1X	No RT Mix	10X
5 μL	10X First Strand Buffer	50 μL
2 μL	100 m*M* dNTPs	20 μL
1 μL	RNase Block Inhibitor	10 μL
1 μL	DEPC dH₂0	10 μL
1X	RT Mix	10X
5 μL	10X First Strand Buffer	50 μL
2 μL	100 m*M* dNTPs	20 μL
1 μL	RNase Block Inhibitor	10 μL
1 μL	Reverse Transcriptase	10 μL

Table 2
Primer Sequences for HIV Coreceptor Genes

Gene	Sequence
CXCR4	
CXCR4-489	5' CCA CCA ACA GTC AGA GGC CAA GGA AGC TGT
CXCR4-1122	5' TCT GTG TTA GCT GGA GTG AAA ACT TGA AGA
CCR2b	
CCR2B-1024	5' TCT CTC GGT GTT CTT CCG AAA GCA CAT CAC
CCR2B-1640	5' CCC TTT GCT CAC CTT TGT CTT TGT CCA GGC
CCR3	
CCR3-239	5' GTA CCA CAT CCT ACT ATG ATG ACG TGG GCC
CCR3-745	5' AGT CTC TTC AAA CAA CTC TTC AGT CTC ATA
CCR5	
CCR5-42	5' GGG TGG AAC AAG ATG GAT TAT CAA GTG TCA
CCR5-601	5' GAA AAT GAG AGC TGC AGG TGT AAT GAA GAC
GADPH	
GADPH-61	5' ATG GGG AAG GTG AAG GTC GGA GTC AAC GGA
GADPH-433	5' AGG GGG CAG AGA TGA TGA CCC TTT TGG CTC

The sets of primers in **Table 2** have been designed specifically to amplify only the gene of choice and have been used successfully in many experiments. The number after the primer name refers to the nucleotide position of the 5' base.

1. Using the following table as a guide, dilute each cDNA sample in DEPC water, depending on the receptor transcript being assayed.

Chemokine Receptor	Dilution
CCR5	1:3
CCR2b	1:3
CCR3	1:3
CXCR4	1:300
GADPH	1:3000

2. Add two drops of mineral oil to each PCR tube. Four PCR tubes are needed for each RNA sample. One tube will receive 10 μL of the RT⁻ template and the other three will receive twofold increments of the RT⁺ template (2.5, 5, and 10 μL). In accordance with the earlier example, if there are nine RNA samples, 36 PCR reactions will be needed.

3. Make a Master PCR Mix:

1X	Reagent	(36+2)X
5 μL	10X PCR Buffer	190 μL
5 μL	200 m*M* dNTPs	190 μL
2.5 μL	Chemokine receptor primer 1	95 μL
2.5 μL	Chemokine receptor primer 2	95 μL
24.5 μL	Molecular biology grade water	931 μL
0.5 μL	Taq DNA polymerase 5U/μL	19 μL

Add 40 μL of Master Mix to each PCR tube.

4. For each RNA sample, add the following amounts of product and water to each PCR tube.

Tube #	Sample	Product	Water
1	RT⁻	10 μL	0 μL
2	RT⁺	2.5 μL	7.5 μL
3	RT⁺	5 μL	5 μL
4	RT⁺	10 μL	0 μL

5. Once all of the cDNA products are added, quickly vortex each tube, and do a quick spin to separate the mineral oil from the PCR reaction.

6. Place the tubes in a PCR machine, and start the following program: 95°C for 30 min, 55 °C for 30 min, 72 °C for 1 h 30 min, 4 °C soak. Repeat for 25 cycles.

3.4. Liquid Hybridization

The oligos are used as probes in the liquid hybridization protocol are identified in **Table 3**.

1. To end-label oligonucleotides, mix the following: 10 pmol of primer in 8.5 μL of ddH₂0, 2 μL of 10X kinase buffer (comes with enzyme), 8 μL of [γ-^{32}P]ATP, and 1.5 μL of T4 polynucleotide kinase. Incubate at 37°C for 1 h. Purify the oligonucleotide from the free nucleotides. Several methods are available *(7)*. The authors use Elutip-d-columns (cat. no. 27370, Schleicher and Schuell). Count the purified probe in a scintillation counter.

Table 3

Probe	Sequence
Fusin-840	5'-CCA GGA GGA TGA AGG AGT CGA TGC TGA TCC-3'
CCR3-513	5'-CAT GGC CAA AAA CCC AGT TAT GCC CCC TGA-3'
CCR2B-1239	5'-TAC AGG TTT CTA TTG TTC AAC AAA CCC TTG-3'
CCR5-81	5'-GGG CTC CGA TGT ATA ATA ATT GAT GTC ATA-3'

2. Pour 6% acrylamide/1X TBE gels. Let the gels cure for at least 1 h before use.
3. Transfer 30 μL of PCR reaction to new tube. Avoid transferring the mineral oil. Add 200,000 counts of labeled oligonucleotide in 10 mL of oligo hybridization buffer to each sample. Vortex the samples, and briefly spin in a microfuge dedicated for use with radioactive materials.
4. Load into a thermocycler dedicated for radioactive materials and run the following program: 95°C for 5 min, 55 °C for 10 min, then cool slowly to room temperature.
5. Add 10 μL of 5X DNA loading buffer to each sample. Vortex the samples and spin briefly. Load 15 μL of each sample onto the gel. Run at 180 V for 1 h and transfer the gel to saran wrap. Expose to PhosphorImager for 1 h or to film overnight.
6. Quantitate each band using the PhosphorImager to check to see if two fold differences in signal strength can be detected.

4. Notes

1. The key to successful use of this protocol is high-quality RNA that is free of genomic DNA. So far, it appears that the chemokine receptors have few, if any, introns; therefore, there is no way to distinguish contaminating DNA from RNA. The RT-negative control will show if any contaminating DNA is present, but the only way to correct a contamination is to retreat the sample with DNase.
2. Preparation of the RNA is best done in microcentrifuge tubes. Larger tubes may used but a loss in recovery should be expected.
3. Before preceding to the cDNA synthesis step, it is good idea to run the RNA out on a RNA denaturing gel *(7)* to check for intact RNA, the presence of detectable genomic DNA, and to confirm the OD reading.
4. The initial dilution for each chemokine receptor has been worked out, depending on the system used, this dilution may have to be modified to ensure a linear response.
5. Extreme care must be given to keep reagents free of contamination. Aliquoting reagents, separate rooms for cDNA synthesis and PCR, the use of ART tips, a clean biosafety hood to set up reactions, and frequent changing of gloves go far in preventing contamination.
6. The probe for the liquid hybridization is effective for at least 2 wk. Radioactive decay should be accounted for when determining the amount of probe needed for 200,000 counts.

References

1. Sattentau, Q. J. and Moore, J. P. (1993) The role of CD4 in HIV binding and entry. *Phil. Trans. Royal Soc. Lond.* **342**, 59–66.
2. Maddon, P. J., Dalgleish, A. G., McDougal, J. S., Clapham, P. R., Weiss, R. A., and Axel, R. (1986) The T4 gene encodes the AIDS virus receptor and is expressed in the immune system and the brain. *Cell* **47**, 333–348.
3. Clapham, P. R., Blanc, D., and Weiss, R. A. (1991) Specific cell surface requirements for infection of CD4 positive cells by human immunodeficiency virus type 1, type 2, and simian immunodeficiency virus. *Virology* **181**, 703–715.
4. Feng, Y., Broder, C. C., Kennedy, P. E., and Berger, E. A. (1996) HIV-1 entry cofactor: functional cDNA cloning of a seven-transmembrane G protein-coupled receptor. *Science* **272**, 872–877.
5. Fauci, A. S. (1996) Host factors and the pathogenesis of HIV-induced disease. *Nature* **384**, 529–534.
6. Carroll, R. G., Riley, J. L., Levine, B. L., Feng, Y., Kaushal, K., Ritchey, D. W., et al. (1997) Differential regulation of HIV-1 fusion cofactor expression by CD28 costimulation of CD4+ cells. *Science* **276**, 273–276.
7. Sambrook, J., Fritsch, E. F., and Maniatis, T. (1989) *Molecular Cloning: A Laboratory Manual, 2nd ed.* Cold Spring Harbor Laboratory Press.

24

Retrovirus-Mediated Gene Transduction of SupT1 Cells

Jen-Tsun J. Lin and Jerome H. Kim

1. Introduction

From a technical perspective, the introduction and stable expression of exogenes in mammalian cells has advanced rapidly in the last few years. Of the gene transduction methodologies, genetic transfer using retroviruses remains the most popular. There are two components of a generic retroviral vector (RV) gene transduction system. The first component is the retroviral vector, which has 5' and 3' long terminal repeats, a packaging site (Ψ site), a selectable marker, the exogene, and a polypurine tract. In many respects, it resembles the retrovirus from which it is derived; however, structural gene coding sequences for *gag*, *pol*, and *env* have been removed or modified. The presence of the Ψ site allows the vector to be "packaged" into a viral particle in the presence of appropriate structural gene products. These products are supplied by the packaging line, which in its simplest form contains genes encoding retroviral Gag, Pol, and Env. The production of infectious virus is prevented because the sequences that permit the encapsulation of viral nucleic acid, the Ψ site, have selectively been deleted. To prevent successful recombination after the introduction of a Ψ site by the retroviral vector containing the exogene, the structural genes are often introduced separately (i.e., as separate coding units) or "poison" sequences are added around the Ψ site of the retroviral vector.

The RV is introduced into a packaging line, the retroviral particle is assembled around the RV RNA as it would around retrovirus wild-type RNA. Supernatant from the packaging line can then be used to "infect" a target cell; the retroviral strategy of reverse transcription, creation of a cDNA, and inte-

From: *Methods in Molecular Medicine, Vol. 17: HIV Protocols*
Edited by: N. L. Michael and J. H. Kim © Humana Press Inc., Totowa, NJ

gration of the cDNA into the host cell genome is accomplished. The presence of a selectable marker allows those cells receiving the exogene to be enriched in the population.

Here, we described an retrovirus-mediated gene transfer protocol that has been used successfully in our hands to introduce the vector containing a selectable marker into the SupT1 cell line.

2. Materials and Reagents
2.1. Plasmid Vectors Used for Transduction

In order to generate a gene-transducing retroviral particle, retroviral vector plasmid must contain the following elements: (1) a packaging signal; (2) the gene of interest; (3) a selectable marker. The three selectable markers that have been used widely in recent years are the neomycin-phosphotransferase gene (*neo*), which confers resistance to Geneticin (Gibco-BRL, Grand Island, NY); the hygromycin-resistance gene (*hyg*), which confers resistance to Hygromycin B (Boeheringer, Indianapolis, IN); and the puromycin-resistant gene (*pur*), which allows cells to survive in Puromycin (Clontech, Palo Alto, CA). The plasmids that are introduced into the packaging cell lines should be purified by CsCl, although those that are purifed by the Quiagen plasmid kit (Quiagen, Chatsworth, CA) are typically comparable.

In these studies we have used pN2-neo, modified to carry the interleukin-7 gene (pN2-IL7, **ref. *1***). In the pN2-IL7 vector the neo resistance gene is upstream of the IL-7 exogene. The IL-7 gene is expressed on a bi-cistronic message; it would alternatively have been possible to insert a second, independent promoter upstream of the IL-7 gene.

2.2. Cell Lines

There are several commercially available packaging cell lines. Of these, we use the GP+E 86 ecotopic packaging cell line and PA317 amphotropic cell lines; both are available from ATCC (Rockville, MD). Fibroblast cell lines are used to determine the titer of the retrovirus generated by the transfected packaging cell lines. Either mouse NIH 3T3 (ATCC) or human HT 1080 cell lines (ATCC) can be used. The SupT1 CD4+ T cell line can be obtained from the NIH AIDS Reagent program.

2.3. Solutions and Reagents for Cell Culture

Trypsin/EDTA (Gibco-BRL); phosphate-buffered saline (PBS, Gibco-BRL). Growth medium for packing cell lines and HT 1080 cell line: Dulbecco's Modified Eagle's Medium (DMEM, Gibco-BRL) supplemented 10% heat-inactivated fetal calf serum (Hyclone, Logan, UT); L-glutamine 2 mM; penicillin-streptomycin (100× stock, Gibco-BRL) (*see* **Note 1**). Growth medium for SupT1 cell line:

RPMI 1640 medium (Gibco-BRL) supplemented with 10% heat-inactivated fetal calf serum (Hyclone, Logan, UT); L-glutamine (2 mM); penicillin–streptomycin (100×) (*see* **Note 1**).

3. Methods
3.1. Generation of Retrovirus

1. On the day prior to transfection, plate 5×10^5 GP+E86 cells onto a 10-cm tissue culture dish. Replace the media 4 h before the transfection. Quiagen-purified retroviral vectors pN2-IL7 are first introduced into the GP+E86 ecotropic packaging line by calcium phosphate coprecipitation. (Mammalian Transfection Kit, Stratagene, La Jolla, CA according to the manufacturer's specifications, *see* **Note 2**).
2. Two days after transfection, virus is harvested, and 1-µL to 1-mL samples of virus-containing medium containing 4 µg/mL polybrene (Sigma, St. Louis, MO) are incubated at 37°C with 1×10^6 PA317 (amphotropic packaging cell line) cells. After 4 h, the medium is removed, and the cells are washed twice with phosphate-buffered saline. The PA317 cells infected with pN2-IL7 are placed in fresh medium and incubated at 37°C.
3. Two days after infection, the PA317 cells are placed in DMEM medium, supplemented with 10% fetal bovine solution (FBS) and Geneticin (G418) at a final concentration of 600 µg/mL (*see* **Note 3**). Neomycin-resistant clones are isolated (after 21–28 d), and the supernatant harvested from the G418-resistant PA317 packaging cells is filtered through a 0.45-µm filter, aliquoted, and stored at –70°C. It is assayed for RV titer and for wild-type virus contamination on the HT1080 cells. Briefly, 5×10^5 HT1080 cells are placed in each well of a 24-well plate. Supernatant from PA317 cells is diluted serially from 10^1 to 10^6. The supernatant is used to infect the HT1080 cells as described above. The cells are selected in G418, and 2–4 wk postinfection, the number of clones is counted in the first nonconfluent well. The dilution at which this happens is designated the "titer" of the packaging line (e.g., if the first nonconfluent well is at 10^4, then the virus titer is 1×10^{-4}/mL). The clone with the highest RV titer is used to infect SupT1 cells (*see* **Note 4**).

3.2. Transduction Protocol

1. 1×10^7 SupT1 cells are infected with supernatant containing 10^5–10^6 colony-forming units (CFUs)/mL of virus in the presence of 4 µg/mL polybrene (Sigma) at 37°C overnight.
2. After 24 h of incubation, the efficiency of transduction is increased by centrifuging the cell–virus mixture at approx 300g for 2 h at 32°C and incubating at 32°C for another 2 h.
3. After the infection the cells are washed once in PBS and cultured in RPMI medium for 2 d. The cells are then maintained in RPMI medium with a concentration of G418 up to 800 µg/mL.

3.3. Detection of Helper Virus in Transduced SupT1 Cell Culture

1. One mL of supernatant harvested from G418-resistant SupT1 cells containing 4 μg/mL polybrene is used to infect 1×10^6 HT1080 cells overnight.
2. Two days after the infection, the HT1080 cells are switched to DMEM with 10% FBS and 600 μg/mL G418. If there is any helper virus present after being vector packaged in the PA317 cells, neomycin-resistant HT1080 colonies will appear 3 wk after G418 selection.

4. Notes

1. All culture media should be filtered through a 0.45-μm filter before use. The fetal calf serum is heat-inactivated at 56°C for 1 h.
2. Calcium phospate coprecipitation (Stratagene [La Jolla, CA], per manufacturer's instructions; **ref. 2**). It is important to mix the DNA slowly with solution provided by the manufacturer. The mixed calcium phosphate precipitate solution should stand at room temperature for at least 20 min before being applied to the cell culture. The precipitated solution should be added, dropwise, onto the cells. The color of the culture media will become pinkish if the pH of the buffered DNA–calcium precipitate is correct. The DNA–precipitate is left in the cell culture for 22 h before being washed away.
3. Stable virus-producing cell lines were generated as described *(3)*. The GP+E86 packaging cell line is used to generate the pseudovirus, and transient transfection of the vector into the GP+E86 cells is used. The supernatant harvested from the transiently transfected ecotrophic GP+E86 cells is then used to infect the amphotrophic PA317 cell line. The stable, vector-producing PA317 cells are selected, colonies are picked and expanded individually.
4. Usually the higher the titer used, the higher the transduction efficiency. However, 1×10^5 CFUs/mL viral titers are sufficient to transduce the target cells. The retrovirus is also temperature-sensitive, therefore careful handling of the viral stocks, to prevent repeated thawing and freezing, is necessary.

References

1. Kim, J. H., Ratto, S., Sitz, K. V., Mosca, J. D., McLinden, R. J., Tencer, K. L., Vahey, M. T., St. Louis, D., Birx, D. L., and Redfield, R. R. (1994) Consequences of stable transduction and antigen-inducible expression of the human IL-7 gene in tetanus toxoid specific T-cells. *Hum. Gene Ther.* **5,** 1457.
2. Chen, C. and Okayama, H. (1987) High efficiency transformation of mammalian cells by plasmid DNA. *Mol. Cell. Biol.* **7,** 2745.
3. Miller, A. D., Law, M. F., and Verma, I. M. (1985) Generation of helper-free amphotropic retroviruses that transduce a dominant-acting methotrexate-resistent DHFR gene. *Mol. Cell. Biol.* **5,** 431.

25

Cloning of HIV Single-Strand DNA Binding Protein from Human Lymphocyte Lambda gt11 Expression Library with [^{32}P]-Oligomers

Sook-Jin Hur and Derhsing Lai

1. Introduction

Lambda gt11 cDNA libraries are routinely used for gene isolation with antibody and oligomer probes *(1–3)*. Briefly, a recombinant DNA library from different types of cells is constructed in a λgt 11 expression vector. The foreign peptides (antigens) are expressed as a β-galactosidase fusion protein in *E. coli*. Because the *lacZ* gene has a strong promoter, the fusion proteins comprise from 0.1–4% of the total *E. coli* proteins *(1–3)*. The expressed fusion antigens are transferred onto nitrocellulose filters and then probed with antibodies to identify the targets containing the specific, cognate epitope.

Here, we used a [^{32}P]-labeled, phosphorothio oligonucleotide (PS), lys 3, a 24-mer complementary to the 3' end of rRNAlys3, which interacts with the HIV primer binding site (PBS), to identify HIV single-strand DNA binding protein(s) from a human lymphocyte λgt 11 expression library *(4–5)*. Several clones were isolated and confirmed by two rounds of screening and enrichment. Two clones bound to the PBS of single-strand DNA specifically by colony hybridization. The putative sequence was amplified by PCR and subcloned into a TA vector (CLONTECH, Palo Alto, CA) utilizing primers specific for a λgt 11 vector. This sequence was obtained by automatic sequencing (ABI, Columbia, MD). This experimental procedure can be also applied in the identification of other DNA or RNA specific binding proteins.

From: *Methods in Molecular Medicine, Vol. 17: HIV Protocols*
Edited by: N. L. Michael and J. H. Kim © Humana Press Inc., Totowa, NJ

2. Methods

2.1. Bacterial Culture Plating

1. Streak *E. coli* Y 1090r– from 25% glycerol stock onto an LB agar (1.5%) plate without $MgSO_4$ containing 100 μg/mL ampicillin and incubate at 37°C overnight.
2. Pick a single colony of *E. coli* Y1090r– and inoculate in LB broth with 0.01 M MgSO4, 0.2% maltose, and 100 μg/mL ampicillin on a shaker at 200 rpm and 37°C until OD_{600} = 2.0.

2.2. Lambda gt 11 Library Titering:

1. Dilution 1: Transfer 2 μL of the library lysate (human lymphocyte cDNA λgt 11 library) into 1 mL of 1× dilution buffer (0.1 M NaCl, 0.01 M $MgSO_4$, 0.035 M Tris·HCl pH 7.5). This is a 1:500 dilution.
2. Dilution 2: Transfer 2 μL of Dilution 1 into 1 mL of 1× λ dilution buffer. Final dilution is 1:25000.
3. Prepare four tubes containing 100 μL of 1× dilution buffer and 200 μL of *E. coli* Y1090r– culture (OD_{600} = 2). Transfer Dilution 2 to each tube with 0 (background control), 2, 5, and 10 μL, respectively.
4. Incubate four tubes at 37°C for 15 min, then add 3 mL of melted LB top agarose (0.7%) with 10 M $MgSO_4$ to each of the tubes. The melted LB agarose can be maintained at 42–45°C.
5. Mix well and immediately pour them onto four 90-mm LB agar-containing $MgSO_4$ plates, respectively. Swirl the plates to allow even spreading of the top agarose.
6. Cool plates at room temperature for 15 min and transfer to 37°C for 7–8 h continuous incubation.
7. Count the plaques (transparent spots) to determine the titer (plaque-forming units [PFU]/mL) of λgt 11 library.
   Formula: PFU/mL = ([# of plaques] [# μL used]) × (dilution factor) × (10^3 μL/mL). Titers calculation: (416/10) × 2.5 × 10^5 × 10^3 (μL/mL) = 1.04 x 10^{10} (PFU/mL) of human lymphocyte λgt 11 library.

2.3. Lambda gt 11 Library Plating

1. Prepare 30 LB agar (1.5%) plates containing 0.01 M MgSO4 and 100 μL/mL ampicillin in 150-mm plates (50–65 mL of LB medium per plate) and store at 4°C.
2. Melt 0.7% top agarose in LB broth (7 mL for each plate) and warm to 42–45°C.
3. Dilute 1 μL of library lysate (=1.04 × 10^7 pfu) in 1 mL of 1× λ dilution buffer (1:1000 dilution).
4. Prepare thirty 15 mL polypropylene centrifuge tubes (Sarstedt, Sarstedt, NC) containing 466 μL of *E. coli* Y1090r– culture (OD_{600} = 2) and 100 μL of 1× λ dilution buffer. Transfer 3 μL (3.12 × 10^4 pfu) of 1/1000 dilution to each tube and incubate tubes at 37°C for 15 min.
5. Transfer 7 mL of top agarose (0.7%) to tube and plaques pour onto the 150-mm LB agar plates prepared in **Step 1**. After the solidification, invert the plates and

incubate at 37°C until plaques reach 1-mm in diameter. Chill the plates at 4°C overnight (total 3.12×10^4 pfu for 150-mm plate).

2.4. Library Screening Using [^{32}P] PS Oligomer

1. Mark the BA-S NC nitrocellulose filters (132 mm) with numbers corresponding to the plates, and soak them in 10 mM isopropyl-β-D-thiogalactopyranoside (IPTG) solution for 30 min at room temperature. Transfer the nitrocellulose filters on the 3M paper to air-dry

2. Place the IPTG-nitrocellulose filter on the top of λgt agarose plates. Use an 18-gage needle (with waterproof ink) to punch three holes on the agar plate through the filter to orient the filter on the plate. Transfer the plates (with filter cover) to 37°C for 2 h.

3. Lift the filters from the plates and let them air-dry at room temperature.

4. Block the filters with 1× binding buffer (25 mM HEPES, pH 7.9, 3 mM MgCl$_2$, 4 mM KCl) with 5% nonfat dried milk, 1 mM phenylmethylsulfonyl fluoride (PMSF), and 1 mM DL-dithiothreitol (DTT) at 4°C for 30 min.

5. Wash the filters with 1× binding buffer with 0.25% nonfat dried milk with 1 mM PMSF, and 1 mM DTT, at 4°C for 15 min and repeat three times.

6. Incubate the [^{32}P]-lys3 probes with filters in 1× binding buffer containing 1 mM DTT, 1 mM PMSF, 0.25% nonfat dry milk, and 10 μg/mL sonicated denatured salmon sperm DNA at 4°C overnight.

7. Wash filters several times with a large amount of 1× binding buffer, 1 mM DTT, 1 mM PMFS, and 0.25% nonfat dry milk (500 mL each time), at least 2 L until the buffer contains no detectable radioactivity.

8. Place the filters on paper to remove excess liquid.

9. Cover the filters with polyvinyl chloride laboratory wrap and expose to X-ray film for 8–24 h.

10. Develop the autoradiographs and identify colonies on the film.

11. Repeat the whole procedure (second-round screening) to confirm the positive plaques at the same position.

12. Align the filters to the plates to select positive clones.

13. Remove the positive clones with a Pasteur pipet by punching through the agar plate and transferring into 0.5 mL of 1× λ dilution buffer with 20 μL of chloroform at 4°C overnight. The λ phage will diffuse into 0.5 mL buffer overnight.

14. Transfer 1 μL of λ phage elution from **step 13** into 2 mL of 1× phage dilution buffer (1:2000 dilution).

15. From 2 mL of λ phage elution (1:2000 dilution), 1 μL of supernatant (200–1000 plaques on a 150-mm plate) is transferred into 15 mL polyprolylene centrifuge tubes containing 466 μL of *E. coli* Y1090r– culture (OD$_{600}$ = 2) and 100 μL of 1× λ dilution buffer. Incubate the tubes at 37°C for 15 min.

16. Add 7 mL of soft agarose (0.75%) into each tube, and pour as top agarose on the agar plate. After the solidification, invert the plate and incubate at 37°C until plaques reach 1–2 mm in diameter (6–8 h).

17. Repeat the same procedure from **steps 1–10** to identify the single colony on the plate.

18. A single clone can be picked, as there are roughly hundreds of plaques on the plate.
19. Pick a single clone with a Pasteur pipet, and transfer it into 0.5 mL of 1 × λ phage binding buffer.
20. Confirm the positive clone by repeating **Steps 14–19** with both lys3 (positive) and negative control oligomers. The whole plate of plaques should be positive with lys3 probe and negative with negative control probe.

2.5. PCR Amplification

1. 5' and –3' oligonucleotide primers for polymerase chain reaction (PCR) amplification of the lambda insert can be purchased from CLONTECH.
2. Standard PCR is performed using –5' and –3' λgt 11 primers. Nine to 20 pmols of both primers are added to 50 µL of PCR Master buffer (2×), 45 µL of H_2O and 1 µL of λ phage elution buffer. Themocycler: 93°C 1 min, 50°C 1 min, 72°C, 2 min for 30 cycles. The final step incubates the mixture at 72°C for 5 min.
3. Run PCR products on 1% agarose TAE gel.
4. PCR products are ligated into TA vector (Invitrogen, CA) at 15°C overnight. Mix: 1 µL 10× ligation buffer; 2 µL TA vector; 5 µL PCR products; 1 µL T4 ligase; and 1 µL water.

2.6. Subcloning the PCR Products

1. Transfer 10 µL of PCR product ligation reaction into 50 µL of competent *E. coli* and keep them on ice for 30 min. Heat shock the competent cells at 42°C for 90 s, then transfer to ice for another 5 min. Add 500 µL of S.O.C. (superoptimal catabolite) solution to each tube of transformed competent cells and shake the tubes at 37°C for 1.5 h. Spread 100 µL of the transformed *E. coli* on an LB agar plate with 100 µg/mL ampicillin at 37°C overnight.
2. Pick a single colony of *E. coli* and incubate it in 5 mL LB broth with 100 µg/mL ampicillin in a shaker with 200 rpm at 37°C for 10–12 h.
3. Prepare the *E. coli* plasmid minipreps DNA purification system (Quiagen) and screen with an appropriate restriction endonuclease to release the inserted PCR product and subject the digestion reaction to electrophoresis on a 1% agarose TAE gel.
4. The insertion can also be sequenced with T7 and SP6 primers.

3. Notes

1. The success of this experiment is based on the low background of the filters after screening with radiolabeled probes. The blocking of filters is an very important step. Here we use 5% nonfat dried milk instead of 20% fetal calf serum to block the nonspecific protein binding sites on the filter. The background is low, and nonfat dried milk is much cheaper than fetal calf serum.
2. The blocking solution (25 mM HEPES, pH 7.9, 3 mM $MgCl_2$, 4 mM KCl with 5% nonfat dried milk, 1 mM PMSF, 1 mM DTT) can be reused several times. We used Complete™ protease inhibitor cocktail tablets (Boehringer Manneheim, Indianapolis, IN), instead of PMSF in later experiments. Complete™ inhibits a large spectrum of proteases.

3. The nitrocellulose filters should remain moist during all steps. If the filters are kept slightly wet, they can be repeatedly washed to reduce background noise. There are many brands of filters. Each brand of filter has its own chemical and physical qualities. For example, the DIG nonradiolabel detection system (Boehringer Mannheim, Mannheim, Germany) works better on the filter from Amersham than S&S. You need to try several brands of filters to optimize hybridization and detection.
4. For the top layer, the use of agarose has been suggested to avoid sticking to the filter during lifting (**step 4** of **Subheading 2.2.**).
5. The probe should contain 1–5 × 10^6 cpm for each incubation and the volume of hybridization fluid should be minimized to barely cover the filters.
6. Remember to label the plates and filters with pen before experiment.
7. An asymmetric, triangular, three-hole system permits the accurate and precise localization of colonies on each plate before lifting the filter (**step 2** of **Subheading 2.4.**). This helps to identify the positive clones on both filter and plate.
8. Always wear clean gloves to handle the filter; the contamination (e.g., oil and grease) on your hands may damage the filter (**step 1** of **Subheading 2.4.**).
9. All LB agar plates should be dry before use (**step 1** of **Subheading 2.2.**). One way to remove the moisture is to open the lid of the LB plates and put them under the bacterial hood for 30 min. Do not overdry.
10. Avoid confluent lysis of phage plaques on the plates (**step 5** of **Subheading 2.2.**). Do not let plaque boundaries overlap. Plaques densities vary between λ phages and their host.
11. Please handle the filters one by one during incubation and washing steps (**step 7** of **Subheading 2.4.**). This will let the solution between filters be removed and circulated. This will help reduce background.
12. You need a smooth top layer, not a ripply, bubbled top layer (**step 5** of **Subheading 2.2.**). You may have less than 10 s to pour the top layer. Practice the pouring of top layer on a blank LB agar plate. The temperature of the lower layer of the LB agar plate will dramatically affect the speed of solidification of the top layer. You can remove bubbles from the top layer by heating before the agar solidifies.
13. It is helpful practice to place the filter on the plate and lift the filter from the plate with the blunt end of a forceps. These are two critical steps of experiment. You should not adjust the position of the filter plate, and you should lift the filter precisely to avoid smearing the plaques on the filter.
14. Ligation reactions can be performed at room temperature in just 5 min by the Rapid DNA ligation kit (Boehringer Mannheim). The result is as good as 15°C overnight ligation.

References

1. Young, R. A. and Davis, R. W. (1983) Efficient isolation of genes by using antibodies probes. *Proc. Natl. Acad. Sci. USA* **80,** 1194–1198.
2. Young, R. A. and Davis, R. W. (1984) Yeast RNA polymerase II genes: Isolation with anitibody probes. *Science* **222,** 778–782.

3. Synder, M., Elledge, S., Sweetser, D., Young, R. A., and Davis, R. W. (1987) λ gt 11: Gene isolation with antibody probes and other applications. *Methods Enzymol.* **154,** 107–128.

4. Lai, D., Guo, H.-G., Gallo, R. C., and Reitz, M. (1996) Possible regulation of HIV replication by a cellular factor binding to the primer site. XI International Conference on AIDS, Abstract A1013.

5. Lai, D., Hur, S.-J., Guo, H.-G., Gallo, R. C., and Reitz, M. (1998) Evidence of regulation of HIV-1 and -2 replications by cellular factor binding to the primer binding site. Submitted.

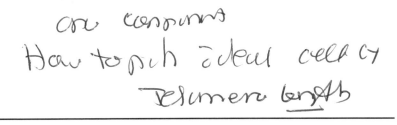

are consumed
How to pick a deal cell by
Telomere length

26

Telomeric Terminal Restriction Fragment (TRF)

Sumesh Kaushal

1. Introduction

Telomeres are protein–DNA structures at the ends of all eukaryotic chromosomes that are maintained by a unique ribonucleoprotein known as telomerase. This highly specialized RNA-dependent DNA polymerase provides a critical solution to the end-replication problem by adding TTAGGG repeats to 3' ends of human chromosomes *(1–3)*. Telomere regulation is both cell cycle and developmentally-regulated, and its control is likely to be complex *(4,5)*. There is gradual telomere shortening with age. This chromosomal pruning is presumed to be regulated by a mitotic clock, by which cell divisions are accounted *(6,7)*. After about 100 cell divisions, a cell reaches its senescence "Hayflick" limit and cell division ceases *(8)*.

Telomere length is maintained in germinal cells (spermatozoa) which constitutively express low levels of telomerase activity *(9)*. Telomerase is usually expressed in 90% of tumor cells *(10,11)* and is induced upon activation in normal cells *(12,13)*. Although a higher level of telomerase activity is observed in majority of tumors, telomere shortening is also seen in tumors undergoing rapid cell division *(14)*.

The common structural feature of eukaryotic telomeres is the presence of GC-rich repeat elements. The basic mammalian repeat element is (TTAGGG)n *(9,15)*. Because telomeric repeats are nonpalindromic and, thus, lack restriction endonuclease sites, restriction enzymes with four-base recognition sites are used to obtain long terminal restriction fragments (TRF) from chromosomal DNA, that are identified by hybridization with radiolabeled (TTAGGG)n probes. Telomeres contain approx 15,000 base pairs (bp) of repeated TTAGGG sequences in newborn humans. With age, somatic cells loose 50–200 bp/cell division, and 30–50 bp with each year of life *(16)*.

From: *Methods in Molecular Medicine, Vol. 17: HIV Protocols*
Edited by: N. L. Michael and J. H. Kim © Humana Press Inc., Totowa, NJ

Recent studies have shown that evaluation of telomere length is relevant to studies of immune system aging. This is especially important in HIV-1 disease, where a high turnover of immune system cells occurs *(17,18)*. As a result of replicative senescence in AIDS patients, shortened telomeres are seen in the CD28–CD8+ subset of T-cells suggesting a rapid expansion of CD8 cells *(19,20)*, whereas relatively stable telomeres are seen in CD4+ cells suggesting a low turnover in the CD4 compartment *(21)*. Since telomere loss is associated with cancer, aging, and replicative senescence in AIDS, telomere analysis is a valuable tool in the understanding of the complicated process of T-cell senescence. Studies designed to evaluate telomere lengths in human T-cell progenitors and subsets of mature T-cells are important since they will explore whether immune system perturbation in HIV disease is in the distal or proximal arm of hematopoiesis.

2. Materials
2.1. Reagents

1. Phosphate-buffered saline (PBS). PBS may be conveniently obtained commercially in sterile bottles. If desired, it may be made using the following recipe and sterile filtered:
   a. 1.15 g anhydrous Na_2HPO_4.
   b. 0.23 g anhydrous NaH_2PO_4.
   c. 9.00 g NaCl.
   d. Distilled H_2O to 950 mL; adjust pH to between 7.2 and 7.4 with either 1 M HCl or 1 M NaOH; add distilled H_2O to 1000 mL.
   e. Filter sterilize by passage through a 0.45 μM pore size filter unit.
2. Ficoll-Hypaque (1.077 g/L; commercially available).
3. CD4 Dynabead M-450 (Dynal Inc. Lake Success, NY).
4. CD8 Dynabead M-450 (Dynal Inc.).
5. Agarose (Gibco-BRL, Gaithersburg, MD).
6. 20X SSC.
7. 0.1 N HCl.
8. Denaturation solution: 1.5 M NaCl, 0.5 M NaOH.
9. Neutralization solution: 1.5 M NaCl, 1.0 M Tris-HCl, pH 8.0.
10. 10% sodium dodecyl sulfate (SDS).
11. TE buffer: 1 mL 1 M Tris-HCl, pH 8.0 (0.01 M), 0.2 mL 0.5 M ethylene-diamine tetra-acetic acid (EDTA), pH 8.0 (0.001 M), 98.8 mL sterile water.
12. DNA loading buffer: 50% glycerol, 0.3% Bromophenol blue, 0.3% xylene cyanol in TE.
13. 10X TBE: 108 g Tris base, 55 g boric acid, 40 mL 0.5 M EDTA, pH 8.0, distilled water in quantity sufficient to bring vol to 1 L.
14. Nylon-1 membrane (Gibco-BRL, Gaithersburg, MD).
15. Quickhyb (Stratagene, La Jolla, CA).

16. DNA STAT-60 (Tel Test Inc., Friendswood, TX).
17. DNA analysis marker system (Gibco-BRL, Gaithersburg, MD).
18. *Rsa*I and *Hinf*I restriction endonucleases (Gibco-BRL).
19. T4 polynucleotide kinase (New England Biolabs, Beverly, MA).
20. Telomeric repeat-specific 18-mer probe (TTAGGG)3.
21. γ^{32}P-ATP (New England Nuclear, Inc., Boston, MA).
22. G-25 Spin column (5 Prime-3 Prime Inc., Boulder, CO).
23. Fetal calf serum (FCS) (Hyclone Labs., Logan, UT).
24. Chloroform.
25. 75% ethanol.
26. Isopropanol.
27. Ethidium bromide, 20 mg/mL solution.

2.2. Apparatus

1. Microcentrifuge.
2. Agarose gel electrophoresis apparatus.
3. Water bath.
4. Power supply.
5. UV-cross linker.
6. PhosphorImager.

3. Methods
3.1. Immunomagnetic Separation of CD4/CD8 Cells

CD4 and CD8 cells are separated by positive selection using M-450 Dynabeads. CD8 cells are separated first, followed by CD4 isolation from CD8-depleted cells.

1. Resuspend Ficoll-Hypaque density gradient separated peripheral blood mononuclear cells (PBMC) (*see* **Note 1**) in 2% FCS/PBS, and chill on ice.
2. Estimate number of target cells and pipet out the required volume of Dynabead M-450 CD8 according to manufacturer recommendations.
3. Add Dynabead M-450 CD8 preparation to cell sample, and incubate at 4°C with gentle shaking for 1–2 h.
4. Isolate rosetted cells by placing test tube in magnetic particle concentrator (MPC) for 2–3 min.
5. Remove the unbound cells from tube while bound cells are attached to the test tube wall by MPC.
6. Save the unbound cell fraction for further isolation of CD4 cells.
7. Wash the isolated cells 4–5 times in 2% FCS/PBS by spin at 500*g* for 10 min.
8. Isolated cells can be now lysed in DNA-STAT or subjected to secondary purification.
9. Isolate the CD4 population in a similar fashion using CD4 specific Dynabead M-450.

3.2. Isolation of Chromosomal DNA

1. Remove supernatant from the cells by centrifugation at 500g for 10 min, lyse cell pellet in DNA STAT-60 (1 mL/5 × 10^6 cells), and homogenize by repetitive pipeting (*see* **Note 2**).
2. Add 0.2 mL of chloroform/1 mL of DNA STAT-60 to lysate, recap the sample tube, shake for 15 s, and let stand at room temp for 2–3 min.
3. Separate organic and aqueous phases by centrifugation at 12,000g for 15 min at 4°C. Carefully remove the upper aqueous phase without disrupting the interphase, and transfer to a fresh tube.
4. Add an equal volume of isopropanol to the aqueous phase, mix, and allow DNA to precipitate for 15 min at room temperature. Centrifuge at 12,000g for 10 min at 4°C. DNA will precipitate as a clear or white pellet at the bottom of the tube.
5. Discard supernatant, wash DNA pellet once with 1 mL of 75% ethanol, and centrifuge at 7500g (max) for 5 min at 4°C. Discard supernatant and air dry DNA pellet at room temperature.
6. Resuspend DNA pellet in TE buffer, pH 8.0. Incubate at 50°C for 15 min to expedite dissolution of DNA. Determine DNA concentration and store samples at 4°C.

3.3. Enzymatic Digestion of DNA

1. Diulte 8 µg of purified genomic DNA in a total of 46 µL of *Rsa*I reaction buffer (50 mM Tris-HCl, 10 mM MgCl$_2$, pH 8.0).
2. Gently mix the contents and add 20 U (2 µL) each of *Hinf* I and *Rsa*I restriction endonucleases.
3. Briefly spin the tube and incubate sample in 37°C H$_2$O bath overnight (*see* **Note 3**).

3.4. Southern Blot Transfer

1. After the overnight restriction digestion, briefly spin the tube and add 2.5 µL of 10X DNA gel loading buffer.
2. Electrophorese the sample overnight at 40 V through a 0.6% agarose gel in 1X TBE buffer containing 0.5 µg/mL ethidium bromide at 4°C.
3. Once the bromophenol dye reaches within 1 cm of the end of the gel end, stop electrophoresis, and photograph the gel.
4. Rock gel in 0.2 N HCl for 10 min at room temperature, followed by denaturation solution for 45 min, and neutralization solution for 30 min.
5. Perform Southern blot transfer to a nylon membrane in 10X SSC buffer for 24 h (*see* **Note 4** and **Chapter 9**).
6. After blotting, UV crosslink nylon membrane at 1200 µJoule in a UV crosslinking device. Wash in 2X SSC for 5 min and let the membrane air dry at room temperature.
7. Cut the mol-wt marker lane from the rest of blot.

3.5. Preparation of Radiolabeled Probe

1. In a screw cap microfuge tube, add 75 ng of (TTAGGG)3 oligonucleotide, 50 µCi of γ-^{32}P ATP, 5 µL of 10X polynucleotide kinase buffer (50 mM DTT, 100 mM

MgCl$_2$, 700 mM Tris-HCl pH 7.6), and 20 U of T4 polynucleotide kinase in a total volume of 50 µL.
2. Briefly spin the contents, and incubate tube at 37°C for 45 min.
3. Stop the reaction by adding 1 µL of 0.1 M EDTA, and purify labeled probe using a G-25 spin column.

3.6. Hybridization

1. Prehybridize the TRF and molecular weight marker blots separately in Quickhyb at 42°C in a water bath for 1 h.
2. Hybridize with 150,000 cpm/mL of labeled probe without carrier DNA at 42°C for 4 h.
3. Wash the blot twice in 2X SSC 0.1% SDS at room temperature for 15 min, followed by a final washing in 1X SSC for 5 min at room temperature.

3.7. Interpretation of Results

1. Realign mol-wt marker to sample blot and exposed to a PhosphorImager screen from 4–12 h (*see* **Note 5**).
2. Scan blot in PhosphorImager (Molecular Dynamics, Inc. Sunnyvale, CA). The point of highest resolution was considered as peak TRF length, and mean TRF was calculated by obtaining the Gaussian distribution above the background from 50 segments drawn across the length of the entire band.
3. Mean TRF values were calculated as $\Sigma(OD_i)/\Sigma(OD_i/L_i)$, where OD$_i$ is the phosphoimager output (arbitrary units) and L$_i$ is the molecular weight of segment at position (i) relative to DNA standards. Sums were calculated over the range of 3–17 kb to obtain mean TRF length (*see* **Note 6**).

4. Notes

1. PBMC from seronegative control subjects can be drawn from volunteers in the laboratory or purchased from blood product vendors. PBMC from seropositive subjects must be collected in accordance with all local and government guidelines for human experimentation.
2. DNA-Stat solutions are corrosive and should be handled with precautions for the use and disposal of hazardous chemicals.
3. The integrity of restriction endonucleases should be assessed periodically with digestions using defined positive and negative control DNA templates.
4. Care should be taken to minimize bubble formation during Southern blotting since this can lead to differential DNA transfer to the nylon membrane.
5. Although storage phosphor imaging devices will greatly facilitate this assay, traditional autoradiography followed by densitometry is a much less costly alternative.
6. To avoid inter assay variation equal amount of DNA was used and samples from same patient were run on same along with a known control sample.

References

1. Blackburn, E. H. (1991) Structure and function of telomeres. *Nature* **350,** 569–573.
2. Shippen, D. E. (1993) Telomeres and telomerases. *Curr. Opin. Genet. Dev.* **3,** 5759–5763.

3. Collins, K. (1996) Structure and function of telomerase. *Curr. Opin. Cell Biol.* **8,** 374–380.
4. Xueli, Z., Kumar, R., Mandal, M., Sharma, N., Sharma, H. W., Dhingra, U., et al. (1996) Cell cycle-dependent modulation of telomerase activity in tumor cells. *Proc. Natl. Acad. Sci. USA* **93,** 6091–6095.
5. Greider, C. W. (1996) Telomere length regulation. *Annu. Rev. Biochem.* **65,** 337–365.
6. Levy, M. Z., Allsopp, R. C., Futcher, A. B., Greider, C. W., and Harley, C. B. (1992) Telomere end-replication problem and cell aging. *J. Mol. Biol.* **225,** 951–960.
7. Harley, C. B. (1991) Telomeric loss: mitotic clock or genetic time bomb? *Mutat. Res.* **256,** 2–6, 271–282.
8. Hayflick, L. (1965) The limited in vitro life time of human diploid cell strains. *Exp. Cell Res.* **37,** 614–636.
9. de Lange, T., Shiue, L., Myers, R. M., Cox, D. R., Naylor, S. L., Killery, A. M. et al. (1990) Structure and variability of human chromosomes ends. *MCB* **10,** 2518–2527.
10. Kim, N. W., Piatyszek, M. A., Prowse, K. R., Harley, C. B., West, M. D., Ho, P. L., et al. (1994) Specific association of human telomerase activity with immortal cells and cancer. *Science* **266,** 2011–2025.
11. Shay, J. W. and Wright, W. E. (1996) Telomerase activity in human cancer. *Curr. Opin. Oncol.*
12. Hiyama, K., Hira, Y., Kyoizumi, S., Akiyama, M., Hiyama, E., Piatyszek, M.A., et al. (1995) Activation of telomerase in human lymphocytes and hematopoietic progenitor cells. *J. Immunol.* **155,** 3711–3715.
13. Nam-ping, W., Levine, B. L., June, C. H., and Hodes, R.J. (1996) Regulated expression of telomerase activity in human T lymphocytes development and activation. *JEM* **183,** 2471–2479.
14. Greider, C. W. and Blackburn, E. H. (1996) Telomere, Telomerase and Cancer. *Sci. Am.* **274(2),** 92–97.
15. Virgina, A. Z. (1995) Telomere: beginning to understand the end. *Science* **270,** 1601–1607.
16. Shay, J. W. (1995) Aging and cancer: are telomeres and telomerase the connection. *Mol. Med. Today* **8,** 378–384.
17. Ho, D. D., Neumann, A. U., Perelson, A. S., Chen, W., Lenord, J. M., and Markowitz, M. (1995) Rapid turnover of plasma virions and CD4 lymphocytes in HIV-1 infection. *Nature* **373,** 123–126.
18. Xiping, W., Ghosh, S. K., Taylor, M. E., Jhonson, V. A., Emini, E. A., Deutsch, P., et al. (1995) Viral dynamics in human immunodeficiency virus type 1 infection. *Nature* **373,** 117–122.
19. Effros, R. B., Allsopp, R., Chiu, C. P., Hausner, M. A., Hiriji, K., Wang, L., et al. (1996) Shortened telomeres in the expanded CD28-CD8+ cell subsets in HIV disease implicate replicative senecence in HIV pathogenesis. *AIDS* **10,** F17-F22.
20. Monterio, J., Batliwalla, F., Oster, H., and Gregersen, P. K. (1996) Shortened telomeres in clonally expanded CD28-CD8+ cells imply a replicative history that is distinct from their CD28+CD8+ counterparts. *J. Immunol.* **156,** 3587–3589.
21. Wolthers, K. C., Wisman, G. B. A., Otto, S. A., de Roda, Husman, A., Schaff, N., de Wolf, F., et al. (1996) T cell telomere length in HIV infection: no evidence for increased CD4+ T cell turnover. *Science* **274,** 1547.

III

HUMORAL IMMUNOLOGY

Opsonize viral particles w/ IgG
↑ IgG FD

27

Serologic Analysis by Enzyme-Linked Immunosorbent Assay (ELISA)

Melissa Krider and Lawrence D. Loomis-Price

1. Introduction

One of the basic requirements for assessing the value of a vaccine candidate is measuring its immunogenicity. This can be done in a variety of ways, with focus on either the humoral or cellular arm of the response, or both. Assay of the humoral response, at minimum, requires the ability to measure changes in antibodies directed against specific antigens. Often, these antigens will be whole proteins. A quick and accurate method for measuring antibody levels against protein antigens is the enzyme-linked immunosorbent assay (ELISA) *(1,2)*. The ELISA assay has been used by vaccine developers for decades and is routinely used for monitoring responses to HIV proteins after infection or vaccination *(3–6)*.

In recent trials of an HIV-1 vaccine, the authors used the ELISA technique to measure antibody levels against the vaccine immunogen, recombinant envelope glycoprotein (rgp160), and another viral antigen, not part of the vaccine (p24) *(7,8)*. Volunteers in this trial were also immunized with a tetanus booster in order to assess the ability to respond to non-HIV based antigens. Responses against tetanus toxoid were also measured by ELISA. In this large (600 patient) Phase II trial, it was convenient to automate many of the assays. For ELISAs, most repetitive manipulations were done using BioMek 1000 workstations. This allowed assay of up to 36 microtiter plates (96-well) per day with a technical staff of only two people. In the procedures that follow, it is assumed that such a workstation is available. If not, it would be possible to perform these assays by hand, especially by running fewer at a time.

From: *Methods in Molecular Medicine, Vol. 17: HIV Protocols*
Edited by: N. L. Michael and J. H. Kim © Humana Press Inc., Totowa, NJ

2. Materials

2.1. Instrumentation

1. BioMek 1000 Automated Laboratory Workstation with Genesis Software (Beckman Instruments, Fullerton, CA).
2. Incubator (Forma Instruments, Marietta, OH).

2.2. Reagents and Consumables.

1. Recombinant proteins rgp160 and p24 (MicroGeneSys, Inc., Meriden, CT).
2. Tetanus toxoid (Connaught, Willowdale, Canada).
3. Standard tetanus antitoxin (National Institute for Biological Standards and Control, Hertfordshire, UK).
4. Human sera were obtained with informed consent from HIV-1-infected patients undergoing vaccine therapy with recombinant envelope vaccine rgp160, (NL4-3, baculovirus, MicroGeneSys) in FDA-approved phase I-and phase II trials *(7,9,10)*. The volunteers were also vaccinated with tetanus toxoid once during the trial. Sera prior to any immunization were compared to those obtained over the course of up to 7 yr of immunization with rgp160. Negative control sera from uninfected individuals were tested individually for reactivity and then pooled.
5. Wash buffer (for gp160 and p24): 2000 mL PBS (Life Technologies, Grand Island, NY), 0.1% Tween (Sigma Chemical Co., St. Louis, MO); make fresh daily. Wash buffer (for Tetanus): 2000 mL PBS, 0.05% Tween; make fresh daily.
6. Blocking solution (for gp160 and p24 only): 1% bovine serum albumin (BSA) (Sigma Chemical Co., St. Louis, MO) in phosphate-buffered saline (PBS). Sterile filter and keep refrigerated up 1 wk.
7. Sample diluent (for gp160 and p24): 10% fetal calf serum (FCS) (heat inactivated) in PBS. Sterile filter and keep refrigerated up to 2 wk. Sample and standard diluent (for Tetanus): 500 mL PBS, 0.1 BSA (Sigma), 0.05% Tween. Sterile filter and keep refrigerated up to 2 wk.
8. pNPP substrate. One 5 mg tablet paranitrophenyl phosphate substrate (Sigma) per 5 mL of DEAE buffer: 114 µL diethanolamine, 0.2 g sodium azide, 0.1 g $MgCl_2 \cdot 6H_2O$ per L of water; pH to 9.8 with HCl. Cover the bottle with aluminum foil (light sensitive) and keep refrigerated up to 1 mo (*see* **Note 1**).
9. Goat antihuman IgG-alkaline phosphatase conjugate (Tago, Inc., Burlingame, CA). Dilute appropriately (typically 1:1000) in conjugate buffer.
10. Conjugate buffer (for gp160 and p24): 500 mL PBS, 0.05% Tween-20, 0.1% BSA. Sterile filter and keep refrigerated for up to 2 wk. Conjugate buffer (for Tetanus): 500 mL PBS, 0.05% Tween-20. Keep refrigerated for up to 2 wk.
11. Stop solution: 3 N NaOH. Keep indefinitely.
12. Tetanus coating buffer: 0.015 M Na_2CO_3 (Sigma), 0.03 M $NaHCO_3$ (Sigma) in water, pH 9.4. Keep refrigerated for up to 1 mo.
13. Coating solution (for gp160): 0.1 µg gp160 per mL of PBS. Coating solution (for p24): 1 µg/mL of PBS. Coating solution (for Tetanus): 0.58 Lf Tetanus toxoid per mL of Tetanus coating buffer. Make fresh daily.

14. Immulon II microtiter plates (flat) (Dynatech Laboratories, Chantilly, VA).
15. Minitubes (1 mL, in strips) (Skatron Instruments, Inc., Sterling, VA). Mminitube racks, pipet tips (250 μL), modular reservoirs (Beckman Instruments, Fullerton, CA).
16. Sterilization filter units (0.2 μm) (Nalge Company, Rochester, NY).

3. Methods
3.1. Use of the BioMek 1000 Workstation

1. Repetitive manipulations of ELISA plates and samples can be efficiently performed using the BioMek 1000. The BioMek can be programmed to perform mixing, pipeting, washing, and reading subroutines. These subroutines can be used in a larger program (called a method) to repeat an ELISA step for many plates or samples. Detailed instructions for use of this instrument are beyond the scope of this chapter; refer to the user's manual for specific instructions.

The following paragraphs briefly describe use of the BioMek 1000 Workstation for a standardized ELISA assay.

2. The BioMek 1000 basically consists of a moving robotic arm, a side-to-side moving carriage (tablet), and various interchangeable tools. These can be used in conjunction with the BioMek peristaltic pump apparatus and BioMek labware. The BioMek tablet has four locations for holding BioMek tip racks, minitube racks, modular reservoirs, and microtiter plates. When a BioMek method runs, the BioMek robotic arm picks up the appropriate tool and moves to a tablet location as programmed.
3. Typical ELISA runs in this laboratory require up to 36 plates; the authors employ three or four BioMek workstations which are manned by 2–4 technical staff. For steps such as washing and conjugating, several plates can be manipulated at once by using several workstations. It is time efficient to start an ELISA step while the previous step is running. BioMeks can be placed inside laminar-flow hoods for steps involving infectious materials.
4. Pipeting: The BioMek pipeting tool will pick up a vertical column of tips from the 8 × 12 rack, and move the tips to a liquid-containing reservoir or rack of minitubes. The pipeting tool will pick up the programmed volume of solution and pipet the solution into a column on a microtiter plate or a column of minitubes in a rack. Empty wells can be interspersed by removing individual tips from the rack of BioMek tips.
5. Washing: The BioMek aspirating tool can aspirate liquid from plates and fill wells (by column) with solution by means of inlet tubing threaded through a peristaltic pump. Inlet tubing is placed in a container of the appropriate wash buffer. Plates are placed on the BioMek tablet and washed by flooding the wells with solution, then aspirating the solution. This should be done at least four times. Inlet tubing and washing tools should be primed with the appropriate liquid before use, and purged with water at the end of the day.

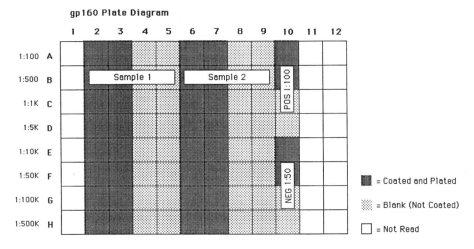

Fig. 1. Typical plate diagram for experiments using rgp160 as plate antigen.

6. Mixing: The BioMek pipetting tool can be used to mix liquids in minitubes by repeatedly picking up liquid from the bottoms of the tubes and dispensing it near the tops of the same tubes (at least four times).

7. Diluting: The BioMek performs serial dilutions by filling columns of minitubes with an amount of diluent determined by the dilution scheme. The minitube rack is manually removed from the tablet, and the first series of patient samples is pipeted manually into the minitubes. The rack of minitubes is returned to the tablet where sample and diluent are mixed. The BioMek pipets a portion of diluted sera from one column of minitubes into the next column, where it is mixed and (a portion) transferred into subsequent columns and mixed. For all assays described, samples are run in duplicate, with corresponding blank (uncoated) wells in duplicate, so each minitube must contain sufficient liquid for four wells.

8. Reading: The BioMek reading tool can be used for measuring optical densities. For these assays, the 405-nm wavelength filter is used.

3.2. Setup

1. Prepare reagents and buffers. Short-lived reagents, conjugates, and ELISA peptides and toxins should be added to buffers or diluent solutions just before use. Concentration calculations should be carried out the day before an experiment.

2. Place the serum samples in order by patient, according to the order in which they will be diluted and plated. Label plate diagrams (refer to **Fig. 1** for an example) to reflect what samples each microtiter plate will contain. Sera identities are checked before an experiment is run, and again as they are returned to the freezer. Control sera from uninfected volunteers must be included with every run.

3. Plates require an overnight incubation with coating antigen, and thus should be coated the afternoon before an experiment.

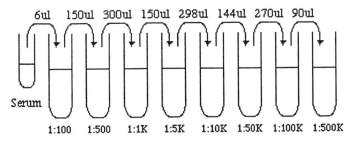

Fig. 2. Typical eight dilution scheme for sera when rgp160 was used as plate antigen.

3.3. ELISA Method

Unless specifically stated otherwise, all steps are run on the BioMek 1000, using methods written to carry out the desired operation.

1. Coating: Coat the Immulon II microtiter plates with 100 μL/well of coating solution. Add the coating solution to a BioMek modular reservoir, and place in the appropriate slot on the BioMek tablet. Place the first two plates and a rack of BioMek tips on the tablet. The BioMek pipeting tool will pick up tips and then aspirate 100 μL of coating solution and pipet the solution into the appropriate column on the microtiter plate. Wells are left uncoated by removing individual tips from the rack of BioMek tips. Repeat for remaining plates. Wrap the plates in cellophane in groups of six and incubate overnight in the dark (*see* **Note 2**).

2. Blocking: After the overnight incubation, add 200 μL of blocking solution to all wells of the microtiter plates. Add blocking solution to a BioMek reservoir and place on the BioMek tablet. Place the first two plates on the tablet. Run a BioMek method that will aspirate the coating solution from the plates and add 200 μL of blocking buffer to each well. Repeat for all plates. Wrap the plates in cellophane, and allow to incubate at room temperature for 2 h (*see* **Note 3**).

3. Tetanus wash: (For Tetanus assay only, after the overnight incubation). Place the inlet tubing in a 2 L container of Tetanus wash buffer. Place the first two plates on the BioMek tablet. Run a BioMek method that will aspirate the coating solution from the plates, then wash the plates four times with Tetanus wash buffer. Repeat for all plates, then place in the refrigerator until they are ready to have serum samples and standards added.

4. Sample dilutions: During the 2 h blocking incubation, prepare the serum dilutions and controls. Serially dilute each patient sample in a rack of minitubes for subsequent transfer to a plate, see **Fig. 2** and **Table 1** for an example. Add sample diluent to a BioMek reservoir and place on the BioMek tablet. Place a numerically labeled rack of minitubes on the BioMek tablet. (Minitubes should be inserted into the minitube rack by column.) The BioMek will add diluent to the minitubes. Remove the rack of minitubes and manually pipet the appropriate amount of each patient sample into the first column of minitubes, starting with the tubes in position A1 and continuing through H8 for the next seven samples. Return the rack to

Table 1
Eight Dilution Schemes for gp160

Dilution factor (cumulative)	Starting diluent volume (μL)	Volume serum or diluted serum transferred (μL)	Ending volume (μL)
1:100	3 × 198	6 (Manually)	600
1:500	3 × 200	150	750
1:1000	2 × 150	2 × 150	600
1:5000	3 × 200	150	750
1:10000	2 × 149	2 × 149	596
1:50000	3 × 192	144	720
1:100000	2 × 135	2 × 135	540
1:500000	2 × 180	90	450

the tablet for the serial dilutions. Minitubes are transferred to an empty rack in horizontal rows before transfer to plates. Cover finished minitube racks with cellophane until they are transferred to the plates (*see* **Note 4**).

5. Standard dilutions: (Tetanus only.) The serially diluted standards for Tetanus are performed much as in **step 4**. After the BioMek adds diluent to the minitubes, the rack of tubes is removed. Antitetanus standard human immunoglobulin is manually added to the first column of minitubes (6.64 μL of 1:8 dilution). The rack is returned to the tablet for the serial dilution with the standards arranged vertically in the first four columns of the rack containing diluted samples.

6. Washing: Wash each plate four times with water, and refrigerate them until ready for plating of samples (*see* **Note 5**).

7. Plating: Mix the previously prepared racks of minitubes, and then transfer 100 μL of diluted sample from the minitubes to a plate. Transfer positive and negative controls from a divided reservoir to the plate at this time. Samples can be transferred to four plates from each rack of minitubes. Wrap the plates with cellophane in groups of four and incubate at 37°C for 1.5 h (*see* **Note 6**).

8. Conjugation: Wash the plates four times with wash buffer and add 100 μL of conjugate in conjugate buffer into each well of the microtiter plate. This can be done in a single method. Wrap the plates in groups of four, and incubate at 37°C for 1.5 h.

9. Development: Wash the plates four times with wash buffer, and add 100 μL of pNPP substrate to each well of the plate. Incubate at room temperature, in the dark, for 15 min. This step is time critical.

10. Reading: Add 50 μL of stop solution to each well, then read the plates at 405-nm.

3.4. Analysis

1. Files from the plate-reader should be directly transferred into an appropriate format, such as a spreadsheet or a database.

2. Using a set of standardized templates and macros, optical density data are grouped with patient sample information.

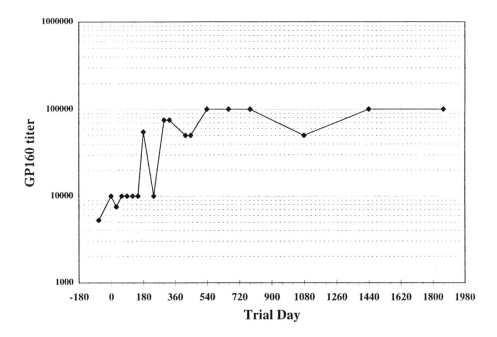

Fig. 3. Example of ELISA data showing response to vaccination over time; plate antigen was rgp160. Sera and secondary concentrations are described in the text. The volunteer was immunized with rgp160 at d 0, 7, 30, 60, and every 60 d thereafter until the trial was completed.

3. Duplicate sample readings are averaged, as are the corresponding blank readings.
4. Blank values (no antigen) are subtracted from the averaged optical density readings:

$$Abs = Abs(Experimental) - Abs(Background)$$

5. An endpoint titer cutoff value is calculated as the average plus twice the standard deviation of all negative control (sera from uninfected controls) readings.

$$Abs > NHS + 2s \quad \text{and also} \quad Abs > 0.20 \, OD$$

6. Patient data are graphed to reflect changes in titer over time (see **Fig. 3** for an example).
7. The experiment is then reviewed by two different individuals for correctness and completeness and incorporated into the analysis database after passing review (*see* **Note 7**).

4. Notes

1. pNPP tablets should not be added to the DEAE buffer until just before use. If many plates are to be run, substrate should be made in batches to minimize time that it sits for 15 min or less.

2. For Tetanus, incubate plates overnight at 4°C.
3. The Tetanus assay has no blocking step.
4. For p24, minitubes are inserted into the racks in columns of six and serum is manually pipeted into the first six minitubes of the first column to give six half-log dilutions. Minitubes are transferred to an empty rack in horizontal rows before transfer to plates. The remainder of the rack can contain the next set of minitubes in rows. Also, manually-diluted controls are added to minitubes by hand, and placed into the rack with the serially diluted samples. For Tetanus, minitubes are inserted vertically into racks. 4 μL of serum are manually pipeted into columns 1, 4, 7, and 10 as there are only three dilutions, with only the 6400 dilution transferred to the plate. Pipet positive and negative controls into the last three tubes of column 10. Note that for transfer to plates, columns 3, 6, 9, and 12 are placed side by side in columns 5 through 8 (rows 1 through 4 will contain standards) of a minitube rack. Columns 9 through 12 can contain up to four more columns of diluted samples.
5. Tetanus plates have already been washed with Tetanus wash buffer.
6. For p24 and Tetanus, positive and negative controls are added to the minitubes, not to a divided reservoir.
7. For tetanus, antitoxin readings are used to plot a standard curve from which concentrations in IU/mL (International Units per milliliter) are determined for each patient sample. Patient data are graphed to reflect changes in IU/mL over time.

References

1. Engvall, E. and Perlmann, P. (1971) Enzyme-linked immunosorbent assay (ELISA) quantitative assay of immunoglobulin G. *Immunochemistry* **8,** 874–879.
2. Butler, J., Spradling, J., Sutter, M., Dierks, S., Heyerman, H., and Peterman, J. (1986) The immunochemistry of sandwich ELISAs—I. The binding characteristics of immunoglobulins to monoclonal and polyclonal capture antibodies adsorbed on plastic and their detection by symmetrical and asymmetrical antibody-enzyme conjugates. *Molec. Immunol.* **23,** 971–982.
3. Weiss, S., Goedert, J., Sarngadharan, M., Bodner, A., Gallo, R., and Blattner, W. (1985) Screening test for HTLV-III (AIDS agent) antibodies. Specificity , sensitivity, and applications. *JAMA* **253,** 221–225.
4. Moore, J., Wallace, L., Follett, E., and McKeating, J. (1989) An enzyme-linked immunosorbent assay for antibodies to the envelope glycoproteins of divergent strains of HIV-1. *AIDS* **3,** 155–163.
5. Viscidi, R., Ellerbeck, E., Garrison, L., Midthun, K., Clements, M.L., Clayman, B., et al. (1990) Characterization of serum antibody responses to recombinant HIV-1 gp160 vaccine by enzyme immunoassay. NIAID AIDS Vaccine Clinical Trials Network. *AIDS Res. Hum. Retrovir.* **6,** 1251–1256.
6. Wintsch, J., Chaignat, C.L., Braun, D.G., Jeannet, M., Stalder, H., Abrignani, S., et al. (1991) Safety and immunogenicity of a genetically engineered human immunodeficiency virus vaccine. *J. Infect. Dis.* **163,** 219–225.

7. Redfield, R. R., Birx, D. L., Ketter, N., Tramont, E., Polonis, V., Davis, C., et al. (1991) A phase I evaluation of the safety and immunogenicity of vaccination with recombinant gp160 in patients with early human immunodeficiency virus infection. *N. Engl. J. Med.* **324,** 1677–1684.
8. Birx, D.L., Ketter, N., and Fast, P. (1996) HIV vaccine development for treatment and prevention, in *Clinical Immunology: Principles and Practice* (Rich, R. R., ed.), Mosby, St. Louis, MO, pp. 764.
9. Birx, D.L. and Redfield, R.R. (1994) Therapeutic HIV vaccines: concept, current status, and future directions, in *Textbook of AIDS Medicine* (Broder, S., Merrigan, T. C. Jr., and Bolognesi, D., eds.), Williams and Wilkins, Baltimore, MD, pp. 693–711.
10. Redfield, R., Birx, D., Ketter, N., Polonis, V., Johnson, S., Davis, C., et al. (1992) Vaccine therapy using rgp 160 in early HIV infection. *AIDS Res. Hum. Retrovir.* **8,** 1333.

28

Quantitative Immunoblotting with Fusion Proteins

Margaret M. Mitchell and Lawrence D. Loomis-Price

1. Introduction

The development of vaccines against HIV-1 is currently hindered by incomplete understanding of correlates of protective immunity *(1–3)*. Experiments are necessary to measure immune responses in sufficiently fine detail that specific protective responses can be discerned from those that are irrelevant or harmful. When vaccines are tested as potential therapeutics, it is further necessary to differentiate induced responses from those associated with the infection itself. Measurement of humoral responses to well-defined antigens particularly lends itself to detailed mapping *(4)*. Small synthetic antigens may be used in ELISA or BIAcore assays *(5–7)*. Larger antigens, such as fusion proteins, may require assays with more specificity, because of the possibility of immune-reactive contaminants. A particularly useful technique in this context is immunoblotting, because contaminating antigens are separated away during the electrophoresis step *(8,9)*. In the authors' laboratory, immunoblots employing fusion proteins of HIV-1 envelope sequences have been successfully used to quantitate new responses post immunization with a vaccine candidate in spite of a substantial baseline response to the whole antigen *(10,11)*. The same technique was used to measure responses against vaccine candidates in small animal models *(12,13)*.

2. Materials

Although it is possible to purchase prepared gels, if a large number are required, it is preferable to prepare them locally to reduce expense and avoid lot-to-lot variability.

From: *Methods in Molecular Medicine, Vol. 17: HIV Protocols*
Edited by: N. L. Michael and J. H. Kim © Humana Press Inc., Totowa, NJ

2.1. Gels

2.1.1. Supplies

1. Electrophoresis unit (lid, cables, magnetic clips, bottom), model AE-6450 (ATTO Corporation, Japan).
2. Inner and outer glass plates, gaskets, spacers, and combs (Bio-Rad, Hercules, CA).
3. Power supply model 1000/500 (Bio-Rad).
4. Multiflex microcapillary tips: nonsterile, RNase/DNase free (PGC Scientifics, Gaithersburg, MD).

2.1.2. Solutions (see **Note 1**)

1. Electrophoresis purity reagents: Tris (Hydroxymethyl) aminoethane, acrylamide/ BIS 29:1 (3.3% C), ammonium persulfate (APS), *N,N,N',N'*-Tetramethyl-ethylenediamine (TEMED), sodium dodecyl sulfate (SDS), bromophenol blue, Coomassie® brilliant blue G-250, glycine, 2-mercaptoethanol (2-ME), low mol-wt standard proteins, (Bio-Rad).
2. Other reagents: glacial acetic acid, glycerol, enzyme grade, Tris-Gly-SDS running buffer Seprabuff™ (Integrated Separation Systems, Natick, MA); Dulbecco's phosphate buffered saline (PBS) (without Ca and Mg), 1X and 10X stock (Gibco-BRL, Gaithersburg, MD).
3. For drying gels: Gel-Dry™ drying solution, cellophane, and Gel-Dry cassettes (top and bottom plus clamps) (NOVEX, San Diego, CA).
4. Tris buffer: 1.5 M, pH 8.8. Add 90.75 g of Tris to 500 mL of water with stirring and pH to 8.8. Store the solution at 4°C. Use within 1 wk.
5. Tris buffer: 0.5 M, pH 6.8. Add 30 g of Tris to 500 mL of water with stirring and pH to 6.8. Store the solution at 4°C. Use within 1 wk.
6. Bis/Acrylamide (*see* **Note 2**): Prepare the solution by adding 73 mL of water directly to the bottle with stirring for 30 min. Filter through a 0.2-μ sterile filter and store sealed and protected from light at 4°C. Use within 1 wk.
7. SDS, 10% (w/v). Store at room temperature for up to 1 mo.
8. Bromophenol blue, 0.2% (w/v). Store at room temperature for up to 1 mo.
9. 4X Sample buffer: Combine 10% SDS , 0.5 M Tris, glycerol, 0.2% bromophenol blue, 2-Beta-mercaptoethanol in the ratio 4.0:2.5:2.0:0.5:2.0 by volume. Store at 4°C for 1 mo.
10. Running buffer: Dissolve two bottles of Seprabuff in 2 L water and take to 20 L total vol in a large carboy. Store at 4°C for 1 wk.
11. Stain: Dissolve 0.25 g of Coomassie blue in 125 mL of methanol. Add 50 mL of glacial acetic acid and 325 mL of water. Store at room temperature indefinitely.
12. Destain: Combine 200 mL of methanol, 200 mL of glacial acetic acid, and 1600 mL of water. Store at room temperature indefinitely.
13. Resolvent (enough for two gels): Combine 5.0 mL of water, 3.75 mL 1.5 M Tris, 6 mL Bis/acryl and 150 μL of 10% SDS to a flask. Degas for 5 min. Add 75 μL APS and 7.5 μL of TEMED simultaneously to the flask after degassing. Pipet immediately.

14. Stacker (enough for two gels): Combine 3.1 mL water, 1.3 mL 0.5 M Tris, 650 μL Bis/acryl, and 50 μL 10% SDS in a flask. Degas for 5 min. Add 25 μL of APS (10%) and 5 μL TEMED simultaneously after degassing. Pipet immediately.

2.2. Blots

1. Instrumentation: PhosphorImager, model 400E (Molecular Dynamics, Sunnyvale, CA).
2. Equipment: Gel holder cassette, fiber pads (sponges), 8 × 11 cm., minitransblot electrophoretic transfer cell (includes lid with cables), Bio-Ice cooling unit, blot absorbent filter paper (thin), blot absorbent filter paper (thick) (Bio-Rad), Protran™ Pure Nitrocellulose Transfer and Immobilization Membrane, 0.2 μ; 33 × 56 cm. (Schleicher and Schuell, Keene, NH), Radtape™ (Integrated Separation Systems); film cassettes with intensifying screens (Sigma, St. Louis, MO), photographic film (Kodak, Rochester, NY), phosphor screen (Molecular Dynamics), Rhomat™ formatted EZ-tape (3M, St. Paul, MN).
3. Reagents (*see* **Note 3**): Methanol, certified A.C.S., Carnation® nonfat dry milk; polyoxyethylene-sorbitan monolaurate (Tween-20); ^{125}I-labeled secondary antibodies (50 μCi, New England Nuclear, Wilmington, DE), anti-MBP (New England Bio-Labs, Beverly, MA) (*see* **Note 4**).
4. Fusion proteins: Proteins consisting of fragments from the HIV-1 envelope fused to the maltose-binding protein of *Escherichia coli* were supplied by MicroGeneSys (Meridan, CT). Fusion proteins are stable indefinitely, several years at least, at –80°C. Once thawed, store at 4°C and use within 2 wk.
5. Sera: Human sera were obtained with informed consent from HIV-1 infected patients undergoing vaccine therapy with recombinant envelope vaccine rgp160, (NL4-3, baculovirus, MicroGeneSys) in FDA approved phase 1 and phase 2 trials *(10,14,15)*. Prior to any immunization, sera were compared to those obtained over the course of up to 7 yr of immunization with rgp160. Negative control sera from uninfected individuals were tested individually for reactivity and then pooled.
6. Transfer buffer: Dissolve 60.6 g of Tris and 280.8 g of glycine in a 20 L carboy containing 16 L of water and 4 L of methanol. Store at 4°C for up to 1 wk.
7. Wash solution: 1X DPBS and 0.2% Tween-20.

3. Methods

Pour gels in batches; make up one or two extra to be safe. At least one gel will be stained and used to confirm proper running of the proteins ("confirmatory gel") and another will be immunostained with a positive control antibody. Plan to run the sera in duplicate.

3.1. Pouring Gels

1. Set up a glass sandwich for each gel that is to be poured, according to the manufacturer's instructions. Be sure the sandwiches are level and the shorter plate is facing outward.

2. Prepare sufficient resolvent for the number of gels to be run, including enough for several extra gels. Add the first four ingredients of the recipe to a plastic Erlenmeyer flask. Degas the solution under vacuum for 5 min. Prepare the 10% APS solution. Add the TEMED and APS simultaneously to the flask after degassing. Upon the addition of APS and TEMED, the solution will start to polymerize, so the pouring of the resolvent (and stacking gel) needs to be efficient.

3. Pipet the resolvent and fill the sandwiches to 1 cm from the lip of the shorter plate. Make sure the top of the resolvent is parallel with the horizontal edge of the small plate. Using a transfer pipet, carefully add 1–2 mm of 1% SDS to cover the top of the gel. Allow 30 min for the resolvent to polymerize.

4. Halfway through the polymerization time of the resolvent, prepare the stacking gel. Combine the first four ingredients of the recipe and degas for 5 min.

5. Pour the unabsorbed SDS off the separation gel. Place a well comb in between the glass plates so that the side with the edges faces outward.

6. Add the TEMED and APS to the stacking gel solution. Pipet the solution against the well comb, dispensing slowly to cover the tops of the wells on the comb. Rearrange the comb so that there are no air bubbles in the stacking gel solution. Add one drop of the 1% SDS solution to the stacking gel and allow to polymerize for 15 min.

3.2. Preparing Antigens

1. Dilute the fusion proteins in 4X sample buffer in small tubes; add PBS as necessary to dilute sample buffer to final 1X concentration. Punch a small hole in the top of the tube.

2. Boil the peptides in gently boiling water for 3 min.

3. Place the molecular weight standards in a 56°C water bath for 10 min.

3.3. Electrophoresis

1. Fill electrophoresis rigs three-quarters full with running buffer.

2. When the stacking gel has polymerized, remove the clips, gasket, and well comb from the glass plates. Number the wells (1–10) on the longer of the two glass plates.

3. Place the gel in the running buffer in the rig with the shorter plate facing inward. Tilt the gel so air bubbles can escape.

4. Insert the cell spacer between the gel and the wall of the rig so that the knobs of the cell spacer are facing outward.

5. Once two gels are in a rig, fill the space between the glass plates with running buffer so the gels stay moist.

6. Load the peptides and standards in the appropriate wells on each gel. Put standards in lanes 1 and 10. The other wells are loaded with fusion proteins.

7. Top off the running buffer between the gels such that the space between the gels is filled with buffer to the top of the tall plates in each rig.

8. Attach the top to the gel rig and plug it into the power source. The leads are color coded and must be attached accordingly.

9. Run the electrophoresis at 150 V for 2 h or until the dye fronts are 0.5 cm from the bottom of the gels.
10. After the run, remove the gels from the rigs. Wedge the two plates apart with a small spatula. It is useful to consistently keep the gel on the shorter of the two glass plates.
11. Cut the gel away from the space bars and stacking gel and discard. Orient the gel by cutting away the bottom right corner. If several gels are run, they may be numbered by using a small pipet tip to punch out holes.
12. Prepare the confirmatory gel. Do not punch holes in this gel. Place in stain for 30–60 min.
13. After staining the confirmatory, rinse it with water and remove all excess stain. Pour destain over the confirmatory so that it is sufficiently covered. Destain for 40–50 min.
14. Once the destaining is complete, rinse the gel with water and then cover with laboratory film. Place at 4°C overnight with gentle agitation.

3.4. Transblotting

1. Place a gel holder assembly unit, along with a stir bar, into each transblot unit. Fill the transblot rigs halfway full with transfer buffer.
2. Cut the thick and thin filter paper and nitrocellulose pieces so that they are slightly larger than the gels. Two of each are needed per gel *(16)*. Soak these with transfer buffer in a small container.
3. Build a transfer sandwich. All the following steps take place in a container filled with transfer buffer. It is important to soak all materials and completely exclude any bubbles. First, place a numbered sandwich holder black side down in the container with transfer buffer. Then place a sponge, a thick and then a thin piece of filter paper.
4. Place a gel on the sandwich with the cut to the left. If more than one gel is run, make sure that the number on the gel corresponds with the number on the sandwich holder.
5. Cover the gel with a nitrocellulose sheet, a thin and thick filter paper, and a sponge. A glass tube may be gently rolled over the gel to remove all the air bubbles between the layers.
6. Seal the sandwich with the clasp and place in the gel assembly holder with the black part of the sandwich holder facing the black part of the gel holder assembly unit.
7. When all sandwiches have been placed in a transblot unit, add an ice pack to each unit and top off with transfer buffer.
8. Stir the solution vigorously on a stir plate.
9. Place the tops on the transblot units so that the electrodes and leads are matching.
10. Transblot for 1.5 h at 100V (*see* **Note 5**).

3.5. Removing Gels and Blots

1. When transblot is complete, turn off the power sources and detach the leads.
2. Half-fill sufficient containers to hold the gels with stain (four gels per container).

3. Remove one sandwich from the gel holder. With the black side up, remove the top sponge, and discard the two top pieces of filter paper.

4. Remove the gel from the nitrocellulose paper, and stain the gel for 30–60 min with gentle agitation.

5. Rinse the gels with water and destain. Follow the same procedure used for the confirmatory.

6. Using a black ball-point pen, number the bottom of the nitrocellulose sheet, and immerse it in 1X DPBS. Wash 3X, 10 min/wash with 1X DPBS. Discard the bottom filter papers.

7. Dry the blots on clean, dry, absorbent paper for 30 min.

8. Store blots in the –20°C freezer until they are required again.

9. Aspirate the water from the gels, and immerse the gels in Gel-Dry solution with agitation for 15 min at room temperature.

10. Wet a cellophane sheet in Gel-Dry solution for 15 s, and place on a plastic panel. Place up to six gels on the panel so that the corners are on the bottom right. Gel-Dry solution can be added to move the gels on the plastic.

11. Wet a second cellophane sheet, and place on top of the gels.

12. Remove excess Gel-Dry and all air bubbles.

13. Secure the frame with two clasps on each side (eitght total per panel), and stand the cassette upright on a piece of absorbent paper at an angle to dry. Allow at least 16 h for the gels to dry.

14. Label the gels in the cassettes. Remove the clasps and the frame, and store the dried gels.

3.6. Immunostaining

1. On the afternoon prior to the staining, set up the appropriate number of small containers half filled with 1X DPBS and 5% milk. As many as 10 nitrocellulose sheets fit in each container. Block the nitrocellulose sheets in this solution overnight at 4°C with gentle agitation.

2. On the next morning, wash the blots twice, 10 min/wash with 1X DPBS. After these two washes, place the nitrocellulose sheets in the apparatus to be used for serum incubation in wash solution (1X DPBS with 0.2% Tween).

3. Incubate the blots with sera diluted appropriately in milk for 3 h at room temperature with moderate agitation (*see* **Note 6**). Incubate at least one blot with a positive control antibody, such as anti-MBP for MBP-fusion proteins. The containers must be sealed to avoid evaporation.

4. Wash the blots three times, 10 min/wash, in wash solution.

5. Incubate the blots with 1 µCi of the appropriate ^{125}I labeled secondary antibody, diluted in milk for 2 h at room temperature with moderate agitation (*see* **Note 7**). Seal the containers to avoid evaporation.

6. Wash the blots three times, 10 min/wash with wash solution.

7. Completely dry on absorbent paper (30–60 min).

8. Fix blots to clean thick filter paper panels with tape, and label with RadTape. Cover with plastic wrap making sure that there are no creases.

9. Expose the panels to photographic film in sealed cassettes at –80°C for 16 h and develop. This step must be carried out in complete darkness.

3.7. Quantitation

1. Blank each phosphorescent screen. Add the ^{125}I-labeled blots 18 h prior to scanning. (The screen blanking time is 7 min.)
2. Place two panels of thick filter paper (that hold the [^{125}I]-labeled blots from the previous day's experiment) face up on the grid side of the phosphorimager cassette. The RadTape with the experiment number on it should be in the upper right hand corner (*see* **Note 8**).
3. After the top part of the phosphorimager cassette has been blanked, place it on top of the blots making sure not to move the panels from the specified coordinates.
4. Leave the cassettes in a cabinet overnight for the 18 h incubation.
5. Allow the scanner to completely warm up according to manufacturer's instructions (at least 30 min).
6. Open the cassettes one at a time, and separate the top part of the screen from the bottom. Take care not to turn the screen towards any light source.
7. Place the screen on the scanner and scan the screens according to the imager's protocol. Fill in the pertinent experimental information.
8. Store the imager information appropriately so that it can be subsequently accessed.
9. Transfer the working file(s) to the workstation.
10. Print a hard copy of the image (use "gray scale").
11. Comparisons between the images on the X-ray film and the images collected by the phosphorimager can be used to determine which bands are of interest. The positive control blot is used at this step to separate specific from nonspecific reactivity.
12. Construct a small template, such as a rectangle that will fit over the bands to be analyzed. It is critical to use the same template for all bands.
13. Use the template rectangle to select all of the bands to be analyzed. Also, select at least one area that is representative of the background of each blot. Multiple rectangles may be needed for a blot due to variations in background.
14. Note the rectangles as they appear on the workstation screen on the hard copy, and match background areas to samples.
15. Use the workstation to quantitate the intensity of each area selected, applying the appropriate background subtraction.
16. Print out the analyzed data and transfer to a working format such as a spreadsheet.

3.8. Example

The data obtained with serial draws from a single volunteer over the course of a Phase 1 vaccine therapy trial are shown in **Fig. 1.** The volunteer was HIV-1 positive at the start of the trial and was immunized multiple times (as often as every 2 mo) with the candidate vaccine. Data from three representative epitopes are shown. Reactivity to one epitope "C41" was strong prior to immunization

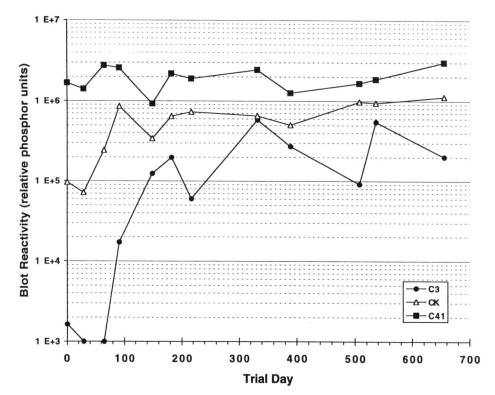

Fig. 1. Representative results obtained with the described quantitative immuno-blotting technique. Reactivity measurable in a volunteer's sera to three different fusion peptides over the course of a vaccine therapy trial are shown. The fusion peptides contained the following HIV-1 envelope sequences, fused to the MBP protein: C41: amino acids (AA) 579–605; CK: AA 735–752; C3: AA 342–405.

and remained constant over the course of the trial. Reactivity to the "CK" epitope was presented prior to immunization but boosted significantly over the course of the trial. Reactivity to the "C3" epitope was not measurable prior to immunization. The volunteer seroconverted to this epitope early in the immu-nization series.

4. Notes

1. All solutions should be of the highest grade available; this will often be called "electrophoresis grade". Water should be deionized and distilled and preferably depyrogenated before use.
2. These reagents are neurotoxic; perform all operations in a hood or well-venti-lated space. Use paper towel to wipe everything down before removing from fume hood.

3. All work with radiation should be done according to appropriate institutional use guidelines, which are beyond the scope of this protocol. At the minimum, all work done with ^{125}I should be carried out behind a lead shield. Proper clothing such as a lab coat, doubled gloves, sleeves, protective eyewear, and a radiation badge and ring should be worn. Dispose of ^{125}I reaction solution and rinses according to appropriate institutional radiation guidelines.
4. ^{125}I-labeled proteins should be kept frozen at −20°C, thawed immediately before use, and used within 30 d.
5. This will vary according to protein size and crosslinking of the gel. It should be optimized for a given set of conditions.
6. Our standard dilution is 1:1000 for human sera, 1:5000 dilution for anti MBP antibody.
7. Because ^{125}I decays, the amount needed per blot must be calculated according to the day of month. Calculate the concentration in μCi/mL, using the following decay equation:

$$\text{conc(day } n) = \text{conc(orig)}/2^{(n/60)}$$

It is very important to use reagent before it decays too far ($n < 30$ d) because unlabeled antibodies will begin to compete significantly and decrease reactivity.
8. For repetitive experiments, placing the panels in standard positions facilitates measurements.

References

1. Birx, D. L., Ketter, N., and Fast, P. (1996) HIV vaccine development for treatment and prevention, in *Clinical Immunology: Principles and Practice* (Rich, R. R. ed.) Mosby, St. Louis, MO, pp. 764–778.
2. Koff, W. C. and Schultz, A. M. (1996) Progress and challenges toward an AIDS vaccine: brother, can you spare a paradigm? *J. Clin. Immunol.* **16**, 127–133.
3. Paul, W. E. (1995) Can the immune response control HIV infection? *Cell* **82**, 127–133.
4. Cason, J. (1994) Strategies for mapping and imitating viral B-cell epitopes. *J. Virol. Methods* **49**, 209–220.
5. Geysen, H. M., Meloen, R. H., and Barteling, S. J. (1984) Use of peptide synthesis to prove viral antigens for epitopes to a resolution of a single amino acid. *Proc. Natl. Acad. Sci. USA* **81**, 3998–4002.
6. Hill, H. and Matsen, J. (1983) Enzyme-linked immunosorbent assay and radioimmunoassay in the serologic diagnosis of infectious diseases. *J. Infect. Dis.* **147**, 258–263.
7. VanCott, T. C., Loomis, L. D., Redfield, R. R., and Birx, D. L. (1992) Real-time biospecific interaction analysis of antibody reactivity to peptides from the envelope glycoprotein, gp160, of HIV-1. *J. Immunol. Methods* **146**, 163–176.
8. Stott, D. I. (1989) Immunoblotting and dot blotting. *J. Immunol. Methods* **119**, 153–187.
9. Towbin, H. and Gordon, J. (1984) Immunoblotting and dot immunoblotting—current status and outlook. *J. Immunol. Methods* **72**, 313–340.

10. Redfield, R., Birx, D., Ketter, N., Polonis, V., Johnson, S., Davis, C., et al. (1992) Vaccine therapy using rgp 160 in early HIV infection. *AIDS. Res. Hum. Retrovir.* **8,** 1333.

11. Loomis, L. D., Deal, C. D., Kersey, K. S., Burke, D. S., Redfield, R. R., and Birx, D. L. (1995) Humoral responses to linear epitopes on the HIV-1 envelope in seropositive volunteers after vaccine therapy with rgp160. *J. Acquir. Immune Defic. Syndr.* **10,** 13–26.

12. Levi, M., Ruden, U., Birx, D., Loomis, L., Redfield, R., Lovgren, K., et al. (1993) Effects of adjuvants and multiple antigen peptides on humoral and cellular immune responses to gp160 of HIV-1. *J. Acquir. Immune Defic. Syndr.* **6,** 855–864.

13. Kaminski, R. W., Loomis, L., Levi, M., Amselem, S., Kersey, K., VanCott, T., et al. (1995) HIV peptide and protein antibody responses elicited by immunization with rgp160 formulated with proteosomes, alum, and/or submicron emulsions. *Vacc. Res.* **4,** 189–206.

14. Birx, D. L. and Redfield, R. R. (1994) Therapeutic HIV vaccines: concept, current status, and future directions, in *Textbook of AIDS Medicine* (Broder, S., Merrigan, T. C. Jr., and Bolognesi, D., eds.), Williams and Wilkins, Baltimore, MD, pp. 693–711.

15. Redfield, R. R., Birx, D. L., Ketter, N., Tramont, E., Polonis, V., Davis, C., et al. (1991) A phase I evaluation of the safety and immunogenicity of vaccination with recombinant gp160 in patients with early human immunodeficiency virus infection. *N. Engl. J. Med.* **324,** 1677–1684.

29

Analysis of Antibody Interactions with HIV-1 Envelope Expressed on the Surface of Acutely Infected H9 Cells

Thomas C. VanCott and Paul L. Hallberg

1. Introduction

Protective antibody responses against HIV-1 have yet to be identified or determined. HIV-1 envelope gp120/gp41 is known to exist as a multimer (tetramers or trimers) on the surface of the virion *(1–4)*. A number of immunoassays have been developed to evaluate HIV-1-specific binding antibody responses using peptides, fusion proteins, and recombinant proteins. Attempts to correlate antibody binding parameters with in vitro HIV-1 neutralization capacity have identified correlations between the presence of V3 antibodies and the capacity to neutralize T-cell line adapted strains of HIV-1. However, no correlation with neutralization of primary HIV-1 isolates and v3 antibodies have been identified *(5)*. Furthermore, binding to monomeric forms of gp120 has shown little correlation with neutralization of the homologous primary HIV-1 indicating that epitope accessibility and tertiary structure of monomeric forms of gp120 differs from quaternary structure of membrane expressed oligomeric gp120/gp41 *(6–8)*.

Acute HIV-1 infection of CD4 T-cell lines (H9, CEM) results in CD4 downregulation and expression of HIV-1 envelope within three to seven days after infection. Sera from HIV-1 infected individuals, volunteers receiving candidate vaccines or epitope-specific monoclonal antibodies can be screened for reactivity against these oligomeric forms of gp120/gp41 *(9–11)*. This assay allows identification of epitopes accessible on the oligomeric forms of gp120/gp41 to perhaps more accurately access potential functional capacity of specific antibody populations. Antibody binding to the surface of infected cells is

From: *Methods in Molecular Medicine, Vol. 17: HIV Protocols*
Edited by: N. L. Michael and J. H. Kim © Humana Press Inc., Totowa, NJ

detected using fluorescent, labeled, secondary antibodies, and fluorescence of individual cells is measured using flow cytometry.

2. Materials
2.1. Equipment

1. Flow cytometer.
2. Falcon test tubes (2058, 12 × 75 mm, Becton-Dickinson Labware, Lincoln Park , NJ).
3. T-75 cm² vented-tissue culture flask (Costar, Cambridge, MA).
4. Hemocytometer with coverslip.
5. Trypan blue.
6. Microscope.
7. Aerosolve™ cannisters (Beckman Instruments, Inc., Palo Alto, CA).

2.2. Reagents and Buffers

1. Culture media (cRPMI): RPMI 1640 (ABI, Columbia, MD), supplemented with 5% heat-inactivated fetal bovine serum (FBS) (Sigma, St. Louis, MO), 1% Pen/ Strep solution (100 U/mL penicillin, 100 µg/mL streptomycin, Gibco, Grand Island, NY), 1% L-Glutamine solution (Gibco).
2. Phosphate-buffered saline (PBS) wash media: PBS, 0.1% BSA, 0.01% Thimero- sal, pH 7.4 (Sigma).
3. H9 cells (AIDS Research and Reference Reagent Program, Rockville, MD).
4. GAH-IgG-PE, Phycoerythrin(PE)-labeled goat antihuman immunoglobulin (Southern Biotechnologies, Birmingham, AL).
5. GAR-IgG-PE, Phycoerythrin(PE)-labeled goat antirabbit immunoglobulin (Southern Biotechnologies).
6. GAM-IgG-PE, Phycoerythrin(PE)-labeled goat antimouse immunoglobulin (Southern Biotechnologies).
7. Monoclonal antibodies (MAbs) to cell surface receptors: Isotype controls (FITC- IgG1, PE-IgG1, PE-Leu-3a (anti-CD4), FITC-HLe-1 (anti-CD45) (Becton- Dickinson, San Jose, CA) (*see* **Note 1**).
8. Monoclonal antibodies to cell surface receptor CD4, PE-OKT4 (OrthoDiagnostic Systems Inc., Raritan, NJ) (*see* **Note 2**).
9. 1% Paraformaldehyde EM-grade, methanol-free solution (EMS, Fort Washington, PA).
10. QC3™ beads (Flow Cytometry Standards Corp, San Juan, PR).
11. Calibrite™ beads (Becton-Dickinson).
12. Normal human serum (NHS), from HIV-1 p24 kits (Coulter Corp., Hialeai, FL).
13. HIV-1 positive serum control (*see* **Note 3**).

3. Methods
3.1. Acute HIV-1 Infection of H9 Cells

1. H9 cells are acutely infected with HIV-1 by mixing 15 × 10⁶ H9 cells with 500 µL viral stock of laboratory-adapted HIV-1 for 60 min at 37°C (*see* **Notes 4** and **5**).
2. Wash cells by centrifuging at 400g for 5 min at 4°C, decanting supernatant, and resuspending in 30 mL of PBS and repeat (*see* **Note 6**).

3. Resuspended cells in 30 mL of cRPMI and transfer to a T-75 vented-tissue culture flask.
4. Feed cultures at d 3 and every subsequent two days with cRPMI (*see* **Note 7**).

3.2. Staining of HIV-1 Infected H9 Cells

1. At peak p24 antigen production (d 3–7) (*see* **Notes 8** and **9**), remove 5×10^6 HIV-1 infected H9 cells, wash two times in PBS wash media, and resuspend at 20×10^6 cells/mL (*see* **Notes 10** and **11**).
2. Remove 20 µL of H9 infected cells (4×10^5 cells) and add together with 20 µL of sera (serum dilutions of 1:50 to 1:500) or MAb (5–50 µg/mL) to a 5 mL Falcon tube and mix thoroughly by vortexing (*see* **Note 12**).
3. Incubate cells and sera together for 1 h at 4°C while mixing (*see* **Note 13**).
4. Wash the cells twice with PBS wash media. Wash cells by centrifuging for 5 min at 400*g* at 4°C, decanting and resuspending in 3 mL of fresh PBS wash buffer (*see* **Note 14**).
5. After the second wash, decant, but do not resuspend in 3 mL of fresh PBS (*see* **Note 15**).
6. Add 10 µL of GAH-IgG-PE into the approximate 200 µL cell suspension and incubate for 30 min at 4°C in the dark (*see* **Note 16**).
7. Wash the cells two times with PBS wash media as in **step 4**, but after decanting, leave the remaining 100–200 µL of buffer in the tube.
8. Fix the cells overnight at 4°C with 1% paraformaldehyde (*see* **Note 17**).

3.3. Acquisition of Data by Flow Cytometry

3.3.1. Setting Flow Cytometer PMT Voltages and Compensation

1. Each of the individual cell samples are analyzed for forward side scatter (FSC), side scatter (SSC), fluorescence-FITC (FL1), and fluorescence-PE (FL2) using a FACscan flow cytometer (Becton-Dickinson) or other commercial flow cytometer (*see* **Note 18**).
2. Flow cytometer detection efficiency and compensation adjustments are validated and normalized prior to each assay by running sets of beads with known fluorescent parameters, such as Calibrite beads and QC3 beads (*see* **Note 19**). In this way, photomultiplier tube voltages are adjusted to yield constant fluorescent signals over time.

3.3.2. Acquisition of Data from HIV-1 Infected H9 Cells

1. Run unstained H9 cells or appropriate uninfected T-cell line cell control and adjust FSC and SSC to ensure that cells of interest can be detected.
2. Draw a gate around the determined viable cell population (*see* **Note 20**).
3. Determine level of autofluorescence for the particular T-cell line used by gating on the appropriate cell population and measuring FL1 and FL2. The level of autofluorescence should be within the first decade of the log scale for both FL1 and FL2 (less than approx 10 mean fluorescence units).

4. Run cells with a positive stain (uninfected H9 cells stained with HLE-1-FITC and L3a-PE) to ensure that flourescence is on scale using parameters selected in **Subheading 3.3.1.**).
5. Establish level of nonspecific binding signal by evaluating uninfected H9 cells stained with representative positive control sera or MAbs (*see* **Note 21**).
6. Check for complete CD4 downregulation in the HIV-1 infected H9 cells (*see* **Note 22**)
7. Establish level of nonspecific binding of negative control sera to infected H9 cells (*see* **Note 23**).
8. Establish appropriate cell flow rate for data acquisition (*see* **Note 24**).
9. Collect data (FITC and PE fluorescence) from 10,000–15,000 cells falling within the defined forward and side scatter profile (gate).
10. Subtract the mean PE fluorescence signal of MAb or sera binding to the uninfected H9 cells from the HIV-1 infected cells (this subtracts nonspecific or specific antibody binding to uninfected H9 cells).
11. Compare all results of test sera or MAbs to negative control MAbs and normal human serum binding to HIV-1 infected H9 cells.

4. Notes

1. Select the appropriate monoclonals for the cell line or type used. For example, the monoclonals, HLe-1(anti-CD45) and Leu-3a(anti-CD4) are appropriate for the assessment of normal baseline expression and function of H9 cell lines. H9 cells are CD3-negative and therefore will not be stained by MAb L4.
2. OKT4 binds to a site on membrane expressed CD4 that is distinct from gp120 so that CD4 can be bound by both gp120 and OKT4 simultaneously.
3. This serum is comprised of several North American HIV-1 sero-positive patients, having a high-titered IgG to gp120 and gp160 of HIV_{IIIB}, $HIV-1_{MN}$, $HIV-1_{RF}$, $HIV-1_{451}$.
4. Various human T-cell lines can be substituted for H9 cells, such as CEM cells shown to exhibit similar levels of HIV-1 envelope expression. Additionally, laboratory-adapted isolates successfully used include $HIV-1_{IIIB}$, $HIV-1_{MN}$, $HIV-1_{RF}$, $HIV-1_{cdc451}$, and $HIV-1_{SF2}$.
5. Uninfected H9 cells should be processed and stained in parallel to the HIV-1 infected cells. Fluorescence signal will function as background, nonspecific binding of various MAbs, or sera to H9 cells.
6. HIV-1 infected cells are centrifuged in contained centrifuge buckets (Aerosolve) to prevent exposure to aerosol created during the centrifugation process. The 50 mL centrifuge tubes are loaded and unloaded into containers within a biosafety laminar flow-hood, located in a BL2+ area or laboratory having negative air pressure.
7. Cells are centrifuged on d 3 at 400g for 10 min, then resuspended in 35–40 mL cRPMI media, and transferred to a T-75 cm^2 vented-tissue culture flask.
8. Peak cell surface HIV-1 envelope expression roughly parallels supernatant p24 concentrations. Time to peak expression varies for the different HIV-1 strains (MN, IIIB, RF, 451) and will have to be optimized for each particular stock. In general, peak expression is obtained between d 3 and 7.

9. Over the course of acute infection, viability of H9 cells diminishes. This may cause problems when staining and during analysis of fluorescence patterns as nonviable cells become more permeable to the fluorescent conjugated antibodies resulting in nonspecific fluorescence. This can be avoided by harvesting and staining cells prior to severe loss in cell viability (>60% viability results in reduced nonspecific staining).

10. The amount of cells harvested will depend upon the size of the particular assay.

11. H9 cells may form large clumps of cells throughout the culture.Syncytia formation (cell fusion) also occurs. For best results, disruption of cell clumps is recommended. Pipet up and down carefully with a 10 mL pipet, and check degree of cell clumping during cell enumeration on hemocytometer. If cell clumping persists, allow cells to settle to bottom of tube and remove upper layer for transfer to another tube.

12. The small volume of cells and sera mixture allows for more limited amounts of reagents to be used.

13. This can either be accomplished using an orbital shaker placed in a 4°C refrigerator or a rack of tubes placed in ice on top of the orbital shaker. It is important to note that placement should be secured, since cells remain infectious.

14. Initially add 1.5 mL of fresh PBS for easier vortexing to resuspend the pellet, then add the remaining 1.5 mL for total volume.

15. After decanting, a small volume of buffer will remain in the tube (approx 100–200 µL).

16. It is important for this and future incubation steps to be performed in the dark to prevent loss of fluorescence efficiency of the fluorescent probe.

17. Incubation of HIV-1 infected cells with 1% paraformaldehyde has been shown to reduce HIV-1 infectivity by greater than five logs *(12)*.

18. Other commercially available flow cytometers can also be used to measure the same experimental parameters. Forward and side scatter are measurements of the size and density, respectively, and allow the operator to analyze only cells of the desired size.

19. Calibrite beads are comprised of three microsphere particles with fluorescence parameters mimicking FITC and PE. The beads are used to adjust instrument settings, check instrument sensitivity, set fluorescence compensation, and monitor instrument performance. QC3 beads are a single population of microsphere particles with both FITC and PE conjugated on the surface. These beads closely resemble human lymphocytes in size and provide additional assurance for instrument performance.

20. Proper gating during analysis is essential for interpretable results. This can be accomplished by initially running uninfected, unstained H9 cells and drawing a gate based on the FSC/SSC signal of the majority of cells. Next, check that these cells are the appropriate cells by analyzing cells stained with anti-CD4 marker. Propidium iodide (PI) can be used to stain viable cells and assist in setting FSC/SSC gate. Care must be taken when using PI due to its high fluorescence intensity and the potential for contamination of the fluidics system. Titrate to find appropriate concentration.

21. Levels of nonspecific binding of antibodies and sera of interest should be evaluated and compared to previous values.

22. The peak of HIV-1 infection is monitored via temporal CD4 down regulation. Once HIV-1 envelope expression becomes detectable by antibody staining, CD4 downregulation may be complete. Using H9 cells, minimal HIV-1 envelope expression is observed prior to complete CD4 downregulation. It is important to measure CD4 expression using a monoclonal antibody outside of the gp120 binding site on CD4. For example, MAb L3a binds to an epitope on CD4, which overlaps the gp120 binding site and may be blocked by gp120 binding to CD4. Therefore, to ensure that CD4 is downregulated and not simply bound to gp120, H9 cells should be stained using a MAb such as OKT4.

23. Levels of nonspecific binding of negative control sera to infected cells is critical to determine if level of nonspecific staining is too high. As mentioned earlier, if acute infection is allowed to proceed for too long, increased nonspecific staining of cells occurs, resulting in background levels which will adversely impact on quality of data.

24. Cell flow rates of 200–400 cells/s are optimal for the collection of data. The flow rate can be adjusted either by the flow cytometer itself or by adjusting the final cell resuspension volume.

References

1. Doms, R. W., Earl, P. L., and Moss, B. (1991) The assembly of the HIV-1 env glycoprotein into dimers and tetramers. *Adv. Exp. Med. Biol.* **300,** 203–219.

2. Earl, P. L., Doms, R. W., and Moss, B. (1990) Oligomeric structure of the human immunodeficiency virus type 1 envelope glycoprotein. *Proc. Natl. Acad. Sci. USA* **87,** 648–652.

3. Pinter, A., Honnen, W. J., Tilley, S. A., Bona, C., Zaghouani, H., Gorny, M., and Zolla-Pazner, S. (1989) Oligomeric structure of gp41, the transmembrane protein of human immunodeficiency virus type 1. *J. Virol.* **63,** 2674–2679.

4. Schawaller, M., Smith, C. E., Skehel, J. J., and Wiley, D. C. (1989) Studies with cross-linking reagents on the oligomeric structure of the env-glycoprotein of HIV. *Virology* **172,** 367–369.

5. VanCott, T. C., Polonis, V. R., Loomis, L. D., Michael, N. L., Nara, P. L., and Birx, D. L. (1995) Differential role of V3-specific antibodies in neutralization assays involving primary and laboratory-adapted isolates of HIV type 1. *AIDS Res. Hum. Retrovir.* **11,** 1379–1391.

6. Moore, J. P., Cao, Y., Qing, L., Sattentau, Q. J., Pyati, J., Koduri, R., et al. (1995) Primary isolates of human immunodeficiency virus type 1 are relatively resistant to neutralization by monoclonal antibodies to gp120, and their neutralization is not predicted by studies with monomeric gp120. *J. Virol.* **69,** 101–109.

7. Moore, J. P. and Sodroski, J. (1996) Antibody cross-competition analysis of the human immunodeficiency virus type 1 gp120 exterior envelope glycoprotein. *J. Virol.* **70,** 1863–1872.

8. Sattentau, Q. J. and J. P. Moore. (1995) Human immunodeficiency virus type 1 neutralization is determined by epitope exposure on the gp120 oligomer. *J. Exp. Med.* **182,** 185–196.

9. Gorse, G. J., Frey, S. E., Newman, F. K., and Belshe, R. B. (1992) Detection of binding antibodies to native and recombinant human immunodeficiency virus type 1 envelope glycoproteins following recombinant gp160 immunization measured by flow cytometry and enzyme immunoassays. The AIDS Vaccine Clinical Trials Network. *J. Clin. Microbiol.* **30,** 2606–2612.

10. Gorse, G. J., Frey, S. E., Patel, G., Newman, F. K., and Belshe, R. B. (1994) Vaccine-induced antibodies to native and recombinant human immunodeficiency virus type 1 envelope glycoproteins. NIAID AIDS Vaccine Clinical Trials Network. *Vaccine* **12,** 912–918.

11. VanCott, T. C., Bethke, F. R., Burke, D. S., Redfield, R. R., and Birx, D. L. (1995) Lack of induction of antibodies specific for conserved, discontinuous epitopes of HIV-1 envelope glycoprotein by candidate AIDS vaccines. *J. Immunol.* **155,** 4100–4110.

12. Sattar, S. A. and Springthorpe, V. S. (1991) Survival and disinfectant inactivation of the human immunodeficiency virus: a critical review. *Rev. Infect. Dis.* **13,** 430–447.

30

Analysis of Antibody–Antigen Interactions Using Surface Plasmon Resonance

Thomas C. VanCott

1. Introduction

Accurate analyses of antibody specificities and affinities are critical to understanding their role in antibody-mediated neutralization of HIV-1 in vitro and their potential activity against HIV-1 in vivo. Multiple immunologic tools currently exist for measuring antibody–antigen interactions to include enzyme immunoassays (EIA), Western blotting, radioimmunoassays, and others. However, these techniques all require some form of protein labeling or secondary antibodies for detection of specific binding interactions. Disadvantages of protein labeling involve potential alterations in protein tertiary structure, while the use of secondary detection antibodies prohibits the measurement of binding interactions in real-time. Recently, instruments utilizing the physical principal of surface plasmon resonance (SPR) (BIAcore™, Pharmacia Biosensor, Piscataway, NJ) *(1–4)* have been developed which allow real-time measurements of protein binding interactions without the use of internal labels or secondary antibodies. Proteins of interest are covalently coupled to a flexible biosensor matrix, and kinetic rate constants can be directly extracted from analyses of association and dissociation binding curves. The relative concentration of immobilized protein can be determined allowing, for example, the comparison of binding efficiency of one antibody against a number of different proteins.

Binding of monoclonal antibodies (MAbs) and polyclonal sera (mouse, rabbit, guinea pig, monkey, human) to both whole HIV-1 proteins (gp120, gp160, p24) and peptides can be measured using SPR *(5–7)*. SPR has been used to characterize the binding kinetics of a HIV-1 gp41-specific neutralizing MAb *(8)* and to demonstrate that the dissociation, but not the association, rate con-

From: *Methods in Molecular Medicine, Vol. 17: HIV Protocols*
Edited by: N. L. Michael and J. H. Kim © Humana Press Inc., Totowa, NJ

stant describing the interaction between HIV-1 gp160 V3-specific MAbs and monomeric gp120 correlates with the ability of the MAb to neutralize the homologous HIV-1 isolate in vitro *(9)*. The ability to control and quantitate biosensor matrix protein concentrations has allowed direct comparisons of antibody reactivity against several antigens. In this way, HIV-1 infected individuals living in Thailand have been serotyped as clade B or E by studying relative binding of their sera to gp160 from clade B or E *(10)*. Furthermore, studies involving antibody and soluble CD4 binding to recombinant forms of gp120 have indicated minimal disruption of tertiary monomeric gp120 structure upon immobilization allowing for more accurate characterization of antibody binding dependence on overall proper protein structure *(11)*. This has allowed more extensive description of the qualitative nature of the binding properties of antibody elicited using various candidate HIV-1 vaccines *(12)*.

Proteins of interest are first covalently linked (immobilized) to the dextran biosensor matrix. Immobilization conditions for each antigen are optimized by conducting a preconcentration step. Once the protein is immobilized, single or multiple antibody interactions can be studied. Bound antibody is dissociated from the matrix (regeneration) allowing the same protein matrix to be used for repeated binding interactions.

2. Materials

2.1. Equipment

1. BIAcore 1000, 2000, or BIAlite™ (Pharmacia Biosensor).
2. BIAcore 1000, 2000, or BIAlite software (Pharmacia Biosensor).

2.2. Reagents and Buffers (see Note 1)

1. HEPES-buffered saline (HBS) running buffer (10 mM N-[2-hydroxyethyl]piperazine-N'-[2-ethanesulfonic acid] [HEPES], 150 mM NaCl, 3.4 mM ethylene diamine tetra-acetic acid (EDTA), 0.05% BIAcore surfactant P20, pH 7.4) (*see* **Note 2**).
2. Sodium formate immobilization buffer: 10 mM sodium formate, pH to 3.5 or pH 3.0 using 1 M HCl.
3. Sodium acetate immobilization buffer (NaAc): 10 mM sodium acetate, pH to 4.0, 4.5, or 5.0 using 1 M HCl.
4. 2-[N-Morpholino]ethanesulfonic acid (*MES*) immobilization buffer: 10 mM adjust pH to 6.0 using 1 M HCl.
5. 400 mM N-ethyl-N'-(3-diethylaminopropyl) carbodiimide hydrochloride (EDC) (*see* **Note 3**).
6. 100 mM N-hydroxysuccinimide (NHS) (*see* **Note 3**).
7. 1 M Ethanolamine (*see* **Note 3**).
8. Borate buffer: 0.1 M borate buffer, adjust pH to 8.5 with 1 M NaOH.
9. 2-(2-pyridinyldithio)ethaneamine hydrochloride (PDEA) activation solution

(80 mM): 4.5 mg of PDEA in 250 μL 0.1 M borate buffer pH 8.5 (*see* **Note 4**).
10. 2-Mercaptoethanol (2-ME): 50 mM 2-ME in 50 mM NaAc, pH 4.5.
11. Regeneration buffers to include HCl, H$_3$PO$_4$, formic acid, NaOH, and MgCl$_2$.

3. Methods

3.1. Immobilization of Ligand

3.1.1. Preconcentration

1. To select optimal ligand immobilization buffer, prepare ligand at an approximate concentration of 10–50 μg/mL at various pH using some or all of the following buffers: sodium formate pH 3.5, NaAc, pH 4.0, NaAc pH 5.0, and MES, pH 6.0 (*see* **Note 5**).
2. Inject 20–30 μL of ligand at each desired pH across an unactivated matrix surface at a flow rate of 5 μL/min (4–6 min injection). Measure binding 30 s after injection and just prior to completion of ligand injection (*see* **Note 6**). Between each ligand injection, inject 5 μL 10 mM HCl to wash matrix of any nonspecifically bound ligand (*see* **Note 7**).
3. Select buffer which yields maximum diffusion signal (from **step 2**) indicating the highest diffusion and concentration of ligand within the biosensor matrix (*see* **Note 8**).
4. Using selected buffer from **step 3**, inject serial dilutions of ligand (20–30 μL at 5 μL/min) across unactivated matrix to determine minimum concentration of antigen with desired diffusion properties (*see* **Notes 9 and 10**).

3.1.2. Immobilization (Amine) (see **Note 11**)

1. Activate biosensor dextran matrix by injecting 35 μL (5 μL/min flow rate) of a 1:1 mixture of EDC and NHS across the matrix (*see* **Note 12**).
2. Inject 30 μL of ligand prepared in selected immobilization buffer across EDC/NHS activated matrix.
3. Deactivate matrix by injecting 30 μL of ethanolamine (*see* **Note 13**).
4. Wash matrix with dilute acid (1 mM HCl) or base (1 mM NaOH) to remove noncovalently bound ligand from the matrix (*see* **Note 14**).

3.1.3. Immobilization (Thiol) (see **Note 11**)

1. Activate biosensor dextran matrix by injecting 10–35 μL (5 μL/min flow rate) of a 1:1 mixture of EDC and NHS across the matrix (*see* **Note 12**).
2. Inject 30 μL of PDEA across matrix placing an active disulfide group in the matrix for coupling to a free thiol group on the ligand.
3. Deactivate matrix by injecting 30 μL of ethanolamine (*see* **Note 13**).
4. Inject 30 μL of ligand prepared in selected immobilization buffer across PDEA matrix to covalently couple ligand to matrix via the ligand free thiol group.
5. Deactivate matrix by injecting 30 μL of 50 mM 2-ME (*see* **Note 15**).
6. Wash matrix with dilute acid (1 mM HCl) or base (1 mM NaOH) to remove noncovalently bound ligand from the matrix (*see* **Note 14**).

3.2 Measurement of Antibody:Antigen Binding Interactions

3.2.1. Antibody:Antigen Interactions

1. Immobilize ligand of interest as described in **Subheading 3.1.** (*see* **Note 16**).
2. Dilute MAbs (0.1–100 µg /mL) or polyclonal sera (1:100) in HBS running buffer (*see* **Note 17**).
3. Set flow rate (rate at which HBS running buffer flows through the biosensor matrix) at 5 µL/min (*see* **Note 18**).
4. Set injection volume at 30 µL (6-min injection).
5. Inject MAb or polyclonal sera across the matrix with immobilized ligand and across a control matrix (*see* **Note 19**)
6. Regenerate matrix using dilute acid (1 m*M* HCl) or base (1 m*M* NaOH) to remove nonspecifically bound antibody from the matrix (*see* **Note 20**).
7. Repeat **steps 2** and **3** for all MAbs and polyclonal sera (*see* **Notes 21** and **22**).

3.2.2. Multiple Sequential Antibody:Antigen Interactions

1. Immobilize ligand of interest as described in **Subheading 3.1.** (*see* **Note 16**)
2. Dilute MAbs (0.1–100 µg/mL) or polyclonal sera (1:100) in HBS running buffer (*see* **Note 17**).
3. Set flow rate (rate at which HBS running buffer flows through the biosensor matrix) at 5 µL/min (*see* **Note 18**).
4. Set injection volume at 30 µL (6-min injection).
5. Inject MAb or polyclonal sera across the matrix with immobilized ligand and across a control matrix (*see* **Note 19**)
6. Inject second MAb or polyclonal sera across the matrix with immobilized ligand. This procedure can be repeated for multiple sequential binding interactions (*see* **Note 23**).
7. Regenerate matrix using dilute acid (1 m*M* HCl) or base (1 m*M* NaOH) to remove nonspecifically bound Ab from the matrix (*see* **Note 20**).
8. Repeat **steps 2** and **3** for all MAbs and polyclonal sera (*see* **Notes 21** and **22**).

3.2.3. Antibody Competition Studies

1. Immobilize MAb of interest as described in **Subheading 3.1.** (*see* **Note 24**)
2. Capture antigen by injecting 30 µL (flow rate 5 µL/min) of gp120 or gp160 at a concentration between 10–50 µg /mL (*see* **Note 25**).
3. Inject 30 µL (flow rate 5 µL/min) of MAb #2 at 5–10 µg/mL (*see* **Note 26**).
4. Regenerate matrix using dilute acid (2.5–10 m*M* HCl) to remove nonspecifically bound MAb from the matrix (*see* **Note 27**).
5. Repeat **steps 2–4** for other MAb combinations (*see* **Note 28**).

3.2.4. Protein Characterization Studies (see **Note 29**)

1. Activate biosensor dextran matrix by injecting 35 µL (5 µL/min flow rate) of a 1:1 mixture of EDC and NHS across the matrix (see Note 12).
2. Inject 30 µL of sCD4 at 20 µg /mL in MES, pH 6.0 at a flow rate of 5 µL/min (*see* **Note 30**).

3. Deactivate matrix by injecting 30 μL of ethanolamine (*see* **Note 13**).
4. Wash matrix with 4.5 *M* MgCl₂ to remove noncovalently bound ligand from the matrix (*see* **Note 14**).
5. Capture gp120/gp160 preparation by injecting 30 μL of gp120/gp160 (10 μg/mL) at a flow rate of 2 μL/min across the sCD4 protein matrix (*see* **Note 31**).
6. Inject 30 μL (flow rate 5 μL/min) of MAb (5–10 μg /mL) or polyclonal sera (1:100) (*see* **Note 32**).
7. Regenerate matrix using 4.5 *M* MgCl₂.
8. Repeat **steps 5–7** to study other MAbs or polyclonal sera.

4. Notes

1. All buffers must be filtered and degassed prior to use. Filter all buffers (0.2 μm) and degas under vacuum (while stirring) for 15–30 min.
2. To reduce nonspecific binding of some polyclonal sera to the dextran matrix, an alternate HBS running buffer may be prepared (10 m*M* HEPES, 300 m*M* NaCl, 5.0 m*M* EDTA, 0.05% BIAcore surfactant P20, pH 7.4)
3. EDC, NHS and ethanolamine are stored at –20°C and should be used within 1–2 h of thawing.
4. Use PDEA buffer within 1 h of preparation.
5. The BIAcore biosensor flow cell is composed of a negatively charged dextran matrix. In order to target and concentrate ligands of interest into this environment, it is necessary to adjust buffer pH to give antigen a positive charge allowing diffusion via electrostatic interactions. Ligands with high isoelectric points (pI > 8.0) will diffuse into the matrix efficiently using MES pH 6.0, while those with lower isoelectric points will require other mentioned buffers. In general, the pH of the immobilization buffer needs to be 1–2 pH units lower than the ligand pI.
6. It is important to record sensorgram baseline approx 30 s after injection. Immediately after ligand injection (<30 s), an alteration in baseline results attributable to refractive index differences between the running HBS buffer and the ligand buffer. After 30 s, this baseline equilibrates and any alterations in signal are directly attributable to diffusion of ligand into the matrix. The signal should be measured just prior to completion of ligand injection and the difference between this signal and the baseline signal measures the amount of ligand diffusion.
7. It is important for signal to return to baseline after each ligand injection. Since the matrix is not activated no ligand should remain within the matrix after conclusion of the injection step. However, depending on physical properties of the ligand, it is common to have some nonspecifically bound ligand remaining within the matrix which can be removed using 10 m*M* HCl.
8. If no diffusion is observed with ligand prepared in each of the immobilization buffers, it may be necessary to increase the concentration of ligand. Repeat **step 1** using higher ligand concentrations.
9. The amount of ligand immobilized depends on both the diffusion of ligand into the dextran matrix (**Subheading 3.1.**) as well as the presence of active groups on the ligand (described in **Subheading 3.1.2.**). Information on diffusion is

obtained from this preconcentration step, however, information on efficiency of covalent coupling may not be determined until the actual immobilization procedure described in **Subheading 3.1.2.** is conducted.

10. Optimal concentration of ligand immobilized within the matrix is dependent upon molecular weight and assay application. For example, for routine screening in which sensitivity is an important consideration, higher concentrations of ligand are desirable, whereas for kinetic applications, lower ligand concentrations are desirable to minimize ligate rebinding to ligand after dissociation. In general, for routine screening, HIV-1 gp120 or gp160 immobilization amounts of 5000–10,000 resonance units (RU) are optimally reactive while for smaller peptides (V3) of 20–30 amino acids, 400–1500 RU are optimally reactive. It is desirable to have preconcentration diffusion values greater than desired immobilization amount owing to the expected less than 100% efficiency in covalent coupling.

11. Multiple chemistries have been used to covalently couple ligand to the biosensor matrix and are described in detail elsewhere *(13–21)*. The two most common coupling chemistries described here involve coupling via amine or thiol groups on the ligand to chemically activated groups within the dextran matrix. HIV-1 gp120, gp160, p24, and several synthetic peptides corresponding to gp160 have successfully been immobilized using amine-coupling chemistries. Several v3 peptides with terminal cysteine amino acids have successfully been immobilized using thiol chemistries.

12. The EDC/NHS injection forms chemically activated NHS-esters within the dextran matrix for covalent coupling to ligand. Altering the volume of EDC/NHS injection alters the time the matrix is in contact with the chemicals and therefore the degree of matrix activation. Fine tuning the amount of ligand immobilized is most efficiently and successfully accomplished by altering injection volumes of EDC/NHS between 5 and 35 µL.

13. Injection of 1 M ethanolamine with high ionic strength serves two purposes. It weakens electrostatic interactions of noncovalently bound ligands, and it deactivates any unreacted activated NHS-ester groups remaining in the dextran matrix.

14. After injection of ligand and matrix deactivation, some noncovalently bound ligand may remain within the matrix and can be removed using 1 mM HCl. This procedure is termed matrix regeneration, requires some optimization work and will be discussed in more detail below (*see* **Note 20**).

15. Injection of 50 mM 2-ME deactivates any unreacted PDEA activated groups remaining in the dextran matrix. Other methods for deactivation have been described elsewhere *(13)*.

16. As discussed in **Note 10**, optimal concentration of immobilized ligand is dependent upon the ligand itself and assay application. For routine screening of MAbs or polyclonal sera, the following concentrations yield high sensitivity: gp120/gp160 (5000–10000 RU), p24 (3000–5000 RU), recombinant CD4 receptor (3000–4000 RU), and synthetic peptides 15–30 amino acids in length (400–1500 RU).

17. Selection of polyclonal sera dilution and concentration of MAb for screening purposes will depend on the nature of the antibody:antigen binding interaction

and will require some optimization. Serum dilutions of 1:50 or 1:100 in HBS running buffer appear to provide good signal-to-noise for polyclonal sera from mice, rabbits, guinea pigs, rhesus macaques, and humans. Lower serum dilutions result in increased nonspecific binding of serum components to the dextran matrix. Levels of nonspecific binding of MAbs or polyclonal sera should be evaluated initially using a blank matrix or matrix with nonspecific protein immobilized. Nonspecific binding signals in the range of 0–20 RU are acceptable background levels. MAbs with affinity constants in the range of 0.1–100 nM can be initially successfully screened at concentrations ranging from 0.1–10 µg /mL.

18. Flow rate can be adjusted between 1–100 µL/min. Slower flow rates allow longer time for interaction between Ab and immobilized antigen leading to both increased specific and nonspecific binding. For lower affinity or avidity protein interactions, decreasing flow rate is recommended to increase sensitivity.

19. Sera and MAbs should be tested initially against a blank or control protein matrix to determine extent of nonspecific binding to the dextran matrix. These values should be subtracted from binding values against ligand of interest. Binding of particular Ab is measured as the difference in RU between a time point taken just prior to Ab injection and a time point taken 30 s after completion of Ab injection.

20. Optimal regeneration buffers for some HIV-1 antigens include: recombinant gp120 and gp160 (60 mM H_3PO_4), oligomeric gp160 (10% formic acid), synthetic v3 peptides (10% formic acid), immunoglobulins (10–50 mM HCl), recombinant sCD4 (4.5 M $MgCl_2$) and p24 (60 mM H_3PO_4). Two factors are important when selecting a regeneration buffer: complete dissociation of bound Ab from antigen and retention of antigen reactivity. These are evaluated by regenerating initially with a weak acid (5 mM HCl) and monitoring both efficiency of matrix regeneration and retention of immobilized ligand reactivity.

21. Computer-driven software allows construction of programs to inject large series of antibodies against up to four separate matrices (each potentially with different antigens of interest). Abs are injected followed by regeneration and washing of the flow cell. Data is summarized in Microsoft Excel (Microsoft, Redmond, WA) spreadsheet format and individual sensorgrams recording each antibody:antigen interaction are recorded for review.

22. Programs can be written to study Ab binding against multiple ligand matrices simultaneously (BIAcore 2000) or sequentially (BIAcore 1000). This allows for relative binding efficiencies against multiple antigens to be determined. For example, binding of polyclonal sera to native and denatured forms of gp120 have been evaluated by immobilizing native and denatured forms of gp120 in adjacent flow cells and injecting antibody across both. Native/denatured gp120 binding ratios are calculated using the following equation: [(gp120 binding in RU)/(denatured gp120 binding in RU)] $*$ [(amt. of denatured gp120 immobilized in RU)/(amt native gp120 immobilized in RU)]. The second part of the equation is a correction for potential concentration differences in the two immobilized proteins.

23. Multiple sequential binding interactions with a single immobilized antigen can be studied. For example, MAbs to the HIV-1 envelope V3 region, sCD4 and a

gp41 MAb can be injected sequentially across a gp160 matrix and three binding interactions can be evaluated. This assay will yield information about epitope mapping, and those MAbs with similar specificities will compete with each other. This assay, however, is not optimal for competition studies since it is difficult to completely saturate the immobilized antigen with competing antibody. The capture assay described below is recommended for competition studies.

24. Monoclonal antibody #1 can be immobilized directly to the dextran matrix as described above. Alternatively, an anti-Ig Ab can be immobilized and used to capture several different MAbs of interest. If anti-Ig Ab is immobilized then a blocking step is required after MAb #1 is captured to block remaining unbound anti-Ig. This is accomplished by an injection of a high concentration of nonspecific Ig (concentration of approx 1 mg/mL).

25. The concentration of antigen (gp120/gp160) to be captured will depend upon the affinity of immobilized MAb #1 for the antigen. In most cases with relatively high affinity MAbs, concentrations of 10–20 μg /mL of gp120/gp160 is sufficient. The amount of antigen captured should be high enough to yield sufficient sensitivity to detect binding by MAb #2 (approx 500–1000 RU). If antigen is in short supply, the flow rate can be reduced to 1 or 2 μL/min instead of increasing the concentration of captured antigen.

26. It is essential to include a negative control MAb in order to measure natural dissociation of captured gp120/gp160 from immobilized MAb #1 to serve as a baseline when calculated the amount of MAb #2 bound.

27. Regeneration of MAb matrices can be accomplished using 2.5–50 m*M* HCl. This will have to be optimized for each individual immobilized MAb.

28. If MAbs #1 and #2 bind to the same epitope then no binding above background will be obtained for MAb #2 since 100% of antigen is bound by MAb #1.

29. This assay has been designed to study and assess reactivity of various HIV-1 envelope glycoproteins to epitope specific MAbs, HIV-1 sera, and sCD4. Preparations of gp120 or gp160 are captured by sCD4 and then bound by various gp160-specific MAbs or HIV-1 sera. Amount of bound Ab to captured gp120 or gp160 is then calculated.

30. Amount of sCD4 immobilized using these conditions may vary between 3000–5000 RU. Higher concentrations of immobilized sCD4 should be avoided since high local sCD4 concentrations may interfere with penetration of multimeric forms of gp160 into the matrix and thereby decrease capture efficiency.

31. The amount of gp120/gp160 captured can be compared to a control gp120/gp160 preparation and assess the relative concentration of sCD4 binding competent gp160 proteins within any given preparation.

32. This assay will determine relative gp160 epitope accessibility/exposure on various gp160 preparations. For example, other surface exposed epitopes on gp160 can be assessed (V3, V1/V2, gp41) to check antigenic structure outside of the sCD4 binding site.

References

1. Altschuh, D., Dubs, M. C., Weiss, E., Zeder, L. G., and Van Regenmortel, M. (1992) Determination of kinetic constants for the interaction between a mono-

clonal antibody and peptides using surface plasmon resonance. *Biochemistry* **31**, 6298–6304.

2. Fagerstam, L. G., Frostell-Karlsson, A., Karlsson, R., Persson, B., and Ronnberg, I. (1992) Biospecific interaction analysis using surface plasmon resonance detection applied to kinetic, binding site and concentration analysis. *J. Chromatog.* **597**, 397–410.

3. Karlsson, R., Michaelsson, A., and Mattsson, L. (1991) Kinetic analysis of monoclonal antibody-antigen interactions with a new biosensor based analytical system. *J. Immunol. Meth.* **145**, 229–240.

4. Sternberg, E., Perssom, B., Roos, H., and Urbaniczky, C. (1991) Quantitative determination of surface concentration of protein with surface plasmon resonance by using radiolabelled proteins. *J. Colloid Interface Sci.* **143**, 513–526.

5. Glaser, R. W. and Hausdorf, G. (1996) Binding kinetics of an antibody against HIV p24 core protein measured with real-time biomolecular interaction analysis suggest a slow conformational change in antigen p24. *J. Immunol. Meth.* **189**, 1–14.

6. Richalet, S. P., Deslandres, A., Plaue, S., You, B., Barre, S. F., and Van, R. M. (1994) Cross-reactive potential of rabbit antibodies raised against a cyclic peptide representing a chimeric V3 loop of HIV-1 gp120 studied by biosensor technique and ELISA. *FEMS Immunol. Med. Microbiol.* **9**, 77–87.

7. VanCott, T. C., Loomis, L. D., Redfield, R. R., and Birx, D. L. (1992) Real-time biospecific interaction analysis of antibody reactivity to peptides from the envelope glycoprotein, gp160, of HIV-1. *J. Immunol. Meth.* **146**, 163–176.

8. Conley, A. J., Kessler, J., Boots, L. J., Tung, J. S., Arnold, B. A., Keller, P. M., Shaw, A. R., and Emini, E. A. (1994) Neutralization of divergent human immunodeficiency virus type 1 variants and primary isolates by IAM-41-2F5, an anti-gp41 human monoclonal antibody. *Proc. Natl. Acad. Sci. USA* **91**, 3348–3352.

9. VanCott, T. C., Bethke, F. R., Polonis, V. R., Gorny, M. K., Zolla-Pazner, S., Redfield, R. R., et al. (1994) The dissociation rate of antibody-gp120 binding interactions is predictive of V3-mediated neutralization of HIV-1. *J. Immunol.* **153**, 449–459.

10. VanCott, T. C., Bethke, F. R., Artenstein, A. W., McCutchan, F. E., McNeil, J. G., Mascola, J. R., Redfield, R. R., and Birx, D. L. (1994) Serotyping international HIV-1 isolates by V3 peptides and whole gp160 proteins using BIAcore. *Methods, a companion to Methods in Enzymol.* **6**, 188–198.

11. VanCott, T. C., Bethke, F. R., Kalyanaraman, V., Burke, D. S., Redfield, R. R., and Birx, D. L. (1994) Preferential antibody recognition of structurally distinct HIV-1 gp120 molecules. *J. Acquir. Immune. Defic. Synd.* **7**, 1103–1115.

12. VanCott, T. C., Bethke, F. R., Burke, D. S., Redfield, R. R., and Birx, D. L. (1995) Lack of induction of antibodies specific for conserved, discontinuous epitopes of HIV-1 envelope glycoprotein by candidate AIDS vaccines. *J. Immunol.* **155**, 4100–4110.

13. BIAcore System Manual, Pharmacia Biosensor, Piscataway, NJ, USA.

14. Gershon, P. D. and Khilko, S. (1995) Stable chelating linkage for reversible immobilization of oligohistidine tagged proteins in the BIAcore surface plasmon resonance detector. *J. Immunol. Methods* **183**, 65–76.

15. Johnsson, B., Lofas, S., and Lindquist, G. (1991) Immobilization of proteins to a carboxymethyldextran-modified gold surface for biospecific interaction analysis in surface plasmon resonance sensors. *Anal. Biochem.* **198,** 268–277.
16. Johnsson, B., Lofas, S., Lindquist, G., Edstrom, A., Muller, H. R., and Hansson, A. (1995) Comparison of methods for immobilization to carboxymethyl dextran sensor surfaces by analysis of the specific activity of monoclonal antibodies. *J. Mol. Recognit.* **8,** 125–131.
17. Johnsson, U., Fagerstam, L., Ivarsson, B., Johnsson, B., Karlsson, R., Lundh, K., Lofas, S., Persson, B., Roos, H., Ronnberg, I., et al. (1991) Real-time biospecific interaction analysis using surface plasmon resonance and a sensor chip technology. *BioTechniques* **11,** 620–627.
18. Masson, L., Mazza, A., and Brousseau, R. (1994) Stable immobilization of lipid vesicles for kinetic studies using surface plasmon resonance. *Anal. Biochem.* **218,** 405–412.
19. O'Shannessy, D. J., Brigham, B. M., and Peck, K. (1992) Immobilization chemistries suitable for use in the BIAcore surface plasmon resonance detector. *Anal. Biochem.* **205,** 132–136.
20. Scouten, W. H., Luoung, J. H. T., and Brown, R. S. (1995) Enzyme or protein immobilization techniques for applications in biosensor design. *Trends Biotechnol.* **13,** 178–185.
21. Stein, T. and Gerisch, F. (1996) Oriented binding of a lipid-anchored cell adhesion protein onto a biosensor surface using hydrophobic immobilization and photoactive crosslinking. *Anal. Biochem.* **237,** 252–259.

31

Measurement of HIV-1 Specific
and Total Antibody Secreting Cells by ELISPOT

Frederik W. van Ginkel, John L. VanCott, Robert Kaminski,
and Thomas C. VanCott

1. Introduction

B-cells play an important role in protection against pathogens, and they secrete specific antibodies in serum and mucosal secretions upon antigenic stimulation contributing to immune exclusion and clearance of pathogens. The frequency of antibody forming cells (AFC) in specific organs is often a reflection of the route of antigen exposure, i.e., systemic, oral, or intranasal, as well as of antigenic load. Enumeration of AFC was originally performed by plaque-forming cell assay measuring lysis of sheep red blood cells. The nature of this assay, that requires coupling of the antigen to sheep red blood cells (SRBC), made detection of various antigen-specific AFC rather cumbersome. However, the development of the enzyme linked immunodetection of AFCs (ELISPOT) combined with the development of standardized lymphocyte isolation techniques enables detection of AFC secreting antibodies specific for many different antigens and derived from various immunologic effector sites *(1–6)*.

2. Materials
2.1. Supplies and Solutions for Tissue Processing

1. 10 cc syringes and 18 gauge needles (Thomas Scientific, Swedesboro, NJ).
2. Surgical scissors and forceps (Hu-Friedy, Chicago, IL).
3. 15- and 50-mL conical tubes (Becton Dickinson, Franklin Lakes, NJ).
5. 200-mm stainless steel screen.
6. 60 × 15 mm petri dishes containing: 8.29 g NH_4CL (0.15 M), 1.0 g $KHCO_3$ (1 mM), 37.2 mg Na_2EDTA (0.1 mM). Add 800 mL H_2O and adjust to pH 7.2–7.4

From: *Methods in Molecular Medicine, Vol. 17: HIV Protocols*
Edited by: N. L. Michael and J. H. Kim © Humana Press Inc., Totowa, NJ

with 1 *N* HCl. Add H$_2$0 to 1 L. Filter sterilize through a 0.2-μm filter, and store at room temperature.

8. Joklik-modified medium (Gibco, Grand Island, NY).
9. Collagenase from *Clostridium histolyticum* Type IV (Sigma, St. Louis, MO).
10. DNase I (Sigma).
11. Ethylenediamine tetra-acetic acid, EDTA (Sigma).
12. Percoll (Pharmacia Fine Chemicals, Pharmacia, Inc., Uppsala, Sweden).
13. Ficoll gradient (Lympholyte M, Cedar Lane Laboratories, Hornby, Canada).
14. Culture media (cRPMI): RPMI 1640 (ABI, Columbia, MD), supplemented with 10% heat-inactivated fetal bovine serum (FBS) (Sigma), 1% Pen/Strep solution (100 U/mL penicillin, 100 mg/mL streptomycin, [Gibco]), 1% L-glutamine solution (200 m*M* [Gibco]).
15. Incomplete RPMI: RPMI 1640 with antibiotics.
16. Hanks balanced salt solution (10X), HBSS (Sigma).

2.2. Supplies and Solutions for ELISPOT

1. Phosphate-buffered saline (PBS), pH 7.2 (Advanced Biotechnologies, Inc., Columbia, MD).
2. Tween-20, polyoxyethylene-sorbitan monolaurate (Sigma).
3. PBS with 0.05% (v/v) Tween-20 (PBS-T).
4. Immulon I flat-bottom plates (Dynatech, Chantilly, VA) or 96-well nitrocellulose plate (Millipore SA, Molsheim, France).
5. Humidified 37°C, 5% CO$_2$ incubator.
6. Alkaline phosphatase (AP)-conjugated or horseradish peroxidase (HRP)-conjugated, affinity purified detection antibodies.
7. BCIP phosphatase substrate solution (Sigma).
8. Agarose type 1 low EEO (Sigma).
9. Alkaline phosphatase gel substrate: mixture of BCIP substrate solution and low melting point agarose (Sigma). Prepare just prior to use (*see* **Subheading 3.2.1.**).
10. 3-Amino-9-Ethyl Carbazole (AEC) (Pierce, Rockford, IL).
11. Dimethyl formamide (DMF).
12. 0.1 *M* sodium acetate buffer, pH 5.2.
13. 30% hydrogen peroxide (H$_2$O$_2$).
14. Filter paper, Whatman no. 1 or equivalent (PGC Scientific, Gaithersburg, MD).
15. Dissecting microscope.

3. Methods
3.1. Collection and Processing of Mouse Cells

The isolation of lymphocytes from (1) the systemic immune compartment, the spleen, (2) the intestinal tract, Peyer's patches (PP) and lamina propria cells, and (3) the respiratory tract, involving lung-derived intraparenchymal cells, and draining lymph nodes of the upper and lower respiratory tract will be described in this section.

3.1.1. Splenocytes

1. Euthanize mice with CO_2 or by cervical dislocation as discussed in Chapter 37 {Collection and processing of mucosal secretions from mice}.
2. Spray exterior of euthanized mice with 70% ethanol.
3. Remove spleens, and place in a 60×15 mm petri dish containing 10 mL of culture media (cRPMI)
4. Prepare splenocyte suspension by gently teasing spleens through a sterile stainless steel screen using the bottom side of a 10-cc syringe plunger (*see* **Note 1**).
5. Disperse clumps in the suspension by drawing up and expelling the suspension through a 10-mL syringe equipped with a 18-gauge needle.
6. Place the single cell suspension into a 15-mL conical tube, and spin at 1500g for 10 min in a Beckman GS6R centrifuge at 4°C.
7. Spleen cells will pellet at the bottom of the conical tube. Discard supernatant with care to not disrupt the pellet.
8. Add 2 mL of sterile ACK lysing buffer to the cell pellet and disperse pellet by drawing up and expelling the suspension through a 5-mL pipet until a single-cell suspension is obtained.
9. After 2 min on ice, wash the cells by filling the conical tube with cRPMI, gently vortex (*see* **Note 2**) followed by centrifugation at 1200 rpm for 10 min to form the cell pellet.
10. Wash cells with cRPMI as in **steps 6** and **7**.
11. Gently vortex to form a single cell suspension and add 10 mL of cRPMI.
12. Place cell suspension on ice for 5 min to allow fibrous tissue debris to settle to the bottom of the tube.
13. Pour off supernatant containing the cell suspension into a new 15 mL conical tube, centrifuge again, and resuspend in a volume suitable for counting (*see* **Note 3**).

3.1.2. Peyer's patches (PP)

1. Prepare mouse for tissue removal as in **Subheading 3.1.**
2. Make an incision from the neck to the lower abdomen with surgical scissors to expose the abdominal cavity.
3. Place the entire small intestine in a 60×15-mm Petri dish containing 5 mL of incomplete RPMI.
4. Excise PP from the small intestinal wall (approx 7 PP/mouse small intestine)
5. Place PP in 6 mL of incomplete RPMI with antibiotics (Pen/Strep) warmed to 37°C containing freshly added collagenase (0.5 mg/mL). The enzyme solution with PP is added to a 10 mL screw-cap glass tube containing a small magnetic stir bar.
6. Incubate for 15 min at 37°C on a magnetic stirrer.
7. Dissociated PP cells are removed by gently pipeting the supernatant. The cells are pelleted by centrifugation (1200 rpm for 10 min), washed in a 50-mL conical tube and resuspended in cRPMI. Keep the cells on ice.
8. Repeat **steps 5** through **7** two more times. For each incubation step, add 6 mL of fresh enzyme solution to undissociated PP tissue. Following each digestion, wash

dissociated PP cells in cRPMI and add isolated PP lymphocytes in the same 50-mL conical tube.

9. Place cell suspension on ice for 5 min to allow fibrous tissue debris to settle to the bottom of the tube.
10. Pour off supernatant containing the cell suspension into a new 15-mL conical tube, centrifuge again, and resuspend in a volume suitable for counting.
11. The average yield of PP lymphocytes is 5×10^6 per mouse.

3.1.3. Lamina Propria Lymphocytes (LPL)

1. Prepare mouse for tissue removal as in **Subheading 3.1.**
2. Make an incision from the neck to the lower abdomen with surgical scissors exposing the abdominal cavity.
3. The peritoneal cavity should be opened, and the intestines should be exposed by carefully dissecting away the mesentery.
4. Remove small intestines from several mice, i.e., the region between the stomach and the cecum.
5. Remove mesenteric and connective tissue.
6. Remove PP from intestines.
7. Open intestines longitudinally and cut into short segments (approx 1 cm in a Petri dish or weighing boat containing RPMI and remove fecal matter by washing the intestines employing a forceps.
8. Wash the intestines for 20 min in PBS containing 1 mM EDTA at room temperature while gently stirring on a magnetic stirrer in a sterilized 125-mL flask to remove intraepithelial lymphocytes (IEL) released in the supernatant.
9. Remove supernatant (can use meshstrainer) to a 50-mL concical tube containing RPMI with antibiotics. Vigorously shake tube for 5 s and remove supernatant and repeat. Repeat **steps 8** and **9**.
10. To isolate LPL from the remaining tissue by enzymatic dissociation, add tissue pieces to a 10-mL screw-cap glass tube containing 0.5 mg/mL collagenase in 10 mL complete RPMI with 5% FCS for 15 min at 37°C.
11. Remove supernatant and centrifuge at 320g for 10 min in a table top centrifuge to collect the LPL and resuspend them in RPMI containing 5% FCS.
12. Repeat **steps 9–11** additional one time.
13. Pool LPLs together and wash one more time.
14. Resuspend the cell pellet in 16 mL of 40% Percoll. 100% Percoll is defined as nine parts of stock Percoll with one part 10X HBSS.
15. Layer 8 mL of 40% Percoll, containing the LPLs, on 2 mL of 75% Percoll.
16. Centrifuge the tubes for 20 min at 20°C and 600–800g.
17. Collect the cells that reside between 75 and 40% Percoll layer.
18. Wash and resuspend cells in cRPMI. Routinely, $1–2 \times 10^6$ LPLs/mouse are obtained using this method.

3.1.4. Intraparenchymal Pulmonary Lymphoid Cells (IPL)

1. Prepare mouse for tissue removal as in **Subheading 3.1.**
2. Attach mouse to a solid backing, e.g., styrofoam with needles.

3. Disinfect exterior of mouse with 70% ethanol.
4. Make an incision from the abdomen to the neck with surgical scissors opening the thoracic cavity exposing the lungs and heart.
5. The diaphragm and sternum should be cut away with special care taken not to puncture or damage the lung or surrounding tissues. The pleural membranes should also be cut so that the lungs are given sufficient area to expand.
6. The walls of the thoracic cavity are pinned to the sides to allow free access to the heart.
7. An incision is made in the left ventricular wall of the heart in order to drain blood from the blood vessels in the lungs by perfusion of 10 mL sterile PBS into the right ventricle. The lungs should turn a white color and fluid should be flowing from the left ventricle incision *(1,2)*.
8. Carefully excise aseptically the tissue from the thoracic cavity containing the heart and lungs.
9. Remove each of the five lobes and cut each lobe into small pieces in RPMI-1640 with 2% FCS.
10. Transfer the pieces (without media) to 10 mL of RPMI-1640 containing 10% FCS, collagenase type 4 at 300 U/mL (Worthington) and DNAse type 1 at 50 U/mL per lung and incubate it at 37°C under constant agitation. Pipet the pieces with a 10 mL pipet every 20 min for 1–1.5 h.
11. Remove the undigested tissue by filtering the digest over a sterile cotton plug in a 10-mL syringe.
12. Wash the resulting cells in RPMI-1640 and resuspend them in cRPMI and centrifuge over a Ficoll gradient (Lympholyte M, Cedar Lane Laboratories) at room temperature for 20 min at 600–800g on a table top centrifuge.
13. Collect the cells at the interface of medium-Lympholyte M and wash them two times with RPMI (10 min at 320g on table top centrifuge)
14. Wash the cells in cRPMI, and count the cells as described in **Note 3**. Routinely $1–3 \times 10^6$ lymphocytes are obtained from naive mice while from immune lungs a total of $5–10 \times 10^6$ are obtained.

3.1.5. Upper Respiratory Tract Associated Lymph Nodes

The draining lymph nodes of the upper respiratory tract are enlarged upon intranasal immunization. A total of three different sets of lymph nodes are associated with the upper respiratory tract and include the submandibular lymph nodes and the superficial and deep cervical lymph nodes.

1. Prepare mouse for tissue removal as in **Subheading 3.1.**
2. Disinfect exterior of mouse with 70% ethanol.
3. Carefully remove skin from the ventricle part of the neck without disturbing underlying tissues. Care should be taken when removing the skin, since these lymph nodes sometimes are attached to the skin. The salivary glands should be visible. Three sets of lymph nodes are associated with the upper respiratory tract i.e., the submandibular lymph nodes, the superficial and deep cervical lymph nodes.

4. The submandibular lymph nodes are located anterior of the salivary glands and can easily be isolated. The superficial cervical lymph nodes are posteriolateral to each of the salivary glands and can be removed without removing the salivary glands. The deep cervical lymph nodes can be found by removing the salivary glands and looking between the sterno-hyoid and sterno-cleido-mastoid muscles. These lymph nodes should be located under these muscles. They are rather small and relatively hard to find in unimmunized mice.

5. Remove lymph nodes and place in a 60 × 15 mm petri dish containing 10 mL of culture media (cRPMI).

6. Prepare lymphocyte suspension by gently teasing lymph nodes through a sterile stainless steel mesh using the bottom side of a 10-cc syringe plunger in order to generate single cell suspension.

7. Disperse clumps in the suspension by drawing up and expelling the suspension through a 10-mL syringe equipped with a 18-gauge needle.

8. Place the single cell suspension into a 15 mL conical tube and spin at 1500g for 10 min in a Beckman GS6R centrifuge at 4°C.

9. Lymphocytes will pellet at the bottom of the conical tube. Discard supernatant with care without disrupting the pellet.

10. Wash cells with cRPMI. No ACK lysis is normally required to remove red blood cells.

11. Gently vortex to form a single cell suspension and add 10 mL of cRPMI.

12. Place cell suspension on ice for 5 min to allow fibrous tissue debris to settle to the bottom of the tube.

13. Pour off supernatant containing the cell suspension into a new 15-mL conical tube, centrifuge again, and resuspend in a suitable volume for counting (*see* **Note 3**).

14. The number of lymphocytes recovered varies between $1–5 \times 10^6$ for naive mice to $5–25 \times 10^6$ for intranasally immunized mice.

3.1.6. Lower Respiratory Tract Associated Lymph Nodes (LRLN)

1. The lung/heart and associated tissue are removed from the thoracic cavity as described in isolation for lung lymphocytes (*see* **Section 3.1.**), but no perfusion of the lungs is needed.

2. The five lung lobes, the esophagus, the thymus, and heart are removed. The remaining amorphous tissue contains the LRLNs (comprised of the hilar and mediastinal lymph nodes also referred to as parathymic lymph nodes).

3. A single cell suspension is obtained by putting this tissue through a stainless steel mesh employing a 5-mL syringe plunger.

4. If needed, red blood cells can be removed by lysis as described for the spleen (**Subheading 3.1.**).

5. The same isolation procedure as described in **Subheading 3.1.**, **steps 8–13** are used to obtain single-cell suspension.

6. The yield in naive mice is approx $0.5–2.0 \times 10^6$ lymphocytes per mouse while the yield in a intratracheal immunized mouse is between approx $3–10 \times 10^6$ lymphocytes.

3.2. ELISPOT Assay

3.2.1. ELISPOT using Agarose gel

1. Dilute antigen, for antigen-specific ELISPOT, or with unlabeled anti-IgG,-IgA, or IgM antibodies for total isotype-specific antibody secreting cells in appropriate coating buffer (*see* **Note 4**) and add 100 µL to the wells of an Immulon I flat-bottom plate. Incubate plates overnight at 4°C.
2. Wash plate two times by filling wells (200 µL/wash) with PBS or RPMI and decant contents (*see* **Note 5**).
3. Add 150 µL of cRPMI containing 10% FCS to each well and incubate 3 h at 37°C to block remaining binding sites
4. Wash plate two times with PBS. Fully aspirate any remaining fluid from the wells by patting bottom of plate with dry absorbent paper (*see* **Note 5**).
5. The cell suspensions should be counted and adjusted to the proper concentration in cRPMI (*see* **Note 3**).
6. Dilute cells to appropriate concentration and add (100 µL/well) to the plate. Starting cell dilution at 1×10^6 cells/well (*see* **Note 6**). Make serial dilutions of cells to load into the wells in order to obtain the best cell concentration to enumerate AFC.
7. Incubate cells for a minimum of 4 h or alternatively overnight at 37°C with 5% CO_2.
8. Wash plates four times with PBS-T. Fully aspirate any remaining fluid from the wells.
9. Add 100 µL of appropriate enzyme conjugated antibodies (AP) to each well. Incubate at 37°C with 5% CO_2 for 1–2 h (*see* **Note 7**).
10. Wash plates three times with PBS-T. Before final aspiration, allow plates to soak in the PBS-T for 10 min to remove any remaining unbound conjugate. Fully aspirate any remaining fluid from the wells. Do two final washes with PBS to remove any residual Tween-20.
11. The BCIP-Agarose gel substrate is prepared by adding 8 mL of the BCIP liquid substrate system (Sigma) to a 15-mL conical. Place this in a water bath to bring the temperature of the substrate up from its storage temperature to approx 80°C. In a separate 15-mL conical, combine 2 mL of dH$_2$O and 0.6 g of low-melt agarose. This solution must then be heated until the agarose melts (usually accomplished with short bursts of 10–15 s in a microwave set on high). Once the agarose melts, indicated by the solution changing from a opalescent to clear solution, the preheated BCIP should be directly added to the agarose solution, vortexed, placed in a multichannel pipetor reservoir and 100 µL quickly added to all the wells of the plates (*see* **Note 8**). Any bubbles that result from dispensing solution must be burst with a 100–200 µL pipet tip before the agarose hardens. The above ratio of solution chemicals is sufficient for one ELISA plate and can be scaled up as needed (*see* **Note 9**).
12. Count blue spots using a dissecting microscope (*see* **Note 10**).

3.2.2 ELISPOT Using Nitrocellulose plates

Although the reagents used with nitrocellulose plates are somewhat different from those routinely used in the ELISPOT using agarose, most of the reagents are interchangeable with exception of the development of spots.

1. Dilute antigen (or anti-mouse-IgG, -IgA, or -IgM antibody for total AFC) to the desired concentration (normally 5 µg/mL), and coat the wells of a 96-well nitro-cellulose-based microtiter plate (Millitier-HA, Millipore Corp.) with 100 µL overnight at 4°C in the appropriate buffer, normally sterile PBS (*see* **Note 4**).

2. The wells are washed twice with 200 µL/well of sterile PBS or RPMI to remove any unbound antigen (or capture antibody for total SFC) that could interfere with spot formation during the cell incubation.

3. Block the wells with 200 µL cRPMI and incubate for 1–2 h at 37°C in a 5% CO_2 incubator.

4. Wash plates twice with PBS or RPMI

5. Add 100 µL/well of serial dilutions of cells, normally starting at 1×10^6 cells/mL (*see* **Note 6**).

6. Incubate for 4 h or overnight at 37°C with 5% CO_2.

7. Wash plates four times with PBS-T. At this point it is not necessary to keep the plates sterile. Flick the plates to remove excess fluid between washing steps and specially following the final wash step and blot dry on a paper towel.

8. Add HRP-conjugated detection antibodies in 100 µL PBS-T containing 0.5% BSA (*see* **Note 11**) and incubate 3 h at room temperature or overnight at 4°C in a humidified chamber.

9. Wash plate three times with PBS-T and two more times with PBS alone to remove the Tween-20 which might interfere with the enzyme reaction.

10. Prepare AEC HRP substrate solution. Prepare a stock solution of AEC by dissolving 0.4 g of AEC in 100 mL of DMF (*see* **Note 12**). Prepare the AEC substrate solution by adding 0.67 mL of AEC stock solution to 10 mL of 0.1 M sodium acetate buffer, pH 5.2 (*see* **Note 13**). Filter the AEC substrate solution using the Whatman no. 1 filter paper. Add 10 µL of 30% H_2O_2.

11. Develop spots by adding 100 µL of the filtered AEC HRP substrate solution to each well and incubate for 15 min to an hour depending on the background versus signal ratio. Stop the reaction by rinsing the plate with water.

12. Count the number of SFC on a dissecting microscope (SZH Zoom Stereo Microscope System, Olympus, Lake Success, NY) (*see* **Note 10**).

4. Notes

1. Alternatively, place 10 mL of cRPMI into a glass homogenizer containing mouse spleens. Move the pestle up and down in the homogenizer until the spleens have been disrupted into single cell suspensions.

2. Overexposure of spleen cells to ACK buffer will significantly reduce the viability of the spleen cell preparation. It is important not to exceed three minutes of incubation on ice in order to maintain optimal viability of the lymphocytes.

3. An average spleen contains approx 1×10^8 lymphocytes. The isolated cells are resuspended in 5–10 mL cRPMI providing an approximate concentration of $1–2 \times 10^7$ cells/mL. A total of 20 mL of these cells are diluted 1:10 in an 0.4% Trypan blue solution (Sigma) which enables one to determine the concentration of viable cells in solution employing a hemocytometer, since live cells exclude

Trypan blue. Normally, over 95% of the cells are viable. A hemocytometer (Hauser Scientific, Horsham, PA) is a graduated microscopic slide of which one large corner square, containing 16 smaller squares, contains a volume of 0.1 mm^3. By averaging the number of cells counted over four large squares (excluding cells located on the demarkation lines located on the right-side and bottom and including cells located on the left side and the top demarkation lines) the number of cells per mL can be calculated by multiplying the number of cells per square with 10^4 and the dilution made in Trypan blue (x10).

4. Coating antigens as well as capture antibodies are normally used at concentrations between 1–10 μg/mL. Buffers commonly used to coat the plates include sterile PBS (pH 7.2–7.4) or carbonate buffer (pH 8.0–9.6). For example, subunit HIV-1 envelope subunit glycoproteins have been used at 5 μg/mL in PBS at pH 7.4.

5. Plates can be washed using multiple techniques. Both manual washing or plate washer (Nunc) have both been found to be sufficient for this purpose. It is important not to wash plates with detergent (Tween-20) containing buffer solution prior to addition of cells.

6. Starting cell concentrations are dependent on the tissue source, antibody isotype, and expected frequency of total and antigen-specific antibody-secreting cells. For example, a high frequency of antigen-specific IgA-secreting cells can be generated in the lamina propria following gut immunization. The frequency of specific IgA-secreting cells may reach several thousand per 10^6 cells. Intranasal immunization can also elicit high levels of antibody-secreting cells in the upper respiratory lymph nodes.

7. For the agarose gel ELISPOT AP-conjugated antibodies were used at the following concentrations to determine antigen-specific or total mouse Ig levels: goat antimouse IgG (1:8,000); goat-antimouse IgA (1:8,000); goat-antimouse IgM (1:4,000) (Southern Biotechnology Associates, Birmingham, AL)

8. The BCIP solution must be preheated so that, when it is added to the agarose solution it does not solidify on contact. This resultant solution must be added to the ELISA wells in a timely fashion for the agarose not to harden in the reservoir.

9. Typically, 100 μL of substrate solution is used in the assay but equal quality results have been achieved when only 50 μL of the solution was added.

10. Cells from unimmunized or uninoculated mice should also be included as controls in the ELISPOT. To decipher positive spots and control for background spots, test cells should also be added to wells without antigen.

11. For the nitrocellulose-based microtiter plate ELISPOT assay, horseradish peroxidase-conjugated antibodies (Southern Biotech Associates) were used at the following concentrations: antimouse IgG (1:3,000); antimouse IgA (1:3,000); antimouse IgM (1:3,000). The antibodies are incubated for 2 h at room temperature or overnight at 4°C. Normally the detection antibodies are directly conjugated with HRP or AP. Alternatively, a biotinylated detection antibody followed by an antibiotin antibody or streptavidin conjugated to the detection enzymes can be used.

12. The AEC stock solution is stable at room temperature for 1 yr.

13. The AEC stock in 0.1 M sodium acetate buffer should be prepared prior to running the assay.

References

1. van Ginkel, F. W., Liu, C., Simecka, J. W., Dong, J-Y, Greenway, T., Frizzell, R. A., et al. (1995) Intratracheal gene delivery with adenoviral vector induces elevated systemic IgG and mucosal IgA antibodies to adenovirus and β-galactosidase. *Hum. Gene Ther.* **6,** 895–903.
2. Hunninghake, G. W. and Fauci, A. S. (1976) Immunological reactivity of the lung. A guinea pig model for the study of pulmonary mononuclear cell subpopulations. *Cell Immunol.* **26,** 89–97.
3. Jackson, R., Fujihashi, K., Xu-Amano, J., Kiyono, H., Elson, C. O., and McGhee, R. J. (1993) Optimizing oral vaccines: induction of systemic and mucosal B-cell and antibody responses to tetanus toxoid by use of cholera toxin as an adjuvant. *Infect. Immunol.* **63,** 4272–4279.
4. Kiyono, H., McGhee, J. R., Wannemuehler, M. J., Frangakis, M. V., Spalding, D. M., Michalek, S. M., and Koopman, W. J. (1982) In vitro immune responses to a T cell dependent antigen by cultures of dissociated murine Peyer's patch. *Proc. Natl. Acad. Sci. USA* **79,** 596–600.
5. Muster, T., Ferko, B., Klima, A., Purtscher, M., Trkola, A., Schulz, P., et al. (1995) Mucosal model immunization against human immunodeficiency virus type 1 with a chimeric influenza virus. *J. Virol.* **69,** 6678–6686.
6. Taguchi, T., McGhee, R. J., Coffman, R. L., Beagley, K. W., Eldridge, J. H., Takatsu, K., et al. (1990) Analysis of Th1 and Th2 cells in murine gut-associated tissues. Frequencies of CD4$^+$ and CD8$^+$ T cells that secrete IFN-gamma and IL-5. *J. Immunol.* **145,** 68–77.

32

Linear Epitope Mapping by the PEPSCAN Method

Lawrence D. Loomis-Price

1. Introduction

The development of vaccine products for the prevention or treatment of HIV requires accurate assessments of the immune response, both humoral and cellular, so that specific responses can be correlated with efficacy. For assay of humoral immunity, a variety of techniques have been developed. The most advanced can pinpoint with high accuracy the epitope for antibodies which bind to continuous stretches of amino acids ("linear" epitopes). Mapping noncontinuous ("conformational") epitopes is significantly more difficult, but continued effort along these lines is warranted since conformational epitopes are dominant in the natural immune response to HIV-1 *(1)*.

Linear epitopes can be mapped using peptides. The precision of epitope mapping depends directly upon the number of peptides made and the degree to which they overlap. The PEPSCAN technique, initially described by Geysen *(2)*, involves the use of an array of unique, overlapping synthetic peptides based on the primary amino acid sequence of an antigen bound to individual pins of a 96-pin block compatible with a standard 96-well microtiter plate. Exposure of the block to serum and the resulting detection of bound antibodies can be used to map linear epitope responses. Several advances have been made in recent years which allows for the rapid, simultaneous synthesis of many peptides in formats suitable for the PEPSCAN procedure *(2)*. The PEPSCAN technique has been used to investigate humoral responses against many HIV-1 proteins, including the envelope and transmembrane proteins from infected patients *(3–5)*, and to monitor humoral immune responses in clinical vaccine studies *(6,7)*.

From: *Methods in Molecular Medicine, Vol. 17: HIV Protocols*
Edited by: N. L. Michael and J. H. Kim © Humana Press Inc., Totowa, NJ

Limitations to the application of this technique include: the large amount of serum required for a single assay, relatively low signal-to-noise ratios, and lack of standardization for the quantitative analysis of the data obtained. The authors have investigated several modifications of the PEPSCAN technique which, in large part, overcome these obstacles. First, exposing peptides to serum in a unique "bath" format significantly reduces background, increases the signal-to-noise ratio, and reduces the amount of serum required. The "bath" technique allows use of the serum at much higher dilutions than previously possible. Antibody reactivities routinely titrate to dilutions of $1:1 \times 10^5$ (human sera) or to $1:1 \times 10^6$ (rabbit sera). Second, use of free "cleaved" peptides which are biotinylated and bound to strepavidin on microtiter plates, reduces variation between amounts of peptide bound and allows for better quantitation of reactivity, as well as reducing background responses.

We have tested these techniques with several HIV strain-specific peptide libraries, defining epitope-specific responses to entire sequences of the HIV-1 envelope protein gp160 from various strains. The sera tested include sera from HIV-positive volunteers (both before and after immunization with envelope products) and sera from gp160 immunized rabbits.

2. Materials
2.1. Synthesis (see Note 1)
2.1.1. Instruments

1. Purchase of appropriate computer-controlled hardware and software for generation of the peptide synthesis schedule and controlling synthesis of peptides is strongly recommended. These are marketed with an LED-based device, such as the PinPAL™ (Craco, Inc., Vienna, VA) (8,9), and PinAID™ (Chiron Mimotopes US, Raleigh, NC), which makes the actual synthesis far easier to accomplish. Trying to do this by hand is time-consuming, tedious, and has a very high error probability (10). A common low-intensity laboratory sonicator (Bransonic model 2200 Ultrasonic Cleaner, Sigma Chemical Co., St. Louis, MO) is helpful for removing peptides from pins for cleavable syntheses. A rocker, orbital shaker, or similar apparatus is used for cleavable peptide synthesis and enzyme-linked immunosorbant assay (ELISA) (Belly Dancer, Stovall Life Science, Inc., Greensboro, NC).

2.1.2. Reagents and Consumables (see Note 2)

1. Peptide support: Peptides are synthesized onto the heads of small "pins" which are purchased on blocks containing 96 pins in an 8×12 pattern designed to match standard 96-well microtiter plates. Pins can be obtained from Chiron Mimotopes. These pins are prederivatized so there is an Fmoc protected amino acid linker (B-Ala for bound-pins and Pro for cleavable pins) ready to start normal peptide synthesis from the C-terminus of the peptide of interest.

2. Amino acids (*see* **Note 3**): Fmoc amino acids with OPfp carboxy activation (ODhbt, for SER and THR) are required. The following protecting groups work well:

Protection	Amino Acids
TRT:	Asn, Gln, His, Cys
But :	Glu, Asp, Ser, Thr, Tyr
Boc:	Lys, Trp
MTR:	Arg (*see* **Note 4**)

Sources for amino acids: Novabiochem (LaJolla, CA), Advanced Chemtech (Louisville, KY), Bachem Bioscience (King of Prussia, PA), Peninsula Laboratories (Belmont, CA).

3. Bulk chemicals: Dimethyl formamide (DMF), and methanol (ACS certified, Fisher, Pittsburgh, PA). These are consumed at a very large rate. Plan on up to 20 L/d of methanol and 10 L/d of DMF (*see* **Note 5**).

4. Deprotection solution: 20% piperidine (*see* **Note 6**) in DMF (HPLC grade, Fisher). Two liters of solution are required per set of five blocks. Dry the solution over about 500 mm^3 of 4 Å molecular sieves for at least 24 h before use, and change the sieves twice a week. If kept properly, this solution can be reused throughout one synthesis (*10*).

5. Wash solution: 0.5% glacial acetic acid in DMF.

6. Coupling solution: 120 mM 1-hydrobenzotriazole hydrate (HOBt) in high purity DMF with the volume controlled by synthesis program. Make this reagent immediately before use.

7. Acetylation reagent (per block of pins): 10 mL high purity DMF, 1 mL acetic anhydride, 0.2 mL diisopropylethylamine. Make this reagent immediately before use.

8. Biotinylation reagent (per block of pins): Dissolve 105 mg HOBt in 13.5 mL DMF (40 mM), add 114 μL N-methyl morpholine (60 mM) and mix, add 166 mg d-Biotin (40 mM) and mix well. A small amount of precipitate is normal. Dissolve 354 mg BOP (Benzotriazol-1-yloxytris-(dimethylamino) phosphonium hexafluorophosphate) in 3.4 mL DMF (40 mM). Combine the two solutions and mix well immediately before use.

9. Deblocking reagent (*see* **Note 7**): 1 L trifluoroacetic acid containing 25 mL phenol, 25 mL 1,2-ethanedithiol, 25 mL water, and 25 mL thioanisol. Cool the cleavage mixture in an ice bath for 5–10 min. Use this reagent immediately after preparation.

10. Cleavage solution: Add 400 mL of filter sterilized, 0.1 M potassium phosphate monobasic, pH 7.4, to 100 mL of acetonitrile (HPLC grade). Store at 4°C, but warm to room temperature before use.

11. Synthesis plates. Polypropylene plates can be obtained from Chiron Mimotopes, or RAM Scientific (Princeton, NJ). Deep well plates are supplied by Chiron Mimotopes. Large and small polypropylene tubes for both synthesis and assays are supplied by Cole-Palmer (Niles, IL).

2.2. ELISA

2.2.1. Instruments

1. Sonicator for disruption bath. This device is required only for the bound-peptide techniques, not for cleaved peptide assays. The sonicator must be a chemically

resistant, high power instrument, with a built-in heater. An example is model HT-5.6, 12 × 12 × 10" ultrasonic bath with heater capable of producing 600 W at 25 KHz (Blackstone Ultrasonics, Jamestown, NY). A normal low-power laboratory sonicator will not work for this application (*see* **Note 8**).

2. Methanol bath (*see* **Note 9**). This is used to heat methanol to boiling for final rinsing and drying of the peptide blocks; it is not required for cleaved peptide assays. A suitable instrument is the SS-5 bath with an AZ-3000 controller (Azonic Technology Inc., San Jose, CA).
3. Plate reader. A spectrophotometer capable of reading 96-well microtiter plate format is required (e.g., UVmax™, Molecular Devices, Sunnyvale, CA).
4. Plate washer. Nunc Immunowash 12-hand plate washer (Fisher Scientific).

2.2.2. Consumables and Reagents

1. Disruption buffer: 20 L PBS (*see* **Note 10**), 1% sodium dodecyl sulfate (SDS), to which 20 mL of 2-mercaptoethanol is added every day. This solution will need to be changed every 2–4 wk depending on level of usage. This buffer is not needed for cleavable peptide ELISAs.
2. Wash solution: Phosphate-buffered saline (PBS) (*see* **Note 10**), 0.1% Tween-20; make fresh solution daily.
3. Blocker (*see* **Note 11**): B-K Buffer (*see* **Note 12**) (for human or monkey serum, well method only): 1 M glucose, 10% glycerol, 10% newborn calf serum (Sigma), and 0.2% sodium azide in PBS. Make this solution weekly.
4. BCB+ buffer (for mouse or rabbit sera for the well method and all sera using the bath method): Five percent casein, 0.5% bovine serum albumin (BSA), 1.0% Tween-20, 2% newborn calf serum, and 0.2% sodium azide in PBS. Casein is dissolved by boiling in 200 mL of 0.1 N NaOH; after cooling, 10X PBS is added along with the other agents, and the pH of the mixture is adjusted to 7.4 before diluting to the appropriate volume.
5. Milk (for cleavable peptide ELISA): Five percent nonfat dry milk in PBS + 0.2% sodium azide. Remake all blockers weekly.
6. PNPP substrate. Dissolve one tablet paranitrophenyl phosphate substrate (Sigma)/ 5 mL DEAE buffer: 114 μL diethanolamine, 0.2 g sodium azide, 0.1 g $MgCl_2 \cdot 6H_2O$/L water and adjust pH to 9.8 with HCl. Cover the bottle with aluminum foil and keep refrigerated. Discard this solution after 1 mo.
7. Strepavidin: Stock strepavidin (Calbiochem, LaJolla, CA) at 1 mg/mL in water is kept frozen in aliquots at –20°C for up to several months. On the day of use, dilute in PBS to 5 μg/mL. Strepavidin is needed only for cleavable peptide ELISA.
8. Immulon II microtiter plates (flat) are supplied by Dynatech Laboratories (Chantilly, VA); alkaline phosphatase labeled, goat F(ab')$_2$ antirabbit and antihuman polyclonal serum is supplied by Biosource International (Camarillo, CA).

3. Methods
3.1. Synthesis

Instructions for carrying out a multiple peptide synthesis are included in the user manuals which accompany the programs designed for this purpose and will not be reproduced here. Instead, the following outline will focus on the technical aspects and decisions which have to be made during peptide synthesis with emphasis on applications to HIV research.

3.1.1. Setting Up

1. Peptide synthesis schedule. Obtain the protein sequence which the peptides are to be synthesized to model in a computer-accessible format. Sequences can be obtained from available databases, such as GenBank (operated by the National Center for Biotechnology Information, http://www.ncbi.nlm.nih.gov), or entered manually.

2. Peptide length and overlap. Peptides of 12 amino acids in length, with eight residue overlap, will locate all linear epitopes in a sequence with a reasonable number of peptides (low redundancy) (*see* **Note 13**) For bound peptide methods, consider making two identical sets of peptides (*see* **Note 14**) For cleavable peptides, add a linker (the amino acids Ser-Gly-Ser-Gly) and biotin on the N-terminus, for a total of 16 AA (17 reactions, including the biotin).

3. Synthesis control peptides. Peptides which can be sacrificed for amino acid analysis as proof of peptide purity are useful for synthesis controls (*see* **Note 15**) as follows:

   Lys-Pro-His-Leu-Arg-Phe-Gly-Ser-Gln-Asp-Ala-Val, and

   Arg-Pro-Tyr-Met-Lys-Phe-Gly-Thr-Asn-Glu-Ala-Val.

   For cleavable peptide syntheses, a dinitrophenol (DNP) pin should be included. After cleavage, this will yield a colored solution with absorbance proportional to the amount of linked DNP still on the pin.

4. Assay control peptides. The following sequences can be used repeatedly in the context of the ELISA to measure reproducibility of the assay:

   Trp-Gly-Cys-Ala-Phe-Arg-Gln-Val-Cys-His-Thr-Thr

   functions well as a positive control (this peptide is positive with nearly all HIV+ sera and highly positive with most) *(11)* and

   Ala-Lys-Ala-Ala-Asp-Ala-Ala-Gln-Ala-Ala-Ser-Ala

   functions well as a negative control.

5. Specific methods. Currently, pins are only available with Fmoc protection. For activation, OPfp pre-activated amino acids work very well (*see* **Note 16**) Dissolve most of the amino acids at 50 mM and use 100 m*M* for those which are kinetically slower to react, including: Cys, His, Ile, Lys, Met, Arg, Trp (*see* **Note 17**)

6. Preparing the blocks (*see* **Note 18**): Label the blocks by etching the plastics with a diamond stylus or a razor blade as the chemicals used in the synthesis and ELISA will obliterate ink. Label the blocks in a consistent location (e.g., in the upper right, over "A1") as orientation is critical for both synthesis and subsequent ELISA. Then remove any pins for peptides that are not being made or are

shorter than the others. This usually occurs at the end of a sequence. DO NOT subject pins to repeated cycles of deprotection in the absence of an amino acid. Simply remove the pin and properly store it until the day that the first amino acid is to be added. Add the amino acid (*see* **Subheading 3.1.2.**) immediately prior to deprotection in piperidine.

3.1.2. Adding Amino Acids

For each amino acid added, one day of synthesis is required; a 12-mer peptide has 12 synthesis days. Because the reaction with the amino acids goes overnight, typically the final wash step will be performed first on any given workday (*see* **Note 19**)

1. Deprotect the N-terminus. Add new pins, if any, at this step. Prewet the pins in DMF for five minutes. Save this solution after use. Move the blocks into the piperidine solution, pins down, but do not agitate at this step. Leave them in the piperidine solution for 1 h.
2. Wash and dry (**steps 3-6** below). For the wash steps, agitate the blocks vigorously through 1–2 L of the following solutions. Be careful to rinse both the top and bottom of the blocks to remove any residual piperidine.
3. DMF/0.5% acetic acid. Rinse the blocks (use the DMF from the prewetting step), and leave in the solution for 5 min (*see* **Note 20**) Discard the solution after use.
4. DMF. Wash vigorously and leave for 5 min. Discard the solution after use.
5. Methanol. Wash vigorously and leave for 3 min. Repeat this step four times total using a progressive wash approach (*see* **Note 19**).
6. Dry. Remove from solvent and dry 30–60 min in a chemical fume hood.
7. Prepare and dispense amino acids (**steps 8–10** below).
8. The computer program guiding your synthesis will tell you how much of each amino acid to weigh out (*see* **Note 21**) Weigh the appropriate amount (a slight excess is acceptable) into polypropylene tubes and store them in a desiccator until needed. Weigh out the HOBt catalyst at the same time.
9. When the blocks are almost through the drying step, dissolve the HOBt completely in the appropriate volume of DMF and vortex to dissolve. Transfer appropriate volumes of DMF/HOB to each of the amino acids, in the order recommended by the manufacturer. It generally takes a couple of minutes for the amino acid to completely dissolve. Certain amino acids are less stable than others and should be dissolved and dispensed as close to being used as possible. Dispense one amino acid while the next is dissolving.
10. Prewet the blocks in DMF for 5 min. Save the DMF solution.
11. React the pins with amino acids (**steps 12–14** below).
12. It is critical to confirm that the blocks and plates are in the proper orientation before proceeding. Putting the blocks in backwards is, unfortunately, a common mistake and will ruin the peptides, even if the error is caught immediately.
13. Very carefully insert the dried blocks into the plates containing the amino acids.
14. Seal the blocks up in a container and let react at room temperature overnight.
15. Wash (**steps 16–18** below). This will be the first step most mornings.

16. Use the DMF from the prewetting step to rinse the amino acids off for 5 min. Some of the amino acids will be discolored via natural degradative reactions.
17. Wash the blocks with methanol four times for 3 min each time with a progressive wash approach (*see* **Note 19**).
18. Dry the blocks for 1 h.

3.1.3. Sequence Termination

1. After the final amino acid has been added, the N-terminus should be capped for use in antibody mapping. For bound peptides, the N-terminus should be acetylated, and for cleavable peptides it should be biotinylated.
2. Deprotect with piperidine: This is done in the same fashion as for amino acid addition.
3. Wash: This is done in the same fashion as for amino acid addition.
4. Acetylation (**steps 5–8** below).
5. Dispense 100 µL of acetylation reagent into each well of a 96-well synthesis plate which will have a pin.
6. Insert the blocks into the plates; prewetting is not necessary.
7. Seal up and leave for 2 h at room temperature.
8. Wash and dry the block according to the post-amino acid procedure.

3.1.4. Biotinylation

1. A linker should be added to separate the peptide from the biotin molecule. This can be accomplished most easily by simply adding four more amino acids (Ser-Gly-Ser-Gly) after the rest of the synthesis is over. The calculations for dispensing will have to be done manually as no existing program currently incorporates this step. Make up these amino acids at 100 µ*M*, as the peptide is now long enough to warrant the higher concentration. Make 10 mL of solution per plate (40.9 mg of HOBt/10 mL DMF).
2. Make up the two components of the biotinylation reagent
3. Prewet blocks for 5 min in DMF.
4. Mix the two components of the biotinylation reagent together.
5. Add 150 µL/well.
6. Place blocks in biotin solution.
7. React overnight at room temperature.
8. Wash the block in DMF and methanol in the same fashion as amino acid addition.

3.1.5. Deblocking

1. The organic protecting groups on all the amino acids are removed at this step. In addition, for cleavable peptides, the bond in the linker is modified by this step so that the peptides can be freed from the solid support.
2. Prepare the cleavage cocktail.
3. Pour the cocktail into a bath and put the blocks in pins down. Do not prewet and do not agitate.
4. Seal the block and let react for 4 h at room temperature.

5. Remove from the deblocking bath and completely immerse the block in methanol for 10 min.
6. Soak in 0.5% acetic acid in 1:1 mixture of methanol:water for 60 min at room temperature.
7. Wash again in water for 5 min.
8. Rinse in methanol and dry. The blocks may be stored dry at 4°C.
9. Before use, pins with bound peptides should be disrupted twice (*see* **Subheading 3.2.3.**). Do not disrupt cleavable peptides.

3.1.6. Cleavage

1. This procedure frees cleavable peptides from the pins (*see* **Note 22**).
2. Thoroughly clean the sonicator.
3. Warm the blocks to room temperature before use.
4. Label 96-deep well plates, one per block.
5. Place 750 μL of cleavage solution into deep well plates. Put blocks into plates. Sonicate each block for 60 min. Maintain sonication bath temperature below 40°C by adding ice or changing the water.
6. Remove the pins from the plates.
7. Remove all solution from wells designated for spectrophotometric analysis, and store at 4°C in cryotubes until the absorbance can be read. The greater the color, the more peptide cleaved off.
8. Cover plate wells with lab film, and store in a zip lock bag at –80°C.
9. Quickly rinse the pins in methanol, and air dry for 5 min. Store in the refrigerator until the peptides have been assayed for activity.
10. Assay peptides by amino acid analysis to determine concentration of peptide.
11. Peptides can be diluted and plated out onto standard 96-well microtiter plates and stored frozen. Once thawed, peptide is usable for 1 wk. Do not refreeze.

3.2. Bound-Peptide ELISA Methods

When the synthetic peptides to be used are bound to a solid phase, the assay procedures used are significantly different from a standard ELISA. Since the antigen is bound to a pin, the nascent sandwich between antigen and antibody also remains attached to the pin. The blocks are moved from solution to solution for the various incubation steps. Washing is done by hand (agitating the block vigorously in a rinse solution). Finally, in order to reuse the peptide, the antibodies must be removed (disrupted). Described below are two variations on the bound-peptide method, one in which the pins are incubated in antibodies contained in 96 well microtiter plates ("well" method) and the other in which the antibodies are contained in larger baths into which many pins are dipped simultaneously ("bath" method).

3.2.1. "Well" Method

1. Block pins in B-K buffer with for 1 h at room temperature.

2. Incubate with sera diluted in blocker overnight at 4°C. For example, use human sera diluted 1:200 in blocker to provide 125 µL antibody solution/well.
3. Wash by vigorously agitating in three changes of wash solution over 15 min.
4. Incubate in labeled antiserum IgG for 2 h at room temperature. For example, use alkaline phosphatase-labeled antihuman antibody, diluted 1:1000 in blocker to with 125 µL/antibody solution per well.
5. Wash as in **step 3**.
6. Develop with the appropriate substrate, prepared according to manufacturer's instructions. For example, use 150 µl of PNPP substrate/well.
7. Allow color to develop and read the results (30–120 min depending on the level of reactivity) using a microtiter plate reader.
8. It is important to not leave the pins in wash solutions or substrate any longer than necessary. As soon as the readings are taken, disrupt the antibodies and clean off the blocks (*see* **Subheading 3.2.3.**).

3.2.2. "Bath" Method

1. Block pins in BCB+ buffer for 1 h at room temperature.
2. Incubate with sera diluted in blocker overnight at 4°C. For example, human sera can be diluted 1:10,000 in blocker. Hold sera in large baths (e.g., 50 mL of diluted serum for an entire block, or 35 mL of diluted serum for a half block). Control pins can be incubated individually by immersing them into minitubes, designed to fit the 96-well format, which will encase a single pin and keep it separate from the rest of the bath.
3. Wash by vigorously agitating in three changes of wash solution over 15 min.
4. Incubate in labeled antiserum IgG for 2 h at room temperature. For example, use 125 µL of alkaline phosphatase-labeled antihuman antibody, diluted 1:1000 in blocker/well. It is also possible to perform this step using a bath, reducing the antibody concentration by 10–50 fold.
5. Wash as in **step 3**.
6. Develop with the appropriate substrate, prepared according to manufacturer's instructions. For example, use 150 µL of PNPP substrate/well.
7. Allow color to develop and read the results (30–120 min depending on the level of reactivity) using a microtiter plate reader (*see* **Fig. 1**).
8. Again, do not leave the pins in wash solutions or substrate any longer than necessary. As soon as the readings are taken, disrupt the antibodies and clean off the blocks (*see* **Subheading 3.2.3.**).

3.2.3. Disruption of Antibody–Peptide Complexes

1. To reuse the pins, the bound antibodies have to be removed and the peptides made available again for binding; this process is called "disruption."
2. Warm the solution in the sonicator to 65°C.
3. Sonicate the blocks for 30 min. The temperature should not rise above 70°C during this process, or the pins may be damaged (or more typically they may fall out of the blocks and be difficult to put back in the correct order).

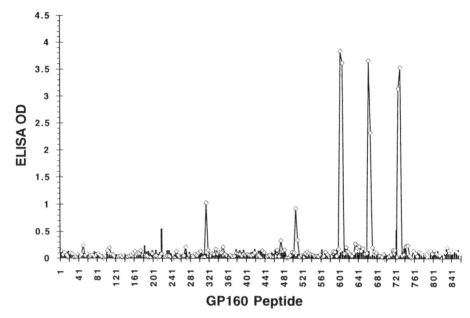

Fig. 1. Reactivity toward the HIV envelope protein gp160 obtained with an HIV+
(-◇-) and HIV– (bars) serum using the bath technique. Peptides were 12 amino acids
in length with eight residue overlaps. Both sera were diluted 1:10,000 in BCB+. Results
shown were obtained after 120 min of ELISA indicator development.

4. Remove the blocks from the sonicator and rinse in hot flowing water for 5–10
   min. They are done when the wash water no longer froths and the pins no longer
   smell of 2-mercaptoethanol.
5. To immediately reuse the pins, rinse them with distilled water and place them
   into blocking solution.
6. If the blocks are not to be reused immediately, boil them in methanol for 2 min,
   dry for 1 h at room temperature (in the chemical hood), and store them double-
   bagged with desiccant at 4°C or below.

3.3. Cleavable Peptide Method

1. This method is more similar to typical ELISA methods in that all incubations
   take place in a single microtiter plate. By far, the most important step for increasing signal-to-noise is the wash step. Manual washing reduces the background
   observed with human sera substantially, compared to commercial plate washers.
2. Plate 50 µL of a 5 µg/mL strepavidin solution per well and dry onto the plate at
   37°C overnight.
3. Wash the plates three times with PBS, 0.1% Tween-20.
4. Dilute peptide to 20–50 µg/mL in PBS and plate 50 µL/well (0.1–0.25 µg/well).
5. Incubate at room temperature for 1 h.

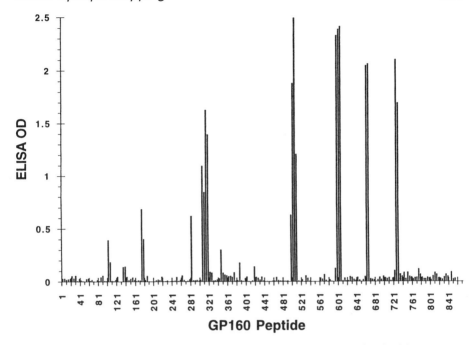

Fig. 2. Reactivity toward the HIV envelope protein gp160 obtained with an HIV+ serum using the cleaved peptide technique. Peptides were 12 amino acids in length with 8 residue overlaps and had a biotin-S-G-S-G linker attached to the N-teminus. Both sera were diluted 1:200 in 5% milk. Results shown were obtained after 45 min of ELISA indicator development.

6. Wash the plates three times with PBS, 0.1% Tween-20.
7. Add 50 μL of sera diluted in blocker (5% nonfat dry milk)/well for 2 h at room temperature. A reasonable serum dilution range is 1:100–1:1000. Sera can be serially diluted to obtain an endpoint titer or screened at one concentration for reactivity.
8. Wash the plates three times with PBS, 0.1% Tween-20.
9. Add 50 μL of labeled anti-IgG (e.g., alkaline phosphatase-labeled antihuman antibody, diluted 1:1000 in blocker)/well for 1 h at room temperature.
10. Wash the plates three times with PBS, 0.1% Tween-20.
11. Develop with the appropriate substrate, prepared according to manufacturer's instructions. For example, use 150 μL of PNPP substrate/well.
12. Allow color to develop and read the results (5–60 min, depending on the level of reactivity) using a microtiter plate reader (*see* **Fig. 2**).

3.4. Analysis

1. The large amount of data generated by this technique demands appropriate computer analysis. Files from the plate-reader should be directly transferred into an appropriate format, such as a spreadsheet or a database.

2. Controls: Positive and negative values are included with each plate. These are mostly a qualitative measure of how well an experiment went. The deterioration of signal obtained from the positive control is a measure of loss of peptide reactivity for the bound methods. Blocks of pins can typically be used at least 20 times, but generally can be used much longer if handled carefully. It is not unusual to have a set last for over 100 experiments.

3. Calculation of cutoff: Since many of the peptides will be unreactive with any given serum, it should be possible to use these unreactive peptides to establish the baseline response. For example, twice the average of the lowest 50% of the responses plus two or three standard deviations will typically establish a reasonable cutoff.

4. Notes

1. Warning: The majority of the reagents used in the synthesis are hazardous. Methanol, which is used in large amounts, is both a contact and vapor toxin and is highly flammable. The synthesis should be performed in an approved chemical safety hood and appropriate protective wear (chemical-resistant gloves, lab coat, and eye protection) should be employed at all times.

2. The organic reagents, including DMF and acetonitrile, will dissolve many common lab materials, including polyethylene microtiter plates, pipets, and tubes. Always use materials made of chemically resistant material such as polypropylene.

3. Abbreviations used: TRT (triphenylmethyl); But (t-butyl); Boc (t-butoxy-carbonyl); MTR (4-methoxy-2,3,6-trimethylbenzene sulphonyl); OPfp (pentafluorophenyl ester); ODhbt, 3,4 dihydro-4-oxo-benzotriazine-3-oxy.

4. PMC or PBC derivatives are even more active.

5. Waste containing these chemicals must be disposed of in accordance with federal and local regulations; means for safe and legal disposal should be arranged before starting any synthesis.

6. Piperidine is a United States Drug Enforcement Agency reportable substance and, as such, has certain restrictions placed on its availability. Orders typically must be written or telefaxed rather than telephoned and must be accompanied by a short statement of intended usage which has been signed by the end user.

7. This solution is toxic, corrosive, noxious, and spontaneously combustible should it come into contact with organic materials such as cloth or paper. Use extreme caution. Do all steps in an approved chemical hood with appropriate protective garments. All solutions must be disposed of appropriately. All materials should either be bagged in the hood for immediate disposal or rinsed or wiped down in the hood before being brought into an open lab.

8. Warning: sonic hazard. This instrument needs to be placed within a sound-damping container or personnel within the immediate vicinity must wear ear protection. The solution used in this bath, which contains 2-mercaptoethanol, produces a noxious odor. If possible, the instrument should be contained within a chemical fume hood.

9. Because of the extreme flammability of boiling methanol, this step requires a specially designed device. This model has the power source and controller located

away from the bath itself (which is kept in a chemical hood). This must be done in a chemical hood and extreme caution must be exercised to avoid producing flame or sparks in the vicinity of the device when it is being operated.

10. Dulbecco's phosphate buffered saline (10X) (PBS, Life Technologies, Grand Island, NY), diluted to 1X and the pH adjusted to 7.4.

11. Every lab has its favorite blocking solutions, and the author's is no exception. The author has found that human and monkey sera have extremely high background reactivity with bound-peptides, probably because of the inability to wash vigorously enough.

12. In the author's hands, the best blocker for reduction of this activity was developed by Birk and Koepsell for immunoblotting *(12)*.

13. The synthesis should be designed to locate all linear epitopes in the region covered with the level of redundancy desired by the investigator. Best estimates available indicate that 90% of linear epitopes include six amino acids or fewer and close to 100% include eight amino acids or fewer *(13,14)*. Larger peptides can be useful to determine semidiscontinuous epitopes, but some precision is lost. The current chemistries available make production of peptides up to 20 amino acids in length possible with very high purity *(15)*. If maximum overlap is used (each peptide of length "N" shares "N-1" amino acids in common with its neighbors), then numerous pins will be positive for each epitope. Although this level of redundancy can be comforting, many more peptides are required than if smaller overlaps are used and the reproducibility of the technique in our hands makes such redundancy unnecessary. Typically, the author synthesizes peptides 12 amino acids in length with eight residue overlap. Although this reduces the number of sequences made by 75% and reveals all epitopes of eight amino acids or smaller, this approach provides for low redundancy. Epitopes of 6–8 amino acids show up on one or two pins.

14. For vaccine studies, the most useful information comes from comparison between reactivity at one time (e.g., prior to immunization) and that at another (e.g., postimmunization). It is hazardous to attempt to compare PEPSCAN data run on different days. Duplicate peptide sets allow comparisons between simultaneously run sera.

15. These include all amino acids that can be detected by standard amino acid analysis techniques such that each can be measured independently. Declining yield with increasing number of synthetic steps can be evaluated by comparing the amounts of arginine versus lysine in the two peptides.

16. The main advantage to this method is its ease of use. These are somewhat more expensive than using the free carboxyl derivatives along with *in situ* activation. The manufacturer reports great success with the latter which also has the advantage of being kinetically more rapid, so that several amino acids can be added per day.

17. A common failure of computer programs governing these syntheses is their inability to allow entry of different amino acid concentrations. However, since they do allow for entry of amino acid formula weights, one can simply double the entered formula weight of any amino acid to double its concentration.

18. Precautions standard to working with peptides should be observed with the pins at all stages of synthesis and use. They should be kept scrupulously clean and dry and preferably in a refrigerated, dark container when not being actively used. Physical contact with the pins themselves should be avoided so as to reduce chemical or proteolytic cleavage.

19. All steps involving the blocks, except for the actual addition of amino acids, occurs in large polypropylene tubs. The wash steps use very large volumes of solvent. This can be reduced by using fresh solvent in a progressive fashion. For example, if four methanol washes need to be done, throw out the wash solution used for the first wash only and save the other three. Use them in the same order the next time washes must be done (the second bath from the first use steps up to be the first bath the second time). Add completely fresh solvent only for the final rinse.

20. Although this step is somewhat controversial, it has worked well in the author's hands. Use only for OPfp derivatives. For *in situ* activation, substitute a simple DMF wash.

21. Store the amino acids in the freezer double-sealed into large bags containing desiccant. Since it is important that these amino acids never be exposed to water, warm them to room temperature before opening the bags and weighing out the contents. The weighing can be done at any convenient time, including the day before, as long as the amino acids are kept dry and shielded from light.

22. Procedures should be done in a laminar flow hood, under sterile conditions. (Bacterial contamination can lead to the breakdown of peptides.)

References

1. Barlow, D. J., Edwards, M. S., and Thornton, J. M. (1986) Continuous and discontinuous protein antigen determinants. *Nature* 322, 747–748.

2. Geysen, H. M., Meloen, R. H., and Bateling, S. J. (1984) Use of peptide synthesis to prove viral antigens for epitopes to a resolution of a single amino acid. *Proc. Natl. Acad. Sci. USA* **81**, 3998–4002.

3. van Tijn, D. A., Boucher, C. A., Bakker, M., and Goudsmit, J. (1989) Antigenicity of linear B-cell epitopes in the C1, V1, and V3 region of HIV-1 gp 120. *J. Acquir. Immune Defic. Syndr.* **2**, 303–336.

4. Pincus, S. H., Messer, K. G., Nara, P. L., Blatner, W. A., Colclough, G., and Reitz, M. (1994) Temporal analysis of the antibody response to HIV envelope protein in HIV-infected laboratory workers. *J. Clin. Invest.* **93**, 2505–2513.

5. Lucey, D. R., VanCott, T. C., Loomis, L. D., et al. (1993) Measurement of cerebrospinal fluid antibody to the HIV-1 principal neutralizing determinant (V3 loop). *J. Acquir. Immune Defic. Syndr.* **6**, 994–1001.

6. Loomis, L. D., Deal, C. D., Kersey, K. S., Burke, D. S., Redfield, R. R., and Birx, D. L. (1995) Humoral responses to linear epitopes on the HIV-1 envelope in seropositive volunteers after vaccine therapy with rgp160. *J. Acquir. Immune Defic. Syndr.* **10**, 13–26.

7. Pincus, S. H., Messer, K. G., Schwartz, D. H., et al. (1993) Differences in the antibody response to human immunodeficiency virus-1 envelope glycoprotein

(gp160) in infected laboratory workers and vaccinees. *J. Clin. Invest.* **91,** 1987–1996.

8. VanAlbert, S., Lee, J., and Carter, J. M. (1992) Amino acid indexer for synthesis of Geysen peptides. Patent application 07/679,990.

9. Carter, J. M., VanAlbert, S., Lee, J., Lyon, J., and Deal, C. (1992) Shedding light on peptide synthesis. *Biotechnology* **10,** 509–513.

10. Carter, J. M. (1994) Epitope mapping of a protein using the Geysen (PEPSCAN) procedure, in *Methods in Molecular Biology*, vol. 36, *Peptide Analysis Protocols*, (Dunn, B. M. and Pennington, M. W., eds.) Humana, Totowa, NJ, pp. 207–223.

11. Wang, J., Steel, S., Montagnier, L., and Sonigo, P. (1986) Detection of antibodies to human T-lymphotropic virus type III by using a synthetic peptide of 21 amino acid residues corresponding to a highly antigenic segment of gp41 envelope protein. *Proc. Natl. Acad. Sci. USA* **83,** 6159–6163.

12. Birk, H. W. and Koepsell, H. (1987) Reaction of monoclonal antibodies with plasma membrane proteins after binding on nitrocellulose: renaturation of antigenic sites and reduction of nonspecific antibody binding. *Anal. Biochem.* **164,** 12–22.

13. Geysen, H. M. (1990) Molecular technology: peptide epitope mapping and the pin technology. *Southeast Asian J. Trop. Med. Public Health* **21,** 523–533.

14. Pinilla, C., Appel, J. R., and Houghten, R. A. (1993) Functional importance of amino acid residues making up peptide antigenic determinants. *Mol. Immunol.* **30,** 577–585.

15. Valerio, R. M., Bray, A. M., Campbell, R. A., et al. (1993) Multipin peptide synthesis at the micromole scale using 2-hydroxyethyl methacrylate grafted polyethylene supports. *Int. J. Peptide Protein Res.* **42,** 1–9.

33

Neutralization of HIV-1 Infection of Human Peripheral Blood Mononuclear Cells (PBMC)

Antibody Dilution Method

John R. Mascola

1. Introduction

Antibodies elicited by passive or active immunization protect against numerous virus diseases. This in vivo protective immunity is often associated with in vitro detection of neutralizing antibodies (NAb) (e.g., polio, measles, influenza, respiratory syncytial virus, yellow fever, dengue, rabies, varicella, hepatitis A, hepatitis B) *(1–7)*. Since human protection from HIV-1-associated disease has not yet been achieved, the role of NAb in protective immunity is not defined. Nonetheless, based on experience with other viruses, it is reasonable to assume that NAb will play an important role in protection against HIV-1.

Virus neutralization assays are designed to measure a reduction in virus infectious titer mediated by exposure to antibody. Initial HIV-1 neutralization assays utilized prototypic virus isolates (e.g., HIV-IIIB) grown in neoplastic T-cell lines (e.g., H9, CEM-SS), and infection was monitored by counting virus induced T-cell syncytia *(8)*. Since T-cell syncytia corresponded to initial infection of a single cell, the fraction of virus neutralized was directly related to a reduction in syncytia. These assays were highly reproducible and demonstrated NAb in the sera of most HIV-infected subjects. However, it was soon appreciated that HIV-1 exhibits a range of biologic phenotypes, and only a minority of strains that are isolated by cultures of human PBMC (primary isolates) will produce syncytia in neoplastic T-cell lines *(9)*. The syncytia inducing (SI) viruses are more often found in late stage HIV-1-infected subjects, whereas non syncytia inducing (NSI) strains tend to be isolated in the asymp-

From: *Methods in Molecular Medicine, Vol. 17: HIV Protocols*
Edited by: N. L. Michael and J. H. Kim © Humana Press Inc., Totowa, NJ

tomatic stage of disease *(10)*. Furthermore, SI virus entry into T-cell lines appears to occur via a different second receptor than entry of NSI viruses into PBMC *(11)*. Since PBMC are permissive for infection of NSI and SI viruses, including genetically diverse HIV-1 strains, several assays have been developed using phytohemagglutinin (PHA)-stimulated PBMC as target cells *(12–14)*. The number of infected PBMC is indirectly measured by assays for virus expression (e.g., reverse transcriptase, p24 antigen). The microtiter plate neutralization assay described below utilizes HIV-1 seronegative donor PHA-stimulated PBMC as target cells and virus infection is assessed by a quantitative ELISA measurement of HIV-1 p24 antigen expressed in PBMC culture supernatants *(15,16)*.

2. Materials

1. Culture media (cRPMI): RPMI 1640 media (ABI, Columbia, MD), supplemented with 15% heat-inactivated fetal calf serum (Intergen, Purchase, NJ), 100 U/mL penicillin, 100 µg/mL streptomycin and 2 mM L-glutamine (each from ABI).
2. cRPMI/IL-2, cRPMI supplemented with 20 U/mL human recombinant IL-2 (Boehringer Manheim, GmbH, Germany).
3. Target cells: Ficoll gradient separated PBMC, from an HIV-1-seronegative donor.
4. The 96-well microtiter boxes—0.5 mL/well (#499-023, PGC Scientific, Frederick, MD).
5. ELISA aspirator: for washing cells in PGC microtiter box (Corning ELISA plate washer - 26305-72, Corning, NY).
6. The 96-well round bottom microtiter plates (Costar, Cambridge, MA).
7. Microtiter plate sealers (Costar, Cambridge, MA).
8. Sorvall microplate carrier: for H-1000B rotor, Sorvall RT 6000D centrifuge (Sorvall Instruments, Wilmington, DE).
9. PHA-P (Difco Labs, Detroit, MI), prepared in sterile distilled water to 1 µg/µL.
10. Pooled normal human serum (NHS) (Sigma, St. Louis, MO).
11. HIV-1 p24 antigen ELISA Kit (Coulter, Hialeah, FL).
12. Coulter HIV-1 extended p24 antigen control (for ELISA standard curve).
13. Vmax ELISA plate reader with Soft Max Pro software (Molecular Devices Corp., Sunnyvale, CA).

3. Methods
3.1. Preparation of PBMC Target Cells

Due to the considerable variation in HIV-1 replication among donor PBMC, individual donor cells are screened on a standard panel of 6 HIV-1 isolates to ensure adequately HIV-1 growth (*see* **Subheading 3.4.**, Pre-Neutralization Titration of Virus Stocks, *see* **Note 1**).

1. Donor PBMC are Ficoll-gradient separated from whole blood or leukophoresis pack by standard procedures.

2. PBMC (20×10^6/vial) are cryopreserved in cRPMI with 10% DMSO and initially placed overnight at $-70°C$, then stored in the vapor phase of liquid nitrogen.

3. For PHA-stimulation, PBMC are thawed quickly in a 37°C water bath and washed in 30 mL of cRPMI. Cells are resuspended in 30 mL of cRPMI/IL-2, transferred to a vented upright T25 flask, and 30 μL of PHA are added (final PHA concentration, 1 μg/mL). PHA is removed after approximately 24 h by a single wash in cRPMI, and cells are again resuspended in 30 mL of cRPMI/IL-2 (*see* **Note 2**). Target cells used in the assay are 3- or 4-d PHA-stimulated PBMC. On the day of the assay, cells are counted and resuspended in cRPMI/IL-2 at 3×10^6/mL. Viability should be greater than 90%.

3.2. Neutralization Assay

Well-characterized infectious virus stocks are important for the accuracy and reproducibility of this assay (see Chapter 1 for methodology of coculture and expansion of HIV-1). Virus stocks should be stored in the vapor phase of liquid nitrogen and pre-titered in the neutralization assay format prior to use. It is important to use the same cryopreserved donor PBMC that will serve as target cells in the neutralization assay (*see* **Subheading 3.4.**). Virus stocks and neutralization plates contain significant amounts of HIV-1 and all work should be carried out in a BL3 laboratory facility or a BL2 facility using BL3 practices. For simplicity of description, the assay described below utilizes serum collected from HIV-1-infected subjects as a source of antibody. Plasma from anticoagulated whole blood can be substituted for serum. Purified polyclonal immunoglobulin, monoclonal antibodies or soluble CD4 can be used with minor alterations in the protocol (*see* **Note 3**).

1. Prior to use, all test sera and control sera (e.g., NHS) are complement depleted by heat inactivation for 40 min at 56°C.

2. Serial dilutions of test sera are made in NHS so that all serum dilutions contain the same amount of human serum proteins. Serial four-fold serum dilutions are aliquoted in quadruplicate wells (25 μL/well) into the 96-well PGC microtiter plate.

3. One aliquot of virus stock is quickly thawed in a 37°C water bath and is diluted in cRPMI/IL-2 to a concentration of 100 TCID50 per 25 μL (*see* **Section 3.4**). Twenty-five microliters of diluted virus stock are added to each serum containing well of the microtiter plate. Care is taken not to touch the serum at the bottom of the wells. After dispensing virus, the microtiter plate is gently tapped against the hood floor to ensure that serum and virus are well mixed in the bottom of the 0.5 mL wells, and the microtiter plate is incubated at 37°C for 30 min (*see* **Note 4**). The final serum concentration is defined as the dilution of serum in the presence of virus, before the addition of cells (e.g., initial 1:4 serum dilution becomes 1:8 with virus). Pooled NHS or individual subject pre-immune sera are used as a control for baseline virus growth. When testing sera from HIV-1-infected subjects, two quadruplicate sets of wells with pooled NHS are used to determine virus growth in the absence of HIV-specific antibody.

4. PHA-stimulated PBMC (50 μL, 1.5×10^5) are added to each well, and the box is again gently tapped against the hood floor to mix PBMC with serum/virus. A loose fitting cover from a 96-well round bottom plate is placed on top of the microtiter plate and the plate is incubated overnight (approx 18 h, *see* **Note 5**).

5. PBMC are then washed three times at 1000 rpm (approx 210g) in the microtiter plate using a plate carrier (*see* **Note 6**). Plates are sealed with an adherent plastic plate sealer (Costar) prior to each wash. Washing removes virus stock p24 antigen and serum anti-p24 antibody (*see* **Note 7**). For each wash, wells are filled to 500 μL with cRPMI (first two washes) or cRPMI/IL-2 (last wash). After each wash, supernatants are aspirated with the Corning ELISA aspirator set to leave 50 μL/well. The cell pellet is not disturbed. After the last wash, 200 μL of cRPMI/IL-2 are added to each well. Cells are resuspended and 220 μL/well are transferred to a round bottom microtiter plate. Plates are inspected daily for uniformity in size of cell pellets and pH of culture media (*see* **Note 8**).

3.3. HIV-1 p24 Antigen Measurement in Culture Supernatants.

Optimal day of collection of culture supernatants is approximated by a preneutralization virus titration as described below (**Subheading 3.4.**). Culture supernatants are generally collected on two or three consecutive days and p24 antigen in control (NHS) wells is determined to reconfirm virus growth kinetics. For the large majority of viruses, p24 antigen is measured on day 4, 5, or 6. Typically, p24 antigen in control wells is 40–200 ng/mL. Coefficient of variation (CV) in quadruplicate control wells is generally under 30%. If CV is greater than 50%, the assay is repeated.

1. 100 μL of culture supernatant are removed from each well and placed into a corresponding microtiter plate with 80 μL of PBS and 20 μL Coulter lysis buffer per well (i.e., final dilution, 1:2). The p24 plate is frozen at –20°C until p24 determination. Fresh cRPMI/IL-2 (100 μL/well) is added if experiment is continued.

2. On the day of p24 determination, plates are thawed and brought to 37°C. Coulter p24 ELISA assay is performed according to the manufacturer's instructions, except that the coulter extended antigen (purchased separately) is used to plot a standard curve (7.8 pg/mL to 4000 pg/mL). The curve is fit with a four-parameter equation using Soft Max Pro, version 1.1.1, computer software, and plates are read on a *V*max ELISA plate reader (Molecular Devices). As the maximum range of the standard curve is 4 ng/mL, most p24 plates are diluted 1:50 to 1:400 in order to be within range of the p24 antigen standards.

3. The ELISA reaction is stopped after 12 min (rather than 30 min). This gives the best range of optical densities for this standard curve.

4. Virus surviving fraction (p24 test serum/p24 control NHS) is calculated and plotted against reciprocal serum dilution. Fifty and 90% serum neutralization titers are calculated by linear regression analysis.

3.4. P24 Preneutralization Titration Of Virus Stocks

Preneutralization virus titration determines the median tissue culture infectious dose ($TCID_{50}$) of the virus stock and allows assessment of virus growth kinetics. $TCID_{50}$ is calculated in order to standardize infectious input (100 $TCID_{50}/25~\mu L$) in the neutralization assay, and growth kinetics are measured to allow optimal timing of p24 antigen determination. HIV-1 p24 antigen in culture supernatant is a measure of virus expression and is an indirect measure of the number of target PBMC infected. Optimal timing of collection of culture supernatants varies among viruses and may vary for individual viruses based on differences in donor PBMC. In order to best approximate the number of PBMC infected, p24 antigen is measured during the linear growth phase of each virus, before peak expression and before secondary waves of infection occur. During this phase of virus growth, there is most likely to be a direct relationship between p24 output and number of PBMC infected. To accurately compare viruses with different growth kinetics, each virus is titered on the same cryopreserved PBMC used in the neutralization assay. The virus titration is done in the neutralization assay format, as described above, except that serial four-fold virus dilutions are pre-incubated with NHS before adding PBMC.

1. Virus stock is diluted in cRPMI/IL-2 (4^0–4^8), and each dilution aliquoted in quadruplicate wells of a PGC microtiter plate (25 μL/well) containing 25 μL of NHS per well. Virus and NHS are incubated for 30 min.
2. Following the neutralization assay format, PBMC are added, incubated overnight, washed three times, and transferred to a round bottom microtiter plate.
3. On days 4, 6, and 8, 100 μL of culture supernatant are collected and replaced with fresh cRPMI/IL-2.
4. p24 antigen ELISA is performed on the day 8 culture supernatant. Wells with ≥ 60 pg/mL are scored as positive for HIV-1 growth, and endpoint virus titer ($TCID_{50}/25~\mu L$) is calculated by the method of Spearman-Karber (*see* **Note 9**).
5. Based on virus $TCID_{50}$, the virus dilution most closely approximating 100 $TCID_{50}/25~\mu L$ is used to measure p24 antigen from days 4, 6, and 8. These data are used to determine the optimal day of collection for each virus in the neutralization assay.

Notes

1. Occasionally donor PBMC replicate HIV-1 very poorly and are not suitable for neutralization assays.
2. Removal of PHA after one day improves susceptibility of PBMC to HIV-1 infection compared to traditional three day PHA-stimulation.
3. The control for baseline virus growth (e.g., NHS versus cRPMI) is substituted as appropriate for different antibody preparations. Likewise, serial dilutions of purified immunoglobulin preparations may be diluted in cRPMI rather than NHS.
4. All 37°C incubations are done in a humidified incubator with 5% CO_2.

5. The optimal time of infection varies among primary viruses. Overnight incubation allows for reproducible maximum infection. We have noted that, compared to one hour infection of PBMC, 18–24 h gives greater infection and greater sensitivity in detection of neutralization.

6. The plate carrier sold with the Sorvall model 6000D centrifuge can be adjusted to fit the microtiter plate by removal of the plate carrier handle.

7. Sera from HIV-1-infected subjects contain variable amounts of anti-p24 antibody which will interfere with detection of p24 by the Coulter ELISA. This can mistakenly be interpreted as evidence of neutralization *(17)*. Three washes dilute the initial 1:4 serum dilution by approximately 10,000-fold. This removes interfering anti-p24 antibody from most sera. In unusual cases, a fourth wash will be necessary. We test each sera for interfering anti-p24 antibody by mock washing sera and cells (no virus) in the neutralization assay format. After three washes, an aliquot of supernatant is spiked with a known amount of p24 antigen, incubated for one hour at 37°C, and tested for p24 by Coulter ELISA. If the amount of p24 detected is significantly less than input, residual serum anti-p24 antibodies are probably present and a fourth wash should be performed in the neutralization assay.

8. Some animal sera (e.g., rabbit sera) may inhibit growth of PBMC compared to NHS or no serum control wells.

9. TCID50 is calculated manually by the Spearman–Karber method *(18)* or by using computer software available from the National Center for Biotechnology Information, National Library of Medicine, National Institutes of Health, Bethesda, MD *(19)*. Since there are 25 μL of virus stock per well in our assay, the calculation gives the $TCID_{50}$ per 25 μL of virus (*see* Chapter 34, Subheading 3.3., for a more detailed description of $TCID_{50}$ calculation). The neutralization assay is performed with 100 $TCID_{50}$ of virus per well. In our hands, virus input substantially less than 100 $TCID_{50}$ results in inconsistent PBMC infection and limits assay reproducibility.

References

1. Hammon, W. McD., Coriel, L. L., and Wehrle, P. F. (1953) Evaluation of Red Cross gamma globulin as a prophylactic agent for poliomyelitis. *JAMA* **151,** 1272–1285.
2. Chen, R. T., Markowitz, L. E., Albrecht, P., et al. (1990) Measles antibody: reevaluation of protective titers. *J. Infect. Dis.* **162,** 1036–1042.
3. Frank, A. L., Taber, L. H., Glezen, P. W., Geiger, E. A., McIlwain, S., and Paredes, A. (1983) Influenza B virus infections in the community and the family: the epidemics of 1976–1977 and 1979–1980 in Houston, Texas. *Am. J. Epidemiol.* **118,** 313–325.
4. Groothius, J. R., Simoes, E. A. F., Levin, M. J., Hall, C. B., Long, C. E., Rodriguez, W. J. (1993) Prophylactic administration of respiratory syncytial virus immune globulin to high-risk infants and young children. *N. Engl. J. Med.* **329,** 1524–1530.
5. Smithburn, K. C. and Mahaffy, A. F. (1945) Immunization against yellow fever. Studies on the time of development and the duration of induced immunity. *Am. J. Trop. Med. Hyg.* **25,** 217–223.

6. Halstead, S. B. (1988) Pathogenesis of dengue: challenges to molecular biology. *Science* **239,** 476–481.

7. Suss, J. and Sinnecker, H. (1991) Immune reactions against rabies viruses-infection and vaccination. *Exp. Pathol.* **42,** 1–9.

8. Nara, P. L. and Fischinger, P. J. (1988) Quantitative infectivity assay for HIV-1 and HIV-2. *Nature* **332,** 469–70.

9. Schwartz, S., Felber, B. K., Fenyo, E. -M., and Pavlakis, G. N. (1989) Rapidly and slowly replicating human immunodeficiency virus type 1 isolates can be distinguished according to target-cell tropism in T-cell and monocyte cell lines. *Proc. Natl. Acad. Sci. USA* **86,** 7200–7203.

10. Tersmette, M., Lange, J. M. A., de Goede, R. E. Y., de Wolf, F., Eeftink-Schattenkerk, J. K. M., Schellekens, P. T. A., Coutinho, R. A., Huisman, J. G., Goudsmit, J., and Miedema, F. (1989) Association between biological properties of human immunodeficiency virus variants and risk for AIDS and AIDS mortality. *Lancet* **1,** 983–985.

11. Feng, Y., Broder, C. C., Kennedy, P. E., and Berger, E. A. (1996) HIV-1 entry cofactor: Functional cDNA cloning of a seven-transmembrane, Gprotein-coupled receptor. *Science* **272,** 872–877.

12. Golding, H., D'Souza, M. P., Bradac, J., Mathieson, B., and Fast, P. (1994) Neutralization of HIV-1. *AIDS Res. Hum. Retroviruses* **10,** 633–643.

13. Hanson, C. V. (1994) Measuring vaccine-induced HIV neutralization: report of a workshop. *AIDS Res. Hum. Retroviruses* **10,** 645–648.

14. D'Souza, M. P., Milman, G., Bradac, J. A., McPhee, D., Hanson, C. V., Hendry, R. M., et al. (1995) Neutralization of primary HIV-1 isolates by anti-envelope monoclonal antibodies. *AIDS* **9,** 867–874.

15. Mascola, J. R., Louwagie, J., McCutchan, F. E., Fischer, C. L., Hegerich, P. A., Wagner, K. F., et al. (1994) Two antigenically distinct subtypes of human immunodeficiency virus type 1: viral genotype predicts neutralization serotype. *J. Infect. Dis.* **169,** 48–54.

16. Mascola, J. R., Snyder, S. W., Weislow, O. S., Belay, S. M., Belshe, R. B., Schwartz, D. H., et al. (1996) Immunization with envelope subunit vaccine products elicits neutralizing antibodies against laboratory-adapted but not primary isolates of human immunodeficiency virus type 1. *J. Infect. Dis.* **173,** 340–348.

17. Mascola, J. R. and Burke, D. S. (1993) Antigen detection in neutralization assays: high levels of interfering anti-p24 antibodies in some plasma (Letter). *AIDS Res. Hum. Retroviruses* **9,** 1173–1174.

18. Hubert, J. J. (1984) *Spearman-Karber Method in Bioassay*, Hunt, Dubuque, IA, pp. 65,66.

19. Spouge. J. (1993) ID-50 software, Version 2. 0. Natl. Ctr. Biotechnol. Inform., Natl. Lib. Med., Natl. Inst. Health. Bethesda, MD.

34

Neutralization of HIV-1 Infection of Human Peripheral Blood Mononuclear Cells (PBMC)

Infectivity Reduction Method

John R. Mascola

1. Introduction

The serum titration neutralization assay described in Chapter 33 utilizes a constant amount of infectious virus and indirectly estimates the antibody-mediated reduction in infectious virus by measuring p24 antigen expressed by human peripheral blood mononuclear cells (PBMC). The assay assumes a direct relationship between expressed p24 antigen and the number of target PBMC infected. Therefore, the optimal time of p24 antigen measurement may vary due to different growth kinetics among viruses. An infectivity reduction assay (IRA) directly measures the effect of antibody on virus endpoint infectious titer. The IRA is more labor-intensive and requires more serum than the antibody titration assay, and it is generally done with a single dilution of antibody. However, it has the important advantage of directly measuring the effect of antibody on virus median tissue culture infectious dose ($TCID_{50}$). In addition, the IRA is unaffected by variation in virus growth kinetics and therefore is theoretically more suitable for comparing neutralization among diverse virus isolates. The assay described below calculates virus $TCID_{50}$ by serially diluting virus stock in quadruplicate wells with phytohemagglutinin (PHA)-stimulated PBMC. Wells are scored positive or negative for HIV-1 infection by measuring expressed p24 antigen after eight days in culture. Results are expressed as the antibody-mediated reduction in virus $TCID_{50}$ (i.e., ratio of virus $TCID_{50}$ in control sera to $TCID_{50}$ in test sera). Thus, a 100-fold reduction in $TCID_{50}$ indicates that 99% of infectious virus has been neutralized.

From: *Methods in Molecular Medicine, Vol. 17: HIV Protocols*
Edited by: N. L. Michael and J. H. Kim © Humana Press Inc., Totowa, NJ

2. Materials

1. Culture Media (cRPMI): RPMI 1640 media (ABI, Columbia, MD), supplemented with 15% heat-inactivated fetal calf serum (FCS) (Intergen, Purchase, NJ), 100 U/mL penicillin, 100 µg/mL streptomycin and 2 mM L-glutamine (all from ABI).
2. cRPMI/IL-2: cRPMI supplemented with 20 U/mL human recombinant IL-2 (Boehringer Mannheim, GmbH, Germany).
3. Target cells: Ficoll gradient separated PBMC, from a HIV-1-seronegative donor.
4. 96-well tissue culture boxes: 0.5 mL/well (#499-023, PGC Scientific, Frederick, MD).
5. ELISA aspirator: Used for washing cells in PGC microtiter box (Corning ELISA plate washer, 26305-72, Corning, NY).
6. 96-well round-bottom microtiter plates (Costar, Cambridge, MA).
7. Microtiter plate sealers (Costar).
8. Sorvall microplate carrier: Used for H-1000B rotor, Sorvall RT 6000D centrifuge (Sorvall Instruments, Wilmington, DE).
9. PHA-P (Difco Labs, Detroit, MI), prepared in sterile distilled water to 1 µg/µL
10. Pooled normal human serum (NHS) (Sigma, St. Louis, MO)
11. HIV-1 p24 antigen ELISA Kit (Coulter, Hialeah, FL).
12. max ELISA plate reader with Soft Max Pro software (Molecular Devices Corp., Sunnyvale, CA).

3. Methods
3.1. Preparation of PBMC Target Cells

1. Donor PBMC are ficoll-gradient separated from whole blood or leukophoresis pack by standard procedures.
2. PBMC (20×10^6/vial) are cryopreserved in cRPMI with 10% dimethylsulfoxide (DMSO) and initially placed overnight at $-70°C$, then stored in the vapor phase of liquid nitrogen.
3. For PHA-stimulation, PBMC are thawed quickly in a 37°C water bath and washed in 30 mL of cRPMI. Cells are resuspended in 30 mL of cRPMI/IL-2, transferred to a vented upright T25 flask, and 30 µL of PHA are added (final PHA concentration, 1 µg/mL). PHA is removed after approx 24 h by a single wash in cRPMI, and cells are again resuspended in 30 mL of cRPMI/IL-2 (*see* **Note 1**). Target cells used in the assay are 3 or 4 d PHA-stimulated PBMC. On the day of the assay, cells are counted and resuspended in cRPMI/IL-2 at 2×10^6/mL. Viability should be >90%.

3.2. Infectivity Reduction Neutralization Assay

Since the IRA measures the affect of antibody on virus $TCID_{50}$, virus stocks are pretitered to ensure an adequate infectious titer (i.e., generally $\geq 10^3$ $TCID_{50}$/25 µL virus stock). Virus stocks and neutralization plates contain significant amounts of HIV-1 and all work should be carried out in a BL3 laboratory facility or a BL2 facility using BL3 practices. For simplicity of description, the assay described below uses serum collected from HIV-1-infected subjects

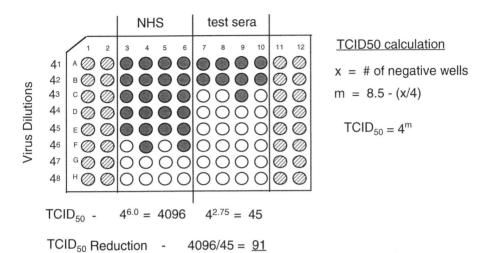

Fig. 1. Example of results of an IRA and Spearman-Karber calculation. Virus TCID$_{50}$ is assayed in NHS and test sera (i.e., neutralizing sera from an HIV-infected patient). Preincubation of virus with NHS resulted in a total of 10 HIV-negative wells after 8 d in culture (i.e., $x = 10$). TCID$_{50}$ is derived from 4^m, where $m = (8.5 - [10/4]) = 6$ and TCID$_{50} = 4^6 = 4096$ (i.e., 4096 TCID$_{50}$ per 25 μL). Likewise, TCID$_{50}$ of virus with test sera resulted in 23 negative wells, $m = [8.5 - (23/4)] = 2.75$ and TCID$_{50} = 4^{2.75} = 45$. Serum-mediated reduction in virus TCID$_{50} = 4096/45$ or 91-fold.

as a source of antibody. Serum is used at a single dilution (1:2). Plasma from anticoagulated whole blood can be substituted for serum. Purified polyclonal immunoglobulin, monoclonal antibodies or soluble CD4 can be used with minor alterations in the protocol (*see* **Note 2**).

1. Prior to use, all test sera and control sera (e.g., NHS) are complement-depleted by heat inactivation for 40 min at 56°C.
2. NHS is aliquoted in eight consecutive rows of the 96-well PGC microtiter box (Rows A-H, 25 μL/well in quadruplicate wells, *see* **Fig. 1**).
3. Test sera is diluted 1:2 in NHS and is similarly aliquoted into the 96-well PGC microtiter box, adjacent to the control NHS (*see* **Fig. 1** and **Note 3**).
4. One amp of virus stock is quickly thawed in a 37°C water bath and eight fourfold dilutions are made (4^1–4^8) in a 96-well microtiter plate (eight replicate wells/virus dilution). Virus dilutions are made in cRPMI/IL2.
5. Starting with the 4^8 virus dilution, each virus dilution (eight replicate wells) is transferred to the corresponding rows of the PGC microtiter box (25 μL virus/well, *see* **Fig. 1**). Care is taken not to touch pipet tips into serum at bottom of wells. After dispensing virus, the microtiter box is gently tapped against the hood floor to ensure that serum and virus are well mixed in the bottom of the 0.5 mL wells, and the microtiter box is incubated at 37°C for 30 min (*see* **Note 4**).

5. PHA-stimulated PBMC (50 µL, 1 x 10^5) are added to each well, and the box again gently tapped against the hood floor to mix PBMC with serum/virus. A loose fitting cover from a 96-well round-bottom plate is placed on top of the microtiter box, and the box is incubated overnight (approx 18 h, *see* **Note 5**).

5. PBMC are then washed and centrifuged three times at approx 210g in the microtiter box using a plate carrier (*see* **Note 6**). Boxes are sealed with an adherent plastic plate sealer (Costar) prior to each wash. Washing removes virus stock p24 antigen and serum anti-p24 antibody (*see* **Note 7**). For each wash, wells are filled to 500 µL with cRPMI (first two washes) or cRPMI/IL-2 (third wash). After each wash, supernatants are aspirated with the Corning ELISA aspirator set to leave 50 µL/well. The cell pellet is not disturbed. After the last wash, 200 µL of cRPMI/IL-2 is added to each well. Cells are resuspended and 220 µL/well is transferred to a round-bottom microtiter plate.

6. Plates are inspected daily for uniformity in size of cell pellets and pH of culture media (*see* **Note 8**). Fresh cRPMI/IL2 (100 µL/well) is replaced on d 4 and culture supernatant is harvested on d 8 for measurement of HIV-1 p24 antigen.

7. On d 8, 100 µL of culture supernatant are removed from each well and placed into a corresponding microtiter plate with 80 µL of phosphate-buffered saline (PBS) and 20 µL coulter lysis buffer/well (i.e., final dilution, 1:2). The p24 plate is frozen at –20°C until p24 antigen determination.

8. On the day of p24 determination, plates are thawed and brought to 37°C. Coulter p24 ELISA assay is performed according to the manufacturer's instructions. Wells with ≥ 60 pg/mL of p24 antigen are scored as positive for HIV-1 infection (*see* **Note 9**).

3. Calculation of $TCID_{50}$

1. Endpoint virus titer ($TCID_{50}$) can be calculated manually by the Spearman-Karber method *(1)* or by using computer software available from the National Center for Biotechnology Information, National Library of Medicine, National Institutes of Health (Bethesda, MD) (Spouge ID_{50}, version 2.0) *(2)*.

2. **Figure 1** depicts an example of IRA results and the Spearman-Karber calculation. Wells are scored as positive for HIV-1 infection based on p24 antigen expression (≥ 60 pg/mL). The $TCID_{50}$ calculation considers the virus dilution factor (fourfold in this example), the number of virus dilutions (i.e., 8) and the total number of negative wells. Since there are 25 µL of virus stock/well, the final calculation gives the $TCID_{50}$ per 25 µL of virus stock.

3. As shown in **Fig. 1**, virus preincubated with NHS has a $TCID_{50}$ of 4096; virus preincubated with test sera from an HIV-infected subject has a $TCID_{50}$ of 45. Thus the serum-mediated reduction in virus $TCID_{50}$ is 4096/45 = 91.

4. The ID_{50} computer software mentioned above will perform the Spearman-Karber calculation. It will also perform a more sophisticated model fit calculation which allows calculation of 95% confidence intervals around the $TCID_{50}$ value. This facilitates statistical comparisons of $TCID_{50}$ values (*see* **Note 10**).

4. Notes

1. Removal of PHA after 1 d improves susceptibility of PBMC to HIV-1 infection compared to traditional 3 d PHA- stimulation.

2. The control for virus $TCID_{50}$ (e.g., NHS vs cRPMI) is substituted as appropriate for different antibody preparations. Likewise, purified immunoglobulin preparations may be diluted in cRPMI rather than NHS.

3. Dilution of test sera in the NHS pool, and direct comparison of virus $TCID_{50}$ in NHS vs test serum, minimizes nonspecific affects of serum proteins on virus $TCID_{50}$. The author has also performed the IRA with pools of sera (i.e., equal volumes of 5 sera from HIV-infected subjects) and demonstrated that serum pools often display a greater magnitude and breadth of neutralization than any individual serum comprising the pool.

4. All 37°C incubations are done in a humidified incubator with 5% CO_2.

5. Overnight incubation allows for reproducible maximum infection. We have noted that, compared to 1 h infection of PBMC, 18–24 h gives greater infection and greater sensitivity in detection of neutralization.

6. The plate carrier sold with the Sorvall model 6000D centrifuge can be adjusted to fit the microtiter box by removal of the plate carrier handle.

7. Sera from HIV-1-infected subjects contain variable amounts of anti-p24 antibody that will interfere with detection of p24 by the Coulter ELISA. This can mistakenly be interpreted as evidence of neutralization *(3)*. Three washes dilutes the initial 1:2 serum dilution by approximately 10,000-fold. This removes anti-p24 antibody from most sera; in unusual cases, a fourth wash will be necessary. The author tests each sera for interfering anti-p24 antibody by mock washing sera and cells (no virus) in the neutralization assay format. After three washes, an aliquot of supernatant is spiked with a known amount of p24 antigen, incubated for one hour at 37°C, and tested for p24 by Coulter ELISA. If the amount of p24 detected is significantly less than input, residual serum anti-p24 antibodies are probably present and a fourth wash should be performed in the neutralization assay.

8. Some animal sera (e.g., rabbit sera) may inhibit growth of PBMC compared to NHS or no serum control wells.

9. The Coulter p24 ELISA kit can reproducibility detect 60 pg/mL of p24 antigen (the standard curve begins at 7.8 pg/mL). The author has found 60 pg/mL on d 8 to be a sensitive marker of HIV-1 infection. Wells rarely turn positive after d 8.

10. Reproducibility experiments in the author's laboratory (i.e., performing virus $TCID_{50}$ in replicates of 10) have shown that $TCID_{50}$ values in one experiment fall within a four- to sevenfold range. Thus, we have defined a 10-fold reduction in $TCID_{50}$ as significant evidence of antibody-mediated neutralization *(4)*.

References

1. Hubert, J. J. (1984) Spearman-Karber Method in *Bioassay.* Hunt, Dubuque, IA, pp. 65,66.
2. Spouge. J. (1993) ID-50 software, version 2.0. National Center for Biotechnology Information, National Library of Medicine, National Institutes of Health, Bethesda, MD.

3. Mascola, J. R. and Burke, D. S. (1993) Antigen detection in neutralization assays: high levels of interfering anti-p24 antibodies in some plasma. *AIDS Res. Hum. Retrovir.* **9,** 1173–1174.

4. Mascola, J. R., Louder, M. K., Surman, S. S., VanCott, T. C., Yu, X-F, Bradac, J., et al. (1996) Human immunodeficiency virus type 1 neutralizing antibody serotyping using serum pools and an infectivity reduction assay. *AIDS Res. Hum. Retrovir.* **12,** 1319–1328.

35

Collection and Processing of Mucosal Secretions from HIV-1 Infected Women

Andrew W. Artenstein and Thomas C. VanCott

1. Introduction

The major route of transmission of the human immunodeficiency virus type 1 (HIV-1) worldwide, like other agents of sexually transmitted disease, is via mucosal surfaces of the genital tract through sexual exposures *(1–4)*. It has been hypothesized that immune responses at these sites may be important determinants of protection against HIV-1 *(1,2,5)*. Because of the potential relationship of mucosal immune responses to protection against HIV-1 infection, an assessment of immune responses at these sites in vaccine trial participants will be critical. Proper collection and processing of specimens from mucosal sites is of vital importance to the measurement of mucosal immune responses. This chapter details the collection and processing procedures of specimens from three distinct mucosal compartments in female subjects. Collection techniques for additional mucosal compartments (e.g. semen, rectal, etc.) can be found in **ref. 6** (*see* **Note 1**).

2. Materials
2.1. Disposable Supplies and Solutions for Collections

1. Phosphate-buffered saline (PBS): 137 mM NaCl, 2.7 mM KCl, 14.1 mM Na$_2$HPO$_4$, and 2.9 mM KH$_2$PO$_4$.
2. Sno-Strips (Akorn, Inc., Abita Springs, LA).
3. Ultrafree-CL centrifugation (low protein binding, 0.22 μm)/transport vial (Millipore, Bedford, MA).
4. Sterile plastic transfer pipet—6 mL (Fisher, Pittsburgh, PA).
5. Sterile specimen containers with screw-on lids (Fisher).

From: *Methods in Molecular Medicine, Vol. 17: HIV Protocols*
Edited by: N. L. Michael and J. H. Kim © Humana Press Inc., Totowa, NJ

6. 10 mL disposable pipet (Costar Corp., Cambridge, MA).
7. PBS premixed with 0.01% sodium azide.
8. Sterile-15 mL Falcon tube (PGC, Gaithersberg, MD).

2.2. Solutions and Reagents for Processing

1. Hemoccult single slides (SmithKline Diagnostics, San Jose, CA).
2. Ultrafree-CL Centrifugation (low protein binding, 0.22 μm)/transport vial (Millipore, Bedford, MA).
3. 1.8-mL sterile Nunc tubes (PGC, Gaithersburgh, MD).

3. Methods

3.1. Collection of Mucosal Secretions

1. Collection/transport tubes and vials should be prepared prior to initiating the actual patient collections. Vaginal lavage fluid will be placed directly into empty Ultrafree-CL vials (Millipore); nasal secretions will be collected in a sterile specimen container with screw-on lid. For endocervical secretions, Ultrafree-CL vials (Millipore) should be preloaded with 0.5 mL of PBS + 0.01% sodium azide solution at room temperature.
2. All collected secretions should be placed on wet ice for transport and should be processed within hours of collection.

3.1.1. Endocervical Secretions (see **Note 2**)

1. The volunteer should assume the lithotomy position with her feet placed in stirrups and the appropriate draping employed. Lighting should be directed to the perianal area.
2. A sterile speculum should be moistened with warm water and inserted into the vagina and secured when adequate visualization of the cervix is accomplished.
3. Two tear flow indicator strips (Sno-strips) should be placed together, grasped with a forceps, inserted approx 3 mm into the cervical os, and removed after secretions have passively accumulated to the "shoulder" of the strips (10–30 s) *(7)*. The strips should be trimmed at the shoulder and placed directly into the preloaded Ultrafree-Cl vial as above.
4. **Step 3** should be repeated with a second pair of strips (*see* **Note 3**).

3.1.2. Vaginal Lavage

1. After the collection of endocervical secretions and with the patient in the lithotomy position, flush 3 mL of PBS over the cervix using a sterile, disposable, plastic transfer pipet (*see* **Note 4**).
2. Using the same pipet, reaspirate the instilled PBS from the posterior fornix of the vagina (where the fluid will pool with the subject in the lithotomy position) and flush over the vaginal wall. Reaspirate the PBS (which now contains vaginal secretions) and place directly into a sterile 15-mL Falcon tube (*see* **Note 5**).

3.1.3. Nasal Wash

1. With the subject sitting in a chair in the upright position and head tilted back, instill 5 mL of PBS into each nostril using a 10-mL disposable pipet.
2. Instruct the subject to hold her breath, not swallow, and attempt to retain the fluid for as long as comfortable, up to 30 s (*see* **Note 6**). The examiner should hold a sterile specimen container near the subject's nose during this time.
3. Tilt the head forward, hold the cup directly under the nose, and have the subject empty the nasal wash into the specimen container.

3.2. Processing of Mucosal Secretions

3.2.1. Endocervical Secretions

1. Remove 10 µL of endocervical secretions, and test for the presence of occult blood (Hemoccult, SmithKline Diagnostics, San Jose, CA); note positive specimens.
2. Centrifuge the Ultrafree-CL centrifugation/transport vial (Millipore) containing the two Sno-strips at 4°C for 15 min at 1500*g* (*see* **Note 7**).
3. Store samples at –80°C in 200-µL aliquots.

3.2.2. Vaginal Lavage

1. Centrifuge the vaginal lavage samples contained within a 15-mL Falcon tube at 4°C for 5 min at 1500*g* (*see* **Note 8**).
2. Remove sample, avoiding any sediment at the bottom of the tube, and transfer to Ultrafree-CL centrifugation tubes.
3. Remove several 10 µL aliquots of vaginal wash, and test for the presence of occult blood (Hemoccult, SmithKline Diagnostics); note positive specimens.
4. Centrifuge Ultrafree-CL centrifugation tubes at 4°C for 15 min at 1500*g*.
5. If the sample is not completely filtered, repeat the centrifugation step (4°C for 15 min at 1500*g*) (*see* **Note 9**).
6. Store samples at –80°C in 500 µL aliquots.

3.2.3. Nasal Wash

1. Transfer the nasal wash from the sterile specimen container into Ultrafree-CL centrifugation tubes using a pipet (*see* **Note 10**).
2. Centrifuge the Ultrafree-CL centrifugation tubes containing the nasal wash at 4°C for 15 min at 1500*g*.
3. If the sample is not completely filtered, then repeat centrifugation step (4°C for 15 min at 1500*g*) (*see* **Note 11**).
4. Store samples at –80°C in 1.5-mL aliquots.

4. Notes

1. Mucosal specimen collection, from various compartments, should be postponed for the following reasons:
   a. Genital tract: if the subject admits to penetrative sexual intercourse or vaginal douching within 72 h of the collection visit; if they were menstruating; or had

an abnormal vaginal discharge or a cervical lesion accompanied by bleeding at the time of the visit.

    b. Nasal: If the subject is experiencing symptoms of an upper respiratory tract infection or nasal allergy.

2. Women who have undergone hysterectomy are generally excluded from study based upon data in animals *(8)* and humans *(9)* that show only negligible quantities of IgA in the absence of the uterus and cervix.

3. Bleeding from the endocervix as a result of Sno-strip insertion is uncommon in our experience; however, if bleeding does occur with the first pair, it is not advisable to insert the second pair of strips.

4. To ensure consistency, it is advisable to keep the order of collection from the two genital compartments uniform; however, it is not clear one specific order is superior to the other.

5. The vaginal washing procedure has been previously calculated to dilute the native secretions approx tenfold *(10)*.

6. The nasal wash procedure is generally well tolerated, although the sensation of fluid in the nose is uncomfortable at first for some subjects. If the fluid can be retained for more than 5 s, it is probably a successful collection. Repeated nasal washes tend to be well tolerated (probably because the subject becomes acclimated to the sensation), however, the effect of repeated nasal washes on levels of mucosal antibody has not been well studied.

7. It is possible that the endocervical sample may not be completely filtered after the initial centrifugation step (this occurs in approx 5–10% of cervical samples) and so an additional centrifugation step (4°C for 15 min at 1500*g*) may be required.

8. A prespin of the vaginal lavage is necessary due to the high viscosity (high mucous content) of the collected sample and allows for more efficient filtration of the wash in the subsequent step.

9. Due to high viscosity, it may be necessary to repeat the centrifugation step for the majority of the vaginal lavage samples. Additionally, if the sample is still not completely filtered after the second centrifugation step, it may be necessary to transfer remaining unfiltered sample to a second fresh Ultrafree-CL centrifugation tube and centrifuge an additional time (4°C for 15 min at 1500*g*).

10. The total amount of nasal wash collected (5–10 mL) should be dispensed as 2-mL aliquots into separate Ultrafree-CL centrifuge tubes. These tubes have 3-mL capacities and using smaller volumes (2 mL) in each tubes will accelerate the filtering step.

11. If a third centrifuge step is required, transfer the remaining nasal wash to a fresh Ultrafree-CL centrifuge tube and centrifuge an additional time (4°C for 15 min at 1500*g*). The majority of the nasal wash collections should be completely filtered after 1–2 centrifugation steps.

References

1. Mestecky, J. and Jackson S. (1994) Reassessment of the impact of mucosal immunity in infection with the human immunodeficiency virus (HIV) and design of relevant vaccines. *J. Clin. Immunol.* 259–272.

2. Miller, C. J., McGhee, J. R., and Gardner, M. B. (1992) Mucosal immunity, HIV transmission, and AIDS. *Lab. Invest.* **68,** 129–145.

3. Piot, P., Plummer, F. A., Mhalu, F. S., Lamboray, J -L., Chin, J., and Mann, J. M. (1988) AIDS: an international perspective. *Science* **239,** 573–579.

4. Padian, N. S., Shiboski, S. C., and Jewell, N. P. (1991) Female-to-male transmission of human immunodeficiency virus. *JAMA* **266,** 1664–1667.

5. Forrest, B. D. (1991) Women, HIV, and mucosal immunity. *Lancet* **337,** 835,836.

6. *DIADS/NIAID Manual for collection and processing of mucosal specimens from AVEG sites.* June 14, 1994.

7. Ashley, R. L., et al. (1994) Protien-specific cervical antibody responses to primary genital herpes simplex virus type 2 infections. *J. Infect. Dis.* **170,** 20–26.

8. Parr, E.L. and Parr, M.B. (1990) A comparison of antibody titres in mouse uterine fluid after immunization by several routes, and the effect of the uterus on antibody titres in vaginal fluid. *Reprod. Fert.* **89,** 619–625.

9. Jalanti, R. and Isliker, H. (1977) Immunoglobulins in human cervico-vaginal secretions. *Int. Arch. Allergy Appl. Immunol.* **53,** 402–408.

10. Belec, L., Meillet, D., Levy, M., Georges, A., Tevi-Benissan, C., and Pillot, J. (1995) Dilution assessment of cervicovaginal secretions obtained by vaginal washing for immunologic assays. *Clin. Diag. Lab. Immunol.* **2,** 57–61.

36

Collection and Processing of Mucosal Secretions from Mice

Robert W. Kaminski and Thomas C. VanCott

1. Introduction

The major route of transmission of the human immunodeficiency virus type 1 (HIV-1) worldwide, like other agents of sexually transmitted disease, is via mucosal surfaces of the genital tract through sexual exposures (1–4). It has been hypothesized that immune responses at these sites may be important determinants of protection against HIV-1 (1,2,5). Development of HIV-1 vaccines which elicit local mucosal immune responses may be critical for an effective preventive vaccine. Specific mucosal immune responses elicited after different routes of mucosal immunization in rodents have been examined previously (6–16). Nasal and oral immunization routes have elicited strong mucosal responses to HIV-1 peptides and whole proteins in mice (7,11,17,18,24). Induction of mucosal and systemic immunity to SIV and HIV-1 antigens in primates has also been obtained using a variety of mucosal routes of vaccine administration (19–22).

Proper collection and processing of specimens from mucosal sites are of vital importance to the measurement of mucosal immune responses. This chapter details the collection and processing procedures of serum and mucosal secretions (vaginal wash, whole saliva, lung wash, intestinal wash, and fecal pellets) from mice.

2. Materials
2.1. Disposable Supplies and Solutions for Collections

1. 1-cc syringes (Thomas Scientific, Swedesboro, NJ).
2. 24-gauge needles (Thomas Scientific).
3. 3-cc syringes (Thomas Scientific).

From: *Methods in Molecular Medicine, Vol. 17: HIV Protocols*
Edited by: N. L. Michael and J. H. Kim © Humana Press Inc., Totowa, NJ

4. Pilocarpine-HCl (lyophilized, [Sigma, St. Louis, MO]).
5. Phosphate-buffered saline (PBS), pH 7.2 (Advanced Biotechnologies, Inc., Columbia, MD).
6. Uniwicks (10 × 25 mm, [Polyfiltronics, Rockland, MA])
7. Catheters (18G × 5.1 cm, [Baxter, Columbia, MD]).
8. Sterile saline 0.9% sodium chloride injection (Abbott Laboratories, North Chicago, IL).
9. Robinul (stock 0.2 mg/mL) (A.H. Robins, Pharmaceutical Division, Richmond, VA).
10. Anesthetic cocktail: 10 mL ketamine (10 mg/mL stock) and 1.5 mL xylozene diluted 1:5 in PBS.
11. Halothane™.
12. Metaphane™.
13. Surgical scissors.
14. Sodium pentobarbital.

2.2. Solutions and Reagents for Processing

1. 4-(2-aminoethyl)-benzenesulfonylfluoride (AEBSF) (Calbiochem, San Diego, CA).
2. Aprotinin (Sigma, St. Louis, MO).
3. Leupeptin (Sigma).
4. Bestatin (B & M, Indianapolis, IN).
5. Lung lavage solution (make fresh daily): 0.2 mM AEBSF, 1 µg/mL aprotinin, 3.25 µM bestatin and 10 µM leupeptin in sterile PBS.
6. Intestinal lavage solution (make fresh daily): 0.2 mM AEBSF, 1 µg/mL aprotinin, 3.25 µM bestatin and 10 µM leupeptin in sterile PBS.
7. ELISA buffer solution: 5% bovine serum albumin (BSA), 5% casein, 0.01% sodium azide in PBS, pH 7.4.

3. Methods

3.1. Euthanasia of Mice

At times during a study, protocol requirements may dictate that the mice be euthanized. There are a number of acceptable ways to sacrifice a mouse, but animal euthanasia guidelines may vary with institutes. A review of the current methods being followed at the institute where one works should be done prior to protocol preparation. Outlined here are three commonly used methods to sacrifice mice. Advantages and disadvantages of these protocols are discussed in **Table 1**.

3.1.1. CO_2 Suffocation

1. Animals are placed in a closed container.
2. CO_2 is pumped in from a canister, or a beaker of dry ice is placed in the container with the animals.
3. Water may be added to the dry ice to produce CO_2 faster.
4. Within 30 s, the mice will be rendered unconscious, but should be left in the container for several additional min to ensure death.
5. Verify death of animal by lack of cardiac pulse.

Table 1
Euthanasia Comparison

Euthanasia method	Advantages	Disadvantages
CO_2 suffocation	Painless, many animals done at once, inexpensive, little to no technical experience required	Abnormal blood gas ratios, blood may clot prior to removal from animal
Cervical dislocation	Painful to animal if not performed properly	Technical experience required
Anesthesia overdose	Painless	Certain anesthesia can affect blood clotting and contaminate the sample; expense of anesthesia

3.1.2 Cervical Dislocation

1. Mouse is held by base of tail.
2. Pencil, large forceps, or other cylindrical object is placed on the neck directly behind the head and ears.
3. Pressure is applied to the cylindrical object in a downward motion to hold the head in place.
4. The tail is then pulled away from the head in a deliberate motion parallel to the body of the mouse until the vertebrae in the neck is dislocated.
5. Verify death of animal by lack of cardiac pulse.

3.1.3. Anesthesia Overdose/Euthanasia Cocktail

1. A cocktail of mouse euthanasia chemicals is administered intraperitoneally (*see* **Note 1**).
2. Dosages are usually based on weight of mouse and manufacturer's directions should be followed.
3. Verify death of animal by lack of cardiac pulse.

3.2. Serum Collection

A number of different techniques exist for collection of whole blood from mice, three of which are described below (cardiac puncture, retro-orbital, and tail bleeding). Each method has distinct advantages in certain situations. The choice of method is dependent on several factors, to include final condition of the mouse, technical ability of investigator, and the amount of sample required. For example, cardiac puncture is used solely at sacrifice and generally yields the highest volume of sample, while retro-orbital bleeding may be done at various time points throughout a study, but yields smaller sample volumes. The requirements of the study must therefore be matched with the method of bleeding to ensure proper treatment of the animals and maintenance of sample integrity.

3.2.1. Cardiac Puncture

1. Sacrifice mice using one of the techniques described in **Subheading 3.1.**
2. Cardiac puncture should be made with a 24-gauge needle attached to a 1-cc syringe. It is possible to collect between 0.7–1.0 cc of whole blood (*see* **Notes 2 and 3**).
3. Whole blood should be placed in a microcentrifuge tube, allowed to coagulate at 4°C or room temperature for 1–2 h, centrifuged at 5000g for 10 min and the supernatant (serum) drawn off. Serum volume should equal approx 1/2 volume of the whole blood collected.
4. Collected serum should be stored at −70°C until assayed.

3.2.2. Retro-Orbital Bleeding

1. Mice are held in one hand by placing the thumb and forefinger behind the ears of the mouse and firmly grasping the scruff on top of the neck. If necessary, the legs can be immobilized with the remaining fingers of the same hand.
2. A glass Pasteur pipet is then placed in the rear corner of the eye and carefully inserted into the retro-orbital process. The pipet is then slowly twisted in place to disrupt the capillary bed and cause the mouse to bleed (*see* **Note 4**).
3. The blood is collected with the Pasteur pipet and then placed in a microcentrifuge tube. It is possible to collect between 0.2–0.8 cc of whole blood (*see* **Note 5**).
4. Whole blood should be placed in a microcentrifuge tube, allowed to coagulate at 4°C or room temperature for 1–2 h, centrifuged at 5000g for 10 min, and the supernatant (serum) drawn off. Serum volume should equal approx 1/2 volume of the whole blood collected.
5. Collected serum should be stored at −70°C until assayed.

3.2.3. Tail Bleeding

1. Mouse is placed in a mouse restrainer with the tail exposed.
2. Approximately 1–2 cm of the tail is cut off from the distal part of the tail.
3. The tail vein will then release the blood freely and should be collected into a microcentrifuge tube (*see* **Note 6**).
4. Whole blood should be placed in a microcentrifuge tube, allowed to coagulate at 4°C or room temperature for 1–2 h, centrifuged at 5000g for 10 min and the supernatant (serum) drawn off. Serum volume should equal approx 1/2 volume of the whole blood collected.
5. Collected serum should be stored at −70°C until assayed.

3.3. Collection of Mucosal Secretions

Collection of vaginal secretions, whole saliva, and fecal pellets can be performed at multiple time points during immunization schedules. Fecal pellets and vaginal secretions are the simplest to collect since no anesthesia is required. Lung and intestinal lavage as described can only be collected at the end of the study after sacrifice.

3.3.1. Vaginal Secretions

1. A microcentrifuge tube containing a 25 × 2 mm uniwick from Polyfiltronics should be weighed and recorded (in mg) (*see* **Note 7**).
2. Instill 25 µL of sterile PBS into vaginal vault of female mouse using a sterile 0–200 µL pipet tip and a micropipet (*see* **Note 8**).
3. Insert a uniwick into the vaginal vault using sterile forceps, and leave in place for approx 30 s (*see* **Note 9**).
4. Remove wick, instill an additional 25 µL into the vaginal vault, and then repeat **step 3** above using the opposite end of the same wick.
5. Place the secretion-saturated wick into a labeled microcentrifuge tube, and store on dry ice immediately. Transfer to –70°C until further processing occurs (*see* **Subheading 3.4.**).

3.3.2 Whole Saliva Collection

1. Inject 50 µl of the anesthetic cocktail intramuscularly (*see* **Subheading 2.1.**) to anesthetize the mouse.
2. Wait until the mouse can be laid on its side without resistance (*see* **Note 10**).
3. Intraperitoneally inject 50 µL of a 0.1 mg/mL solution of pilocarpine-HCl diluted in PBS and lay the mouse on its side on an absorbent surface (*see* **Note 11**).
4. Place a Pasteur pipet (or other similar collection device) into the lower part of the mouth. Adjust the position of the pipet regularly to aid in collection. Each mouse will yield approx 0.2 mL saliva (*see* **Notes 12, 13** and **14**).
5. Immediately after collection is complete or sufficient volume is collected, intraperitoneally inject 0.1 mL of a 1:10 solution of robinul diluted in PBS. This will stop fluid secretion and revive the mouse (*see* **Note 15**).
6. After collection is completed, inject 250 µL subcutaneously of sterile saline into the mouse to rehydrate (*see* **Note 16**).
7. Store sample on dry ice and transfer to –70°C until assayed.

3.3.3. Lung Lavage (see **Note 17**)

1. Euthanize the mouse with CO_2 or by cervical dislocation (*see* **Subheading 3.1.**).
2. Spray exterior of euthanized mouse with 70% ethanol.
3. Make an incision from the neck to the lower abdomen with surgical scissors and expose the thoracic cavity.
4. The diaphragm and sternum should be cut away with special care taken not to puncture or damage the lung or surrounding tissues. The pleural membranes should also be cut so that the lungs are given sufficient area to expand.
5. Nodes and glands should be dissected away from the trachea, and the tissues covering the trachea should be removed.

6. A plastic catheter should be placed into the trachea by inserting the catheter needle bevel side up next to the anterior section and as proximal to the mouth as possible. After the needle is inserted and the catheter is inside the trachea, the needle should be pulled back inside of the plastic catheter sheath, but not out of the catheter (this is done in an effort to keep the flexible plastic catheter rigid to facilitate proper placement). The catheter should then be gently advanced into the trachea until it is adjacent to the bifocation of the lungs (*see* **Note 18**).

7. The elasticized trachea tissue should fit around the larger diameter of the catheter and seal the junction of the catheter and the trachea preventing contamination and fluid loss (*see* **Note 19**).

8. After the catheter is secured in the trachea, a 1-cc syringe filled with lung lavage solution should be attached to the end of the catheter using the leur locks and 1 cc slowly injected, watching the lungs inflate.

9. Once the lung lavage solution has filled the lungs, the plunger of the syringe should be withdrawn slowly to collect lavage fluid (*see* **Note 20**).

10. After the first 1 cc has been collected, **repeat steps 8** and **9** so that a total of 2 cc has washed the lungs.

11. Approximately 1.8 mL of lung fluid secretions can be collected. This fluid should be stored at 4°C until processed (*see* **Note 21**) (*see* **Section 3.4.C**).

3.3.4. Intestinal lavage (see **Note 17**)

1. Euthanize mouse with CO_2 or by cervical dislocation (*see* **Subheading 3.1.**).

2. Spray exterior of euthanized mouse with 70% ethanol.

3. Make an incision from the neck to the lower abdomen with surgical scissors and expose the abdominal cavity.

4. The peritoneal cavity should be opened and the intestines exposed by carefully dissecting away the mesentery.

5. Locate the duodenum (differentiated from the jejunum and ileum by its color, texture, and shape) that is distal to the stomach. In the area where the duodenum ends and the jejunum begin, remove approx 10 in. of the small intestine containing the jejunum and ileum. Once removed, this section of the small intestine must be kept moist with sterile saline or PBS.

6. Insert a flexible plastic catheter into one end of the intestine and thread about 1–2 in. of intestine onto the catheter with the catheter's needle pulled into the sheath to maintain rigidity but reduce chance of intestinal perforation.

7. The intestines can then be secured to the catheter by simply placing the thumb and forefinger of one hand on the intestinal section threaded on the catheter and applying slight pressure (*see* **Note 22**).

8. The needle should then be removed from the sheath and a 3-cc syringe prefilled with 2 mL of gut lavage solution should be attached to the catheter via the leur lock.

9. The opposite end of the intestine should be placed into a 1.8-cc microcentrifuge tube. The gut lavage solution should then be slowly instilled so as not to cause a rupture which may occur if an excess amount of pressure is exerted on the intestinal wall (*see* **Note 23**).

10. The sample should be stored on wet ice until processed (*see* **Note 21**) (*see* **Subheading 3.4.**).

3.3.5. Fecal Pellets

1. Collect approx 0.1 g of fecal pellets/cage of five mice, which is the equivalent of 12–15 individual pellets (2–3 pellets/mouse) into a microcentrifuge tube (*see* **Note 24**).
2. Store samples at −70°C until processed (*see* **Section 3.4.E.**).

3.4. Processing of Mucosal Secretions

3.4.1. Vaginal Secretions

1. Weigh frozen vaginal secretion samples consisting of a microcentrifuge tube containing a secretion saturated uniwick. Calculate weight of sample collected by computing the numerical difference between the pre- and postsample weight.
2. 800 µL of ELISA dilution buffer is added to each tube and allowed to thaw at 4°C (*see* **Note 25**).
3. Each sample is then vortexed and centrifuged at 5000g for 15 min (*see* **Note 26**).
4. Samples are then diluted in suitable ELISA buffer solution and run (*see* **Note 27**).
5. Additional processing such as sterile filtering may be required for assays involving cell culture.

3.4.2. Whole Saliva

1. Saliva samples are thawed and diluted in appropriate buffer for immunoassays.
2. Additional processing such as sterile filtering may be required for assays involving cell culture.

3.4.3. Lung Lavage

1. The lung fluid collected (approx 1.8 cc in lung lavage solution) *(6)* should be spun at 1500g for 10 min at 4°C to remove any tissue and cellular debris.
2. The supernatant is collected and aliquoted.
3. The fluid sample should be stored at −70°C until assayed.
4. Additional processing such as sterile filtering may be required for assays involving cell culture.

3.4.4. Intestinal Lavage

1. The intestinal fluid collected (approx 1.8 cc in intestinal lavage solution) *(6)* should be spun at 1500g for 10 min at 4°C to remove any tissue and cellular debris.
2. The supernatant is collected and aliquoted.
3. The fluid sample should be stored at −70°C until assayed.
4. Additional processing such as sterile filtering may be required for assays involving cell culture.

3.4.5. Fecal Pellets

1. Add 1 mL PBS/1% sodium azide solution to 0.1 g of fecal pellets (*see* **Notes 28** and **29**).

2. Let sample stand at room temperature for about 10 min to allow pellets to be saturated with sodium azide solution.
3. Vortex vigorously for 10–15 min or until solution is homogenous (*see* **Note 30**).
4. Spin in microcentrifuge at 10,000g for 10–15 min.
5. Store supernatants at –70°C until ready to test by ELISA.
6. Additional processing such as sterile filtering may be required for assays involving cell culture.

4. Notes

1. For example sodium pentobarbital at 60 mg/kg can be administered intraperitoneally.
2. Care must be taken to allow blood flow into the syringe to proceed at a reasonable rate. An excessive amount of negative pressure in the syringe will cause either the heart cavity to collapse or the needle to suction the side of the heart wall. Both situations will result in little to no blood collection.
3. Maximum efficiency of blood collection is achieved when the puncture site is located in the ventricles.
4. If the animal is not to be sacrificed after the procedure, a gauze pad should be placed on the eye and firm pressure applied to stop the bleeding.
5. Mice can be bled on a regular schedule without sacrificing the animal using this method. Care must be taken not to take an excess of whole blood. If a large quantity is going to be taken (i.e., volume >0.2 mL), then the fluid must be replaced with subcutaneous injections of sterile saline.
6. If permitted by current animal handling guidelines, a heat lamp may be used or the tail may be immersed in warm water prior to tail bleeding to increase the flow rate of the collected whole blood.
7. Use of uniwicks for collection of vaginal secretions has been adapted from **ref. 6**.
8. Option of anesthetizing mice prior to procedure. Alternatively, mice may be anesthetized with a inhalant anesthetic (Halothane or Metaphane) prior to collection to facilitate a secure hold on the animal.
9. The uniwick can be manipulated once inside the vaginal vault by gently moving the wick around to ensure optimal contact with mucosal surfaces.
10. If a lesser amount of anesthetic is used, the mouse may not be completely immobilized. In this instance, the mouse should be restrained behind the ears with one hand while the other is manipulating the pipet into the mouth. If the mouse is not adequately anesthetized, the saliva secreted into the mouth may be ingested prior to collection or may be ingested from the collection vessel.
11. Pilocarpine will cause all of the mouse excretory systems to release; urination usually precedes salivation.
12. Volume range of saliva collected is 75–250 µL. Most success in resuscitating the animal is found when the volume collected is limited to approx 100 µL. With this technique, all mice should salivate.
13. This procedure must be done with extreme care if the mouse is not to be sacrificed. Saliva should be removed immediately from the mouth as salivation begins. The excess fluids secreted can easily go into the trachea and drown the mouse or

cause a respiratory infection. Such respiratory infections generally result in the death of a mouse 7–10 d postprocedure.

14. Greatest success has been found when pipet tip is placed directly on the front teeth of mouse, thus allowing sample to be withdrawn but eliminating the possibility of disrupting the mucosal lining of the mouth.

15. Robinul should be administered within 5 min of the injection of pilocarpine.

16. This procedure should be undertaken immediately after administration of robinul (approx 30 s).

17. The protocol for collection of lung and intestinal washes has been adapted from **refs.** *10* and *23*.

18. Care must be taken at this point to ensure that the needle edge is not being exposed and is safely placed in the sheath. The lungs can not be severed or loss and contamination of sample will occur.

19. Alternatively, the insertion could then be sealed by tying a string around the trachea, pressing the inside wall of the trachea against the exterior wall of the catheter. The knot should be made tight to prevent fluid from being introduced from the surrounding area and contaminating the sample.

20. The lungs can also be gently massaged and slight pressure applied to facilitate the delivery of the fluids into the syringe.

21. Since lung and intestinal lavage are only collected at the single time point at sacrifice, it is critical to also collect these lavage samples on control mice to serve as negative controls for immunoassays.

22. Alternatively, the intestine can be secured to the catheter by tying a thread around the intestine and catheter.

23. At times, the fluid must be coaxed through the intestine. This is accomplished by gently massaging the intestine with the thumb and forefinger at sites where the fluid is not flowing. The entire intestine should be monitored during this procedure to identify leaks and ruptures.

24. Collection of dry pellets from a cage containing five mice results in a pooled sample. Alternatively, since mice may excrete fecal pellets when first handled, individual fecal pellets can be obtained in this manner.

25. The ELISA buffer solution listed in **Subheading 2.2** has yielded data with signal:noise; alternate buffers can be used for this step. However, they should be optimized prior to use.

26. Uniwicks have been manufactured with material that adsorbs fluid rather than absorbing sample. This allows approx >90% of the collected sample to be retrieved from the wicks *(6)*. Soaking the wicks in buffer solution allows the samples to be eluted into the buffer solution. This procedure is enhanced by vortexing the samples to produce a homogenous solution of sample and buffer solution. Centrifugation is an additional sample retrieval enhancement step which forces the sample off the wick. Maximum sample retrieval is obtained when these soaking, vortexing, and centrifugation steps are used in combination.

27. Estimation of a starting dilution of sample must take into account the following factors:

a. The vaginal vault is instilled with a total of 50 µL.
b. The dilute collected sample is then diluted again when the fluid is retrieved from the wick via centrifugation.
c. The sample may be diluted a third time during whichever immunoassay is employed to measure total or specific antibody titers. For example, a typical collection results in a final accumulated volume of 65-85 µL, 50 µL of which is the PBS that was originally instilled. Therefore, 15–35 µL is the normal range of vaginal secretions collected.
28. A 0.01% Thimerasol solution may be alternatively used if sodium azide solution disrupts assay which may potentially occur when using HRP-conjugated antibodies in enzyme immunoassays.
29. The protocol for processing of fecal pellets has been adapted from **ref. *16***.
30. This may require extra vortexing if the samples were not allowed to stand long enough in **step 2** of **Subheading 3.4.5.**

References

1. Mestecky, J. and Jackson, S. (1994) Reassessment of the impact of mucosal immunity in infection with the human immunodeficiency virus (HIV) and design of relevant vaccines. *J. Clin. Immunol.* **14,** 259–272.
2. Miller, C. J., McGhee, J. R., and Gardner, M. B. (1993) Mucosal immunity, HIV transmission, and AIDS. *Lab. Invest.* **68,** 129–145.
3. Piot, P., Plummer, F. A., Mhalu, F. S., Lamboray, J. L., Chin, J., and Mann, J. M. (1988) AIDS: an international perspective. *Science* **239,** 573–579.
4. Padian, N. S., Shiboski, S. C., and Jewell, N. P. (1991) Female-to-male transmission of human immunodeficiency virus. *JAMA* **266,** 1664–1667.
5. Forrest, B.D. (1991) Women, HIV, and mucosal immunity. *Lancet* **337,** 835,836.
6. Haneberg, B., Kendall, D., Amerongen, H. M., Apter, F. M., Kraehenbuhl, J. P., and Neutra, M. R. (1994) Induction of specific immunoglobulin A in the small intestine, colon-rectum, and vagina measured by a new method for collection of secretions from local mucosal surfaces. *Infect. Immunol.* **62,** 15–23.
7. Muster, T., Ferko, B., Klima, A., Purtscher, M., Trkola, A., Schulz, P., et al. (1995) Mucosal model of immunization against human immunodeficiency virus type 1 with a chimeric influenza virus. *J. Virol.* **69,** 6678–6686.
8. O'Hagan, D. T., Rafferty, D., McKeating, J. A., and Illum, L. (1992) Vaginal immunization of rats with a synthetic peptide from human immunodeficiency virus envelope glycoprotein. *J. Gen. Virol.* **73,** 2141–2145.
9. O'Hagan, D. T., McGee, J. P., Holmgren, J., Mowat, A. M., Donachie, A. M., Mills, et al. (1993) Biodegradable microparticles for oral immunization. *Vaccine* **11,** 149–154.
10. Orr, N., Robin, G., Cohen, D., Arnon, R., and Lowell, G. H. (1993) Immunogenicity and efficacy of oral or intranasal Shigella flexneri 2a and Shigella sonnei proteosome-lipopolysaccharide vaccines in animal models. *Infect. Immunol.* **61,** 2390–2395.
11. Staats, H. F., Nichols, W. G., and Palker, T. J. (1996) Mucosal immunity to HIV-1: systemic and vaginal antibody responses after intranasal immunization with the HIV-1 C4/V3 peptide T1SP10 MN(A). *J. Immunol.* **157,** 464–472.

12. Abraham, E. and Shah, S. (1992) Intranasal immunization with liposomes containing IL-2 enhances bacterial polysaccharide antigen-specific pulmonary secretory antibody response. *J. Immunol.* **149,** 3719–3726.
13. Vajdy, M. and Lycke, N. Y. (1992) Cholera toxin adjuvant promotes long-term immunological memory in the gut mucosa to unrelated immunogens after oral immunization. *Immunology* **75,** 488–492.
14. Langermann, S., Palaszynski, S., Sadziene, A., Stover, C. K., and Koenig, S. (1994) Systemic and mucosal immunity induced by BCG vector expressing outer-surface protein A of Borrelia burgdorferi. *Nature* **372,** 552–555.
15. Vadolas, J., Davies, J. K., Wright, P. J., and Strugnell, R. A. (1995) Intranasal immunization with liposomes induces strong mucosal immune responses in mice. *Eur. J. Immunol.* **25,** 969–975.
16. VanCott, J. L., Staats, H. F., Pascual, D. W., Roberts, M., Chatfield, S. N., Yamamoto, M., et al. (1996) Regulation of mucosal and systemic antibody responses by T helper cell subsets, macrophages, and derived cytokines following oral immunization with live recombinant Salmonella. *J. Immunol.* **156,** 1504–1514.
17. Bukawa, H., Sekigawa, K., Hamajima, K., Fukushima, J., Yamada, Y., Kiyono, H., et al. (1995) Neutralization of HIV-1 by secretory IgA induced by oral immunization with a new macromolecular multicomponent peptide vaccine candidate. *Nat. Med.* **1,** 681–685.
18. Lowell, G. H., Kaminski, R. W., VanCott, T. C., Slike, B., Kersey, K., Zawoznik, et al. (1997) Nasal immunization with HIV gp160 plus proteosomes, emulsomes and/or cholera toxin B subunit to induce serum, intestinal, lung and vaginal antibodies. *J. Infect. Dis.* **175,** 292–301.
19. Lehner, T., Bergmeier, L. A., Panagiotidi, C., Tao, L., Brookes, R., Klavinskis, et al. (1992) Induction of mucosal and systemic immunity to a recombinant simian immunodeficiency viral protein. *Science* **258,** 1365–1369.
20. Lehner, T., Bergmeier, L.A., Tao, L., Panagiotidi, C., Klavinskis, L.S., Hussain, L., et al. (1994) Targeted lymph node immunization with simian immunodeficiency virus p27 antigen to elicit genital, rectal, and urinary immune responses in nonhuman primates. *J. Immunol.* **153,** 1858–1868.
21. Marx, P. A., Compans, R. W., Gettie, A., Staas, J. K., Gilley, R. M., Mulligan, M. J., et al. (1993) Protection against vaginal SIV transmission with microencapsulated vaccine. *Science* **260,** 1323–1327.
22. Lubeck, M. D., Natuk, R. J., Chengalvala, M., Chanda, P. K., Murthy, K. K., Murthy, S., et al. (1994) Immunogenicity of recombinant adenovirus-human immunodeficiency virus vaccines in chimpanzees following intranasal administration. *AIDS Res. Hum. Retrovir.* **10,** 1443–1449.
23. Orr, N., Arnon, R., Rubin, G., Cohen, D., Bercovier, H., and Lowell, G. H. (1994) Enhancement of anti-Shigella lipopolysaccharide (LPS) response by addition of the cholera toxin B subunit to oral and intranasal proteosome-Shigella flexneri 2a LPS vaccines. *Infect. Immunol.* **62,** 5198–5200.
24. VanCott, T. C., Kaminski, R. W., Mascola, J. R. Kalyanaraman, V., Wassef, N., Alving, C, et al. (1998) HIV-1 neutralizing antibodies in the genital and respiratory tracts of mice intranasally immunized with oligomeric gp160. *J. Immunol.* **160,** 2000–2012.

IV

CELLULAR IMMUNOLOGY

37

Lymphocyte Proliferation Assay

Karl V. Sitz and Deborah L. Birx

1. Introduction

The lymphocyte proliferation assay is used as an in vitro surrogate, similar to the in vivo delayed-type hypersensitivity assay, to assess the overall quality and character of the cellular arm of the immune response. The lymphocyte proliferation assay is used to assess congenital immune deficiencies, transient immune compromised states, and more recently, the progressive immune deficiency of HIV infection (*see* **Note 1**) *(1–19)*.

This assay is used to assess the ability of peripheral blood mononuclear cells (PBMCs) (**Note 2**) to proliferate in response to various nonspecific (mitogen) and specific (recall antigen) stimuli. These stimuli trigger a complicated series of events that ultimately leads to cell division. Although cell division may be determined by simple microscopic enumeration of cells before and after stimulation, this technique is both labor intensive and error prone. Therefore, the incorporation of [^{3}H]-labeled thymidine into newly synthesized DNA has become a standard surrogate measurement of proliferation (*see* **Note 3**). A flow chart (**Fig. 1**) depicts the steps involved in this assay.

This assay may be slightly modified for the following studies: T-lymphocyte epitope mapping, assessment of cytokine production, evaluation of growth enhancing and inhibiting factors, evaluation of crossreactivity between different protein sequences, assessment for prior exposure to infectious agents, study of the requirements for signal transduction, and evaluation of factors related to apoptosis.

From: *Methods in Molecular Medicine, Vol. 17: HIV Protocols*
Edited by: N. L. Michael and J. H. Kim © Humana Press Inc., Totowa, NJ

Proliferation Assay Flow Diagram

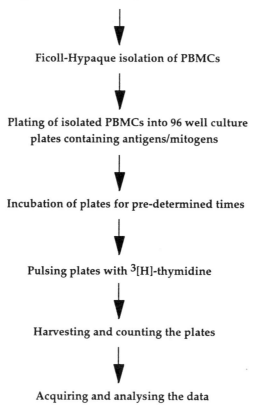

Venipuncture to obtain heparinized whole blood

Ficoll-Hypaque isolation of PBMCs

Plating of isolated PBMCs into 96 well culture
plates containing antigens/mitogens

Incubation of plates for pre-determined times

Pulsing plates with ^{3}[H]-thymidine

Harvesting and counting the plates

Acquiring and analysing the data

Fig. 1. Proliferation assay flow diagram.

2. Materials (*see* Note 4)

2.1. Ficoll-Hypaque Isolation of PBMC

1. Heparinized whole blood or blood collected in acid citrate dextrose (ACD) tubes (**Subheading 3.1.** and *see* **Note 5**).
2. Phosphate-buffered saline. PBS may be conveniently obtained commercially in sterile bottles. If desired, it may be made using the following recipe and sterile filtered:
   a. 1.15 g anhydrous Na_2HPO_4.
   b. 0.23 g anhydrous Na_2HPO_4.
   c. 9.00 g NaCl.
   d. Distilled H_2O to 950 mL; adjust pH to between 7.2 and 7.4 with either 1 M HCl or 1 M NaOH; add distilled H_2O to 1000 mL.
   e. Filter sterilize by passage through a 0.45 μM filter unit.

3. Ficoll-Hypaque solution (1.077 g/liter; commercially available).
4. Complete medium (*see* **Note 6**):
   a. RPMI 1640 medium.
   b. 2 m*M* L-glutamine.
   c. 100 U/mL penicillin.
   d. 100 mg/mL streptomycin.
   e. 50 m*M* 2-mercaptoethanol.
   f. 5% heat-inactivated (56°C for 30 min) normal human AB serum.
5. 50 mL conical centrifuge tubes.
6. Low-speed centrifuge.
7. Trypan Blue, 0.4%.
8. Hemocytometer.

2.2. Culture Procedure

1. PBMC suspension (*see* **Note 7**).
2. Complete medium.
3. Selected mitogens and/or antigens (**Figs. 2** and **3** and **Note 8**).
4. 96-well U-bottom tissue culture plates (**Note 9**).
5. Incubator with temperature, CO_2 and humidity controls.

2.3. Pulse and Harvesting Procedure

1. ^{3}H-labeled methyl thymidine, 50–75 mCi/mL.
2. Semi-automated multiwell harvester with recommended filter paper.
3. Scintillation fluid.
4. Liquid scintillation counter.

2.4 Data Analysis

1. Computer with spreadsheet or database software.

3. Methods (*see* Note 4)

3.1. Ficoll–Hypaque Isolation of PBMC

1. Using standard venipuncture techniques, withdraw 10–15 mL of whole blood into a heparinized syringe, green top (sodium heparin) tube (**Notes 2** and **5**), or ACD tube. To heparinize a syringe, draw 0.25 mL of sodium heparin (1000 U/mL) into the syringe, coating the inner surface prior to venipuncture.
2. Invert the tubes or syringe several times after drawing to mix the heparin throughout the blood sample. It is critical to prevent clotting, since clotting activates the cellular components and also depletes lymphocytes.
3. Pipet 10–15 mL of heparinized whole blood into a 50-mL tube.
4. Add an equal volume of PBS and gently mix.
5. Underlay with Ficoll–Hypaque; slowly and carefully pipet 10 mL of Ficoll–Hypaque into the very bottom of the 50-mL conical tube containing the blood/PBS mixture, taking care to maintain a perfect interface between the blood/PBS mixture and the Ficoll (*see* **Note 10**).

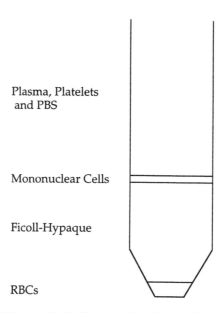

Fig. 2. Ficoll-Hypaque density gradient.

6. Balance the tube(s) in enclosed centrifuge containers, place in the centrifuge, and spin at 900g (2000 rpm for Beckman GH-3.7 rotors) for 20–30 min at 22°C. Make certain that the centrifuge brake is "OFF," otherwise the interface will be disrupted.
7. A representation of how the specimen will appear post-centrifugation is given in **Fig. 2**.
8. Using a 10-mL pipet, carefully aspirate the clear, yellow, plasma/PBS component to a level just above the mononuclear cell interface. Care should be taken to remove as much of the plasma/PBS, with contaminating platelets, as possible while not losing mononuclear cells. The diluted plasma may be saved for future antibody studies if desired.
9. Using a 5-mL pipet, aspirate the cloudy mononuclear cell interface being careful not to aspirate up much of the Ficoll layer. Transfer these cells into a new 50-mL conical tube and add approx 40 mL of PBS (*see* **Note 11**).
10. Balance the tubes in the centrifuge containers; place in the centrifuge; and centrifuge at 400g (1300 rpm for Beckman GH-3.7 rotors) for 10 min at 22°C.
11. Discard the supernatant, either by pipet or single-motion pouring, taking care to not disturb the mononuclear cell pellet.
12. Resuspend the pellet by gentle vortexing.
13. Add 10 mL of PBS to the 50-mL tube and re-mix.
14. Take a 20-µL aliquot of cells and mix with 20 µL of trypan blue. Count the number of viable and dead cells using a hemocytometer.
15. Add approx 40 mL of PBS and repeat **steps 10–12**. These washing steps are used to remove residual Ficoll, platelets, and other serum components.
16. Add an appropriate volume of complete medium to achieve a final concentration of 1×10^6 PBMCs/mL.

	1	2,3,4	5,6,7	8,9,10	11	12
A	PBS Only	PBS Only	PBS Only	PBS Only	PBS Only	PBS Only
B	PBS Only	100,000 PBMC PHA-L 5 ug/ml Sample #1	100,000 PBMC PWM 2.5 ug/ml Sample #1	100,000 PBMC ConA 20 ug/ml Sample #1	100,000 PBMC Medium Only Sample #1	PBS Only
C	PBS Only	100,000 PBMC PHA-L 2.5 ug/ml Sample #1	100,000 PBMC PWM 1.25 ug/ml Sample #1	100,000 PBMC ConA 10 ug/ml Sample #1	100,000 PBMC Medium Only Sample #1	PBS Only
D	PBS Only	100,000 PBMC PHA-L 1.25 ug/ml Sample #1	100,000 PBMC PWM 0.625 ug/ml Sample #1	100,000 PBMC ConA 5 ug/ml Sample #1	100,000 PBMC Medium Only Sample #1	PBS Only
E	PBS Only	100,000 PBMC Medium Only Sample #1				PBS Only
F	PBS Only					PBS Only
G	PBS Only					PBS Only
H	PBS Only	PBS Only	PBS Only	PBS Only	PBS Only	PBS Only

Fig. 3. Mitogen plate.

17. Gently mix the PBMC/complete medium and place the tube in the 37°C, 5% CO_2, 95% humid incubator with the cap loosened until ready to plate.

3.2. Culture Procedure

1. Dilute the chosen mitogens and antigens to 2× the final desired concentration using complete medium. The range of final desired concentrations should always

	1	2,3,4	5,6,7	8,9,10	11	12
A	PBS Only	PBS Only	PBS Only	PBS Only	PBS Only	PBS Only
B	PBS Only	100,000 PBMC HIV-1 gp160 5 ug/ml Sample #1	100,000 PBMC HIV-1 p24 5 ug/ml Sample #1	100,000 PBMC HIV-1 nef 10 ug/ml Sample #1	100,000 PBMC Medium Only Sample #1	PBS Only
C	PBS Only	100,000 PBMC HIV-1 gp160 2.5 ug/ml Sample #1	100,000 PBMC HIV-1 p24 2.5 ug/ml Sample #1	100,000 PBMC HIV-1 nef 5 ug/ml Sample #1	100,000 PBMC Medium Only Sample #1	PBS Only
D	PBS Only	100,000 PBMC HIV-1 gp160 1.25 ug/ml Sample #1	100,000 PBMC HIV-1 p24 1.25 ug/ml Sample #1	100,000 PBMC HIV-1 nef 2.5 ug/ml Sample #1	100,000 PBMC Medium Only Sample #1	PBS Only
E	PBS Only	100,000 PBMC Medium Only Sample #1	100,000 PBMC Tetanus toxoid 6.25 LF/ml Sample #1	100,000 PBMC Candida albicans 1:100 Sample #1		PBS Only
F	PBS Only					PBS Only
G	PBS Only					PBS Only
H	PBS Only	PBS Only	PBS Only	PBS Only	PBS Only	PBS Only

Fig. 4. Antigen plate.

be experimentally determined by titration of actual reagents with control PBMC samples.

2. A sample 96-well U-bottom plate diagram is shown in **Figs. 3** and **4**.
3. Add 0.1 mL of the appropriate antigens and mitogens by Eppendorf repeater pipet to each well following a specific protocol, similar to the examples above.
4. Remove the PBMC from the incubator. Gently mix the tube to thoroughly resuspend the PBMC, then add 0.1 mL (100,000) of cells by repeater pipet to each designated well of the 96-well plates.

5. Remaining cells may be cryopreserved for future study.
6. Place the plates into a 37°C, 5% CO_2, 95% humid incubator for the predetermined incubation periods. This is often 2–3 d for the mitogen plate and 6–7 d for the antigen plate (*see* **Note 12**).

3.3. Pulse and Harvesting Procedure

1. At the end of the incubation period, and at a standard time prior to harvesting the plate (6–18 h), add 1.0–1.5 mCi (20 mL of 50–75 mCi/mL in complete medium) of [³H]-labeled methyl thymidine to each well of the assay (*see* **Note 13**).
2. Place the plates back into the incubator for the remaining 6–18 h.
3. At the end of the [³H]-thymidine pulse, harvest the plates onto filter paper using a semi-automated multiwell harvester. Follow the directions specified by the manufacturer (*see* **Note 14**).
4. The filter paper containing bound DNA may be dried using either ethanol or by moderate microwave heating.
5. Once the filter paper is dry, transfer the filter paper into a scintillation container appropriate to the automated scintillation counter that is being used. Add scintillation fluid to the scintillation container(s) as specified by the counter system.
6. Count the samples in the scintillation counter according to the program's specification with a desired variability of <2%.

3.4. Data Analysis (see Note 15)

1. If possible, import the raw data into a spreadsheet or database to allow for more automated analysis.
2. Determine the mean and standard deviation of the wells representing background proliferation (wells containing only cells and complete medium).
3. Determine the mean and standard deviation of all series of replicate experimental stimulations.
4. Data are routinely presented in the following ways:
   a. Simple enumeration of both baseline and experimental counts per minute (cpm) with associated standard deviation or standard error of the mean.
   b. Net stimulation: subtraction of the background mean from the experimental mean.
   c. Stimulation index: division of the experimental mean by the background mean.

4. Notes

1. A complete discussion of the diseases associated with defects in lymphocyte proliferation is beyond the scope of this text. These are more fully discussed in **ref. *20***.
2. Although PBMCs are described in these methods, other sources of lymphocytes, such a lymph node homogenates and bone marrow aspirates, may also be used when available.
3. This methodology deals exclusively with [³H]-thymidine incorporation. Other, nonradioactive, techniques involving fluorescence labeling and flow cytometric enumeration of cells may also be used but are beyond the scope of this text.

4. The lymphocyte proliferation assay is dependent on culture sterility. Contaminating bacteria or fungi will adversely affect the interpretation of the results. It is therefore imperative that sterile materials and sterile technique be used up to the harvesting step. Although antibiotics are often added to culture medium, contamination by mycoplasma and fungi will not be avoided unless scrupulous aseptic technique is used. If contamination problems occur, it is wise to check the incubators, water baths, hoods, and other equipment for potential colonization.

5. When working with infectious material appropriate measures must be undertaken to minimize the risk of infection of laboratory workers. Details of these measures may be obtained from CDC and OSHA recommendations and are beyond the scope of this text.

6. Complete medium should be freshly made in quantities that will be used in < 1 mo; otherwise, pH changes and potential degradation of serum components and antibiotics may ensue. Antibiotics may be omitted if the mononuclear cell source is sterile and scrupulous sterile technique is observed. 10% normal human AB serum or 10–20% fetal calf serum (FCS) may be required for more fastidious long term cultures. Since serum components may contain factors that cause stimulation or inhibition of culture growth, it is imperative to screen several lots of various sera at different concentrations in order to determine the lot/concentration that provides maximal growth with minimal background stimulation. Once a desirable lot is identified it should be purchased in a quantity sufficient to be used throughout the experimental period; once the serum is heat-inactivated, aliquots should be stored at –20°C or lower temperature until ready to be used.

7. It is critical to use PBMC of high viability. PBMC that have been freshly isolated from blood samples that are less than 24 h old are usually highly viable (>95%). Cryopreserved PBMC may contain slightly fewer viable cells but if the cryopreservation and thawing techniques are performed correctly; cryopreservation should not adversely affect proliferative capacity. However, care must be taken in interpretation of experiments in which PBMC of low viability are used since damaged cells and cellular debris may inhibit proliferative responses.

8. Depending on the goal of the experiment a variety of mitogens and/or antigens may be tested in the proliferation assay. **Figs. 3** and **4** simply depict panels that have been recently utilized in our laboratory. Once the mitogens/antigens are selected it is imperative that preliminary titration experiments be performed to determine the antigen concentration that causes peak specific proliferation in an aliquot of control cells (if known and if available) under the identical experimental conditions (i.e., fresh or cryopreserved cells). Because individual variation may occur, it is often wise to bracket the wells containing the optimal concentration with wells that contain 2× and 1/2× the optimal concentration.

9. U-bottom (round bottom) wells allow cells to better physically associate with other cells in the culture. This is usually an advantage when dealing with moderate numbers of cells (1×10^5) with a relatively low precursor frequency for the stimulus, as occurs in most PBMC assays. Assays that use rapidly dividing cell lines often prefer flat-bottom wells that allow expansion without crowding.

10. As an alternate technique, the blood/PBS mixture may be overlaid into a 50-mL conical tube containing 10 mL of Ficoll-Hypaque. Slowly and carefully, pipet the blood/PBS mixture onto the top of the Ficoll, letting the liquid run down the side of the tube at a 45° angle, again maintaining a perfect interface between the two. Experience with this technique is critical to maintaining an interface; novices often find the underlaying technique (**Subheading 3.5.**) easier to perform.

11. PBS should be in at least 3× excess during the initial wash, otherwise the cells may not be pelleted due to contaminating Ficoll.

12. The optimal period of incubation depends on a combination of the strength of the stimulus, the precursor frequency of the responding cells, and potential toxicity associated with the stimulus. Each stimulus may have different optimal incubation times for maximal proliferation, which must be determined experimentally for novel stimuli. In general, as a compromise, all mitogens may be placed on the same plate with a 2–3-d incubation period and all antigens may be placed on another plate with a 6–7-d incubation period. Because of potential problems with evaporation from the outside wells of the plate, particularly those incubated for greater than five days, it may be preferable to fill the outside wells with PBS and use only the interior wells for culture of cells (as demonstrated in **Figs. 3** and **4**).

13. The optimal length of pulsing with [³H]-thymidine is usually between 6–18 h. Although 6 h may give excellent results for a large subpopulation of proliferating cells, 18 h of pulsing may give more consistent incorporation for more weakly proliferating cells. Although the length of pulsing is often determined by convenience of laboratory schedule, it must be consistent over the course of an experimental protocol.

14. In general, the harvester aspirates each individual well of the plate onto a specified region of filter paper and lyses the cells using distilled water. Once the cells lyse, the DNA, with incorporated [³H]-thymidine, is bound to the filter paper while unincorporated [³H]-thymidine is washed away.

15. A detailed discussion of the statistical considerations and quality control issues involved in the lymphoproliferative assay is beyond the scope of this text. An excellent review of these topics is found in **refs. 20** and **21**.

5. References

1. Ballet, J. J., Couderc, L. J., Rabian, H. C., Duval, R. C., Janier, M., Danon, F., Clauvel, J. P., and Seligmann, M. (1988) Impaired T-lymphocyte-dependent immune responses to microbial antigens in patients with HIV-1-associated persistent generalized lymphadenopathy. *AIDS* **2**, 291–297.
2. Cooper, D. A., Tindall, B., Wilson., E. J., Imrie, A. A., and Penny, R. (1988) Characterization of T lymphocyte responses during primary infection with human immunodeficiency virus. *J. Infect. Dis.* **157**, 889–896.
3. Hoy, J. F., Lewis, D. E., and Miller, G. G. (1988) Functional versus phenotypic analysis of T cells in subjects seropositive for the human immunodeficiency virus: a prospective study of in vitro responses to Cryptococcus neoformans. *J. Infect. Dis.* **158**, 1071–1078.

4. Hofmann, B., Jakobsen, K. D., Odum, N., Dickmeiss, E., Platz, P., Ryder, L. P., Pedersen, C., Mathiesen, L., Bygbjerg, I. B., Faber, V., et, al. (1989) HIV-induced immunodeficiency. Relatively preserved phytohemagglutinin as opposed to decreased pokeweed mitogen responses may be due to possibly preserved responses via CD2/phytohemagglutinin pathway. *J. Immunol.* **142,** 1874–1880.

5. Krowka, J. F., Stites, D. P., Jain, S., Steimer, K. S., George, N. C., Gyenes, A., Barr, P. J., Hollander, H., Moss, A. R., Homsy, J. M., et, al. (1989) Lymphocyte proliferative responses to human immunodeficiency virus antigens in vitro. *J. Clin. Invest.* **83,** 1198–1203.

6. Reddy, M. M. and Grieco, M. H. (1989) Cell-mediated immunity to recombinant human immunodeficiency virus (HIV) antigens in HIV-infected populations. *J. Infect. Dis.* **159,** 120–122.

7. Ridley, D. J., Houk, R. W., Reid, M. J., and Boswell, R. N. (1989) Early lymphocyte transformation abnormalities in human immunodeficiency virus infection. *J. Clin. Immunol.* **9,** 119–124.

8. Wahren, B., Rosen, J., Sandstrom, E., Mathiesen, T., Modrow, S., and Wigzell, H. (1989) HIV-1 peptides induce a proliferative response in lymphocytes from infected persons. *J. Acquir. Immune Defic. Syndr.* **2,** 448–456.

9. Borkowsky, W., Krasinski, K., Moore, T., and Papaevangelou, V. (1990) Lymphocyte proliferative responses to HIV-1 envelope and core antigens by infected and uninfected adults and children. *AIDS Res. Hum. Retroviruses* **6,** 673–678.

10. Pedersen, C., Dickmeiss, E., Gaub, J., Ryder, L. P., Platz, P., Lindhardt, B. O., and Lundgren, J. D. (1990) T-cell subset alterations and lymphocyte responsiveness to mitogens and antigen during severe primary infection with HIV: a case series of seven consecutive HIV seroconverters. *AIDS* **4,** 523–526.

11. Schellekens, P. T., Roos, M. T., De, W. F., Lange, J. M., and Miedema, F. (1990) Low T-cell responsiveness to activation via CD3/TCR is a prognostic marker for acquired immunodeficiency syndrome (AIDS) in human immunodeficiency virus-1 (HIV-1)-infected men. *J. Clin. Immunol.* **10,** 121–127.

12. Tacket, C. O., Baqar, S., Munoz, C., and Murphy, J. R. (1990) Lymphoproliferative responses to mitogens and HIV-1 envelope glycoprotein among volunteers vaccinated with recombinant gp160. *AIDS Res. Hum. Retroviruses* **6,** 535–542.

13. Teeuwsen, V. J., Siebelink, K. H., de, W. F., Goudsmit, J., Uytde, H. F., and Osterhaus, A. D. (1990) Impairment of in vitro immune responses occurs within 3 months after HIV-1 seroconversion. *AIDS* **4,** 77–81.

14. Johnson, J. P., Hebel, R., and Shinaberry, R. (1991) Lymphoproliferative responses to mitogen and antigen in HIV-infected children. AIDS Res Hum Retroviruses **7,** 781–786.

15. Gorse, G. J., Belshe, R. B., Newman, F. K., and Frey, S. E. (1992) Lymphocyte proliferative responses following immunization with human immunodeficiency virus recombinant GP160. *The NIAID AIDS Vaccine Clinical Trials Network Vaccine* **10,** 383–388.

16. Kelker, H. C., Seidlin, M., Vogler, M., and Valentine, F. T. (1992) Lymphocytes from some long-term seronegative heterosexual partners of HIV-infected individuals proliferate in response to HIV antigens. *AIDS Res. Hum. Retroviruses* **8,** 1355–1359.

17. Bansal, A. S., Moran, A., Potter, M., Taylor, R., Haeney, M. R., and Mandal, B. K. (1993) Lymphocyte transformation responses to phytohaemagglutinin and pokeweed mitogen in patients at differing stages of HIV infection: are they worth measuring? *J. Clin. Pathol.* **46,** 846–848.

18. Daftarian, M. P., Diaz, M. F., Creery, W. D., Cameron, W., and Kumar, A. (1995) Dysregulated production of interleukin-10 (IL-10) and IL-12 by peripheral blood lymphocytes from human immunodeficiency virus-infected individuals is associated with altered proliferative responses to recall antigens. *Clin. Diagn. Lab. Immunol.* **2,** 712–718.

19. Pontesilli, O., Carlesimo, M., Varani, A. R., Ferrara, R., Guerra, E. C., Bernardi, M. L., Ricci, G., Mazzone, A. M., D'Offizi, G., and Aiuti, F. (1995) HIV-specific lymphoproliferative responses in asymptomatic HIV-infected individuals. *Clin. Exp. Immunol.* **100,** 419–424.

20. Fletcher, M. A., Klimas, N., Morgan, R., and Gjerset, G. (1992) in *Manual of Clinical Laboratory Immunology,* 4th ed. (Rose, N. R., et. al., eds.) American Society for Microbiology, Washington, D. C., pp. 213–219.

21. James, S. P. (1996) in *Current Protocols in Immunology* (Coligan, J. E. et. al., eds.) Wiley, New York, pp. 7. 10.

38

HIV-1-Specific Cytotoxic T-Cell Assays

Josephine H. Cox

1. Introduction

Cytotoxic T-cells (CTL) provide the basis of protective immunity in many viral infections by appearing early in the immune response and becoming involved with the elimination of virus by lysis of infected cells. A considerable amount of evidence suggests that CTL may be an especially important component of the host defense against HIV-1 *(1,2)* . Strong CTL activity is seen early during the course of infection *(3,4)*, in nonprogressor individuals, some of whom have been infected for a decade or more with HIV-1 *(5,6)* and also in some HIV-1 exposed sex workers *(7)* and babies *(8,9)* who remain HIV-1-negative.

Freshly isolated peripheral blood mononuclear cells (PBMC) from HIV-1-infected persons can mediate the lysis of target cells expressing a variety of HIV-1 proteins *(10,11)*. However, some sort of in vitro stimulation/expansion of CTL precursor cells is generally required. In such cases, CTL responses can be stimulated to most HIV-1 antigens—nef, gag, pol, vif, and env *(12–14)*. The rationale for in vitro stimulation (IVS) is to allow the specific stimulation of a small population of cytotoxic T precursor cells which may be circulating in blood at the time of draw, but are undetectable by the CTL assay. Incubation of cells in vitro allows for the amplification of this population to a level at which CTL activity, if present, is detectable. Depending on the method of in vitro stimulation, and the source of PBMC, both CD8+ and CD4+ CTL can be induced.

In HIV-1 infected persons, the majority of these CTL are major histocompatibility (MHC) class I-restricted, CD8+ cells that recognize antigen that has been processed by the endogenous route *(15)*. The in vitro stimulation and expansion of CD8+ HIV-1 specific CTL as well as target cell recognition by CD8+ CTL require that processed antigen in the form of 9–10 amino acid

From: *Methods in Molecular Medicine, Vol. 17: HIV Protocols*
Edited by: N. L. Michael and J. H. Kim © Humana Press Inc., Totowa, NJ

length peptides, bound to MHC class I molecules, are presented on the surface of antigen-presenting cells. In addition to MHC class I restricted CTL, it is possible to generate HIV-1 specific CD4+ CTL. These cells generally recognize antigen processed by the exogenous route. CD4+ HIV-1 envelope-specific CTL lines have been reported after in vitro stimulation of PBMC of HIV-1-seronegatives and HIV-1 seropositives immunized with HIV-1-envelope proteins *(16–18)*. The in vitro stimulation and expansion of CD4+ HIV-1 specific CTL as well as target cell recognition by CD4+ CTL requires that processed antigen in the form of 10–15 amino acid length peptides, bound to MHC class II molecules, are presented on the surface of antigen-presenting cells.

Recognition of the complex of antigen-specific peptide and MHC class I molecule by CD8+ CTL leads to a cascade of events culminating in the destruction (lysis) of the virally infected cell or tumor cell. In the CTL assay described below, CTL and sodium ^{51}chromate (^{51}Cr)-labeled target cells expressing the MHC class I molecules and peptides of interest are incubated together. Lysis of target cells by CTL is measured by the release of the ^{51}Cr into the supernatant. Likewise, ^{51}Cr-labeled target cells expressing MHC class II and antigen can be lysed by CD4+ CTL.

Transformed (immortalized) human B cell lines make ideal target cells for CTL assays, since they express abundant MHC class I and II molecules and can process antigen by both the exogenous and endogenous routes. In addition, transformed human B cells readily bind both MHC class I- and II-restricted peptides allowing for fine tuning of antigen specificity. Described below are methods for detection of CTL in fresh PBMC and from PBMC stimulated in vitro.

2. Materials
2.1. Effector and Target Cells

1. Effector cells are PBMC-isolated by standard Ficoll-Hypaque procedure (*see* Chapter 37, Subheading 3.1.). For testing CTL activity against a single antigen along with controls, 10–15 mL of whole blood are generally required or 15×10^6 isolated PBMC. For each additional antigen, approx 5 mL of blood are required or 5×10^6 isolated PBMC. Where possible, fresh PBMC should be used. However, if longitudinal studies are being performed, cryopreserved PBMC can be used in order to compare different study dates.
2. The most suitable target cells for use in CTL assays are autologous B lymphoblastoid cell lines (BLCL); the method for transforming B cells is described in **Subheading 3.1.** Once established, BLCL can be maintained in continuous culture for multiple passages. The critical requirements are that the BLCL should be in log phase and have a viability of 70–80% before use in the CTL assay.

2.2. Solutions and Reagents

1. Complete medium (CM): For culture of the BLCL target cells, preparation of the effector cells and all assay procedures, RPMI 1640 media supplemented with 2% L-glutamine, 1% penicillin/streptomycin, 10% heat-inactivated fetal calf serum (FCS), and 2.5% HEPES buffer are used. All reagents can be obtained from Gibco-BRL (Gaithersburg, MD). For in vitro stimulation, it is better to use RPMI 1640 media supplemented with 2% L-glutamine, 1% penicillin/streptomycin, 2.5% HEPES buffer, and 5–10% heat-inactivated pooled normal donor serum (CM-NHS). Medium should be warmed to 37°C before use in all procedures described below. All solutions should be sterile filtered before use and proper sterile technique should be used in setting up the assay.

2. Epstein Barr Virus (EBV) for transformation of B cells: Supernatant from B95-8 cells serves as a good source of EBV. The B95-8 cells can be obtained from the American Type Culture Collection (Rockville, MD) (ATCC # CRL-1612). Supernatants can be harvested from cells growing in log-phase and stored at –70°C (*see* **Note 1**).

3. Cyclosporin A (Sigma, St. Louis, MO): Cyclosporin A is first dissolved in 100% ethanol at 5 mg/mL and the stock is then diluted 1:10 in CM. The 0.5 mg/mL stock should then be sterile filtered and can be stored in aliquots at 4°C. Final concentration for use in B cell transformations is 2 µg/mL.

4. Leighton slant tubes (PGC Scientific, Gaithersburgh, MD): 10 mL capacity tubes for tissue culture have a large surface area for cell expansion and are better for examination of cells under the microscope.

5. Vaccinia recombinants: Vaccinia recombinants expressing a variety of HIV-1 antigens can be obtained from the AIDS Research and Reference Reagent Program Catalog (McKesson BioServices, Rockville, MD), now available on-line at http://www.niaid.nih.gov/reagent. Methods describing the construction, characterization and maintenance of vaccinia recombinants are contained in Current Protocols in Molecular Biology *(19)*. The titer of a vaccinia recombinant stock is given as a plaque forming units (PFU), the titers can range anywhere from 1×10^8/mL to 1×10^{11}/mL. Virus stocks are provided as cell-free or cell-associated virus. Vaccinia virus is a very hardy virus; stocks of the virus should be stored at –70°C. Freeze-thawing of the virus does not appear to be a problem, provided that the stocks are vortexed vigorously to break up clumps. Strict biosafety regulations for using vaccinia recombinants in the laboratory should be followed, including, in some cases, a requirement for personnel to be immunized.

6. Peptides: Peptides can be obtained from several commercial sources. For CTL recognition, it is best to have the C-terminal ends made with a free acid (OH). Lyophilized peptides should be made up in distilled water at a concentration of 1–5 mg/mL, aliquots can be stored at –20°C; some peptides loose activity after repeated freeze thaw cycles. The choice of peptide is entirely dependent on the HIV-1 antigen of interest and of the MHC of the patient (*see* **Note 2**).

7. Paraformaldehyde (PFA) (Sigma): A 1.5% (w/v) solution is made up by dissolving 1.5 g of PFA in 100 mL of PBS (Ca- and Mg-free PBS). Heat, but do not boil,

stirring until the PFA dissolves. The cooled solution should be sterile filtered and can be kept at 4°C.

8. Sodium chromate, $Na_2{}^{51}CrO_4$ (^{51}Cr), (NEN, Dupont, Boston, MA or Amersham Life Science, Arlington Heights, IL): The concentration should be adjusted to 1 mCi/mL in sterile phosphate-buffered saline (PBS). The half-life of ^{51}Cr is 27.7 d. Stocks can be used for up to 6 wk after their calibration date. Generally the isotope should be stored at 4°C. Proper training in safety and handling of radio chemicals is required.

9. 10% sodium dodecyl sulfate (SDS) (Gibco-BRL): SDS can be made in PBS and sterile filtered or can be purchased ready-made and sterile. Stock SDS has a long shelf life at room temperature.

10. Interleukin-7 (IL-7). Available from Genzyme (Boston, MA) or R & D Systems (Minneapolis, MN).

11. Interleukin-2 (IL-2) (Boehringer Mannheim, Indianapolis, IN).

2.3. Equipment

The release of ^{51}Cr from lysed target cells can be measured either by a gamma scintillation counter or a liquid scintillation counter.

3. Methods
3.1. Transformation of B Lymphocytes

1. Separate PBMC by standard Ficoll-Hypaque procedure (*see* Chapter 38, **Subheading 3.1.**). Five to ten milliliters of whole blood are required or $5–10 \times 10^6$ isolated PBMC (frozen PBMC can also be used). Prepare the PBMC at a concentration of between 5 and 10×10^6 cells/mL in CM. Place 1 mL of the cells in a 10-mL slant tube (*see* **Note 3**)

2. Add one vial of EBV containing supernatant (in 1 mL volume), 2 mL CM and 2 µg/mL Cyclosporin A (4 mL total). The culture is incubated for 7 d at 37°C in a humidified CO_2 incubator, after which 1 mL of medium is removed and a further 1 mL of EBV-containing supernatant along with fresh Cyclosporin A is added. The tube is incubated for an additional 7–14 d, after which the culture medium should become acidic and the cells should form macroscopic clumps. Clumps generally appear after 2–3 wk. Occasionally, the culture will appear static and will not start forming clumps until 6–8 wk after initiation of the culture.

3. The cells should be expanded at this stage by splitting 1:2 or 1:3 in CM and transferring the cells to larger volume flasks as necessary and then cryopreserving the cells. The cell line can be continuously maintained in 75 cm^2 flasks by splitting the cells 1:3 once or twice a week (*see* **Note 4**). Confirmation of the immortalization of the cells is best assessed by the continued growth of the cells in culture.

3.2. Target Preparation
3.2.1. Vaccinia-Infected BLCL

1. Centrifuge 30 mL of the patient's BLCL, resuspend the pellet in 5 mL of CM and count the number of viable cells. Viability of the EBV-transformed cells should be >70%.

2. Dispense $2–5 \times 10^6$ BLCL into 15-mL centrifuge tubes (one tube should be set up for each test antigen, e.g., vaccinia-gp160 envelope, control vaccinia and uninfected control target cell). Pellet the cells, discard the supernatant, and add vaccinia virus at a concentration of 5–10 PFU/cell, and adjust the volume to give a final concentration of 5×10^6 BLCL/mL. Therefore, for 5×10^6 cells, 5×10^7 virus is needed in a total volume of 1 mL. Incubate for 1 h at 37°C in a CO_2 incubator. The tubes should be shaken every 15 min to increase infectivity. Loosen caps slightly to allow for air exchange.

3. After 1 h, wash the cells with CM, and then resuspend the cells at a concentration of 2×10^6 cells/mL in CM. Make sure gas exchange can take place by loosening the caps of the tubes, and incubate for 5 h at 37°C in a CO_2 incubator. Alternatively, the cells can be infected overnight (i.e., 10–16 h). In this case, however, it is best to reduce the virus input to 5 PFU/cell for the first hour of infection. After removal of excess vaccinia virus by washing with CM, the cells can be placed in 10 mL of CM and incubated overnight in a 25 cm^2 flask. Stocks of vaccinia can vary somewhat, and it is best to check the titer of the recombinants and their specificity in-house to ensure optimum viability and infection of the target cells (*see* **Note 5**).

4. Postinfection, count the cells and dispense 1×10^6 viable cells into a labeled 15-mL tube and centrifuge. Decant supernatant, add 100 µCi ^{51}Cr/1×10^6 target cells, and 10% v/v of fetal bovine serum (FBS). Incubate at 37°C for 1 h. Wash three times with CM using approx 10 mL each wash and finally adjust the cell concentration to 5×10^4 cells/mL in CM. This is the dilution of BLCL used for plating.

3.2.2. Peptide-Pulsed BLCL

If only one or two peptides are being tested, 1×10^6 BLCL in 1 mL of CM are incubated with the required amount of peptide for 1 h (the concentration would have to be determined empirically, however, the ranges are generally between 0.1–100 µg/mL, with 1–10 µg/mL usually optimal). The BLCL are then labeled as described above and after washing, the cell concentration is adjusted to 5×10^4 cells/mL in CM and are ready for plating. If multiple peptides or several dilutions of a single peptide are being tested, it is best to first label the cells with ^{51}Cr, complete the washing procedure, and adjust the BLCL concentration to 1×10^5/mL. Fifty microlitres of the required peptide in CM is added to the plate at 4 times the required concentration; thus, for a final concentration of 1 µg/mL the peptide stock should be made up at 4 µg/mL. Add 50 µL of the labeled BLCL and incubate 1 h at 37°C. Effector CTL are added as described below (**Subheadings 3.3.** and **3.4.**).

3.3. Preparation of Effector PBMC: Fresh-Unstimulated PBMC

1. After Ficoll-separation, count cells and adjust the concentration of PBMC to 1×10^6 cells/mL. In order to partially purify the PBMC population, adherent macrophages can be removed by placing the PBMC suspension in a 75 cm^2 tissue culture

flask and incubating the cells at least 1 h at 37°C. The flask should be laid down flat in the incubator.

2. Postincubation, collect the PBMC and dispense into a 15-mL centrifuge tube. Gently rinse the flask with an additional 3 mL CM avoiding disturbing the adherent macrophages, and add to remaining cells. Pellet the cells, decant the supernatant, and resuspend the pellet in 500 μL of CM.

3. Count the PBMC and adjust the concentration to 5×10^6 cells/mL; this concentration is for the effector:target (E:T) ratio of 100:1, assuming that 5×10^3 target cells are used per well. If 15×10^6 PBMC were provided for the assay, there should be plenty of cells to perform all of the required dilutions to give E:T ratios of 100:1, 50:1, 25:1, and 5:1. Stepwise dilutions of the PBMC are performed in CM medium to generate aliquots of cells at 2.5, 1.25, and 0.25×10^6, respectively, for the required E:T ratios. The dilutions are usually performed in dilution tubes, using CM. Each E:T incubation is performed in triplicate. Therefore, a minimum of 300 μL of each concentration of PBMC is required for each target cell (*see* **Note 6**).

3.4. Preparation of Effector PBMC: In Vitro Stimulated PBMC

Several methods are available for antigen-specific stimulation of HIV-1-specific CTL. All of these methods have been published *(16,18,20–23)*. The methods are described below. The author has found them to be reproducible for expanding (CM-NHS) CTL, including quantitative measures of CTL precursors. For all in vitro stimulations, it is best to use CM with 5–10% pooled NHS. For expansion of CTL, a population of stimulator cells (HIV-1 antigen expressing cells) and responder cells (PBMC containing precursor CTL) is required. During the IVS, stimulator and responder cells are cocultured and the expanded CTL are harvested and assayed against appropriate target cells.

3.4.1. Expansion of HIV-1-Specific CTL Using Vaccinia Virus-Infected or Peptide-Pulsed BLCL

This protocol is based on the method originally described by Van Baalen et al *(20)*.

1. Centrifuge at least 5×10^6 (and up to 2×10^7) autologous BLCL from each culture, and infect with required vaccinia recombinant at 5–10 PFU/cell as described in **Subheading 3.2.** Combinations of 2–3 recombinants can be used. In this case, the PFU/cell of each recombinant generally should not exceed 5 PFU/cell.

2. After 1.5 h of infection, wash the cells once with sterile PBS. Pellet the cells, and fix with 1.5% w/v PFA in PBS at a concentration of 1×10^7 cells/mL for 15 min at room temperature (*see* **Note 7**). Wash cells once with PBS, and decant supernatant.

3. Incubate cells at 1×10^7 cells/mL in 0.2 *M* glycine in PBS (sterile-filtered) at room temperature for 15 min; wash once with PBS, and decant the supernatant.

4. Resuspend the fixed infected BLCL (stimulator cells) at a concentration of about 5×10^6/mL in sterile PBS. Stimulator cells can be prepared the day before the in vitro restimulation protocol and can be stored for up to 1 mo at 4°C.

5. Fresh or cryopreserved PBMC can be used for the responder population. Plate PBMC and stimulator cells at a ratio of 5:1 at a concentration of 2–4 × 10^6 cells/mL in CM-NHS in a 24-well plate, T25, or T75 flasks depending on the number of cells available. Interleukin-7 (IL-7) is added at 100–300 U/mL on d 0 and interleukin-2 (IL-2) is added at 10 U/mL on d 7.

6. There are drawbacks to using B cells as stimulator cells, most notably because of the high background CTL responses to vaccinia and EBV specific antigens (*see* **Note 8**). An alternative to using vaccinia-infected BLCL as the source of stimulator cells is to use BLCL pulsed with known MHC class I restricted HIV-1-peptides (peptides are added at 10–20 µg/mL) or BLCL transfected with HIV-1 antigens *(16)*. Peptide pulsed or transfected stimulator BLCL are fixed by gamma-irradiation (3000 rads), PFA or UV irradiation (*see* **Note 7**) and mixed at a 1:10 ratio with responder PBMC. IL-7 and IL-2 are added as in **Subheading 3.4.1., step 5**.

7. The cultures are incubated for 12–14 d before testing for CTL activity. Cultures should be checked for changes in acidity of the medium and for visible aggregates of cells, indicating cell proliferation and activation (*see* **Note 9**). On the day of the assay, the cells are harvested, washed, and resuspended in CM. Cells are counted and prepared as in **Subheading 3.3., step 3**.

3.4.2. Expansion of HIV-Specific CTL Using Vaccinia-Infected PBMC

As an alternative to using fixed vaccinia-infected BLCL as the source of antigen presenting cells for stimulation of HIV specific CTL, the patient's own PBMC can be used; these do not need to be fixed *(23,27)*.

1. One fifth of the available patient PBMC are infected with required vaccinia recombinant at 5–10 PFU/cell as described above (**Subheading 3.2.**). Combinations of 2–3 recombinants can be used; in this case the PFU/cell of each recombinant generally should not exceed 5 PFU/cell.

2. After 1.5 h infection, wash the cells once with 10 mL of CM and resuspend cells at a concentration of approx 2 × 10^6 PBMC/mL. These autologous stimulator cells are then mixed at a ratio of 1:5 with the responder PBMC as decribed in **Subheading 3.4., steps 5-7**.

3. As with the use of B cells as stimulator cells, this method can generate vaccinia-specific CTL as well as HIV-1-specific CTL (*see* **Note 8**).

3.4.3. Bulk Culture of HIV-1-Specific CTL

For bulk culture CTL recognizing whole virus, the method originally described by Gotch et al. *(21)* can be used.

1. Take 1/5th (20%) of the total number of PBMC and stimulate with 10 µg/mL PHA (or concentration just below the plateau of proliferation depending on the prep of PHA) in wells of a 24-well plate at 1–2 million cells/mL/well. Put the other 4/5th (80%) of the cells into a small flask at 1–2 million cells/mL in CM-NHS and leave in incubator overnight.

2. After 16–18 h, wash the PHA-blasted cells twice and then add to cells in flask and adjust the concentration to 1–2 million cells/mL. Incubate for six more days and assay for CTL on d 7. Alternatively, purified human IL-2 (10 U/mL) can be added on d 7 and assay for CTL on d 14.

3. If frozen cells are used for this assay, thaw the cells late afternoon, wash twice with CM-NHS, and then put in a small flask at 1 million/mL to recover overnight before stimulating with 10 μg/mL of PHA. Leave the PHA on 6–8 h, then wash and add to the unstimulated cells in the flask.

4. The cultures are incubated for 7–10 d before testing for CTL activity. On the day of the assay, the cells are harvested, washed, and resuspended in CM. Cells are counted and prepared as in **Subheading 3.3., step 3**.

3.4.4. Limiting Dilution Cultures of HIV-1 Specific CTL

Precursor frequencies of HIV-1 epitope specific CTL can be determined by performing limiting dilution analysis of (LDA) isolated PBMC. The IVS is performed in 96-well plates, with 24 replicates of responder PBMC plated at different dilutions and a fixed number of stimulator cells.

1. PBMC are resuspended at fourfold dilutions starting at 1.6×10^6 PBMC/mL and down to 2.5×10^3 PBMC/mL. One hundred microliters of each of these dilutions is added to 24 replicate wells of a 96-well microtiter plate. If more PBMC are available, a greater number of dilutions or more replicates can be set up.

2. BLCL stimulator cells, either peptide-pulsed or vaccinia-infected fixed BLCL (as described above) are resuspended at a concentration of 2.5×10^5/mL. One hundred microliters are added to each well containing PBMC. Autologous irradiated PBMC (3000 rad) are added at 1×10^4/mL to provide T-cell help and lymphokines. On day 3, IL-2 is added at 10 U/mL.

3. After 10–14 d (*see* **Note 9**), a multichannel pipet is used to resuspend the effector cells in each well and 50–100 μL of cells are removed and assayed for cytotoxicity against the targets of interest.

3.4.5. Expansion of HIV-1-Specific CD4+ CTL

The in vitro stimulation protocol for the generation of HIV-1-specific CD4+ CTL is described in Chapter 42. On the day of the assay the CD4+ cells are harvested, washed and resuspended in CM. Cells are counted and prepared as in **Subheading 3.3., step 3**.

3.5. Plating of Effectors and Targets

1. In a 96-well U-bottomed microtiter plate, dispense 100 μL of each effector cell concentration in triplicate. For example, place 100 μL of effectors for the 100:1 ratio for BLCL target #1 into wells C1–3, for the 50:1 ratio into wells D1–3, etc. For BLCL target #2, place 100 μL of effectors for the 100:1 ratio into wells C4–6, for the 50:1 ratio into D4–6, etc.

2. Dispense 100 μL of the appropriate BLCL target cells, adjusted to 5×10^4 cells/mL

to every well containing effector cells. Dispense 100 μL of BLCL target cells in wells A1–3 and H1–3 for target #1, A4–6 and H4–6 for target #2, etc. To row A, add 100 μL of sterile 10% SDS. Addition of 10% SDS lyses the target cells and releases all the ^{51}Cr from the target cells, the ^{51}Cr released from the SDS treated cells is used to calculate the maximum release (max). To row H add 100 μL of CM. The ^{51}Cr released from these wells is used to calculate the spontaneous release (spon). For LDA experiments, 24 replicate wells of each target and effector are set up along with spon and max wells; volumes should be adjusted to 200 μL/well by adding CM.

3. Incubate microtiter plate (with lid on) for 4–6 h at 37°C. Six hours is usually recommended for peptide-pulsed target cells, 4 h for vaccinia-infected target cells.

3.6. Harvesting the Assay Plate

1. Remove the plate from the incubator. Supernatant fluid is harvested using the Skatron Harvesting System (the manual supplied with the harvester gives very clear directions). The principal of this system is that supernatant from individual wells is absorbed onto a cartridge with a filter disk on the end closest to the cells; the latter prevents transfer of cells to the cartridge. The cartridge is then removed from the plate leaving the filter disk in the plate. The cartridge is placed in a macrowell tube and the tube is placed in the gamma counter for detection of ^{51}Cr (*see* **Notes 10** and **11**).

2. The level of CTL activity as denoted by the percent specific lysis (% lysis) of labeled BLCL targets is determined by the following formula:

$$\% \text{ lysis} = \frac{\text{mean test cpm} - \text{mean spon CPM}}{\text{mean max cpm} - \text{mean spon CPM}} \times 100$$

CPM = counts/minute (mean CPM is usually average of three replicates), test cpm = cpm released by the BLCL target cells in the presence of effector cells, spon = cpm released by the BLCL target cells in the absence of any effector cells (*see* **Note 12**), and max = cpm released by the target cells in the presence of SDS.

3.7. Data Analysis

The combined use of whole HIV-1 virus, recombinant vaccinia viruses containing HIV-1 genomic sequences, and peptides provides a comprehensive screen for detection of antigen-specific cytotoxic responses after immunization or infection.

1. Most gamma counters can be programed to calculate the percent specific lysis (percent of lysis). This value alone can suffice as a measure of CTL activity or nonparametric tests, such as Kruskall-Wallis or Wilcoxon tests, which can be used to determine significant statistical differences between slopes of response curves at different E:T ratios and different groups of patients and controls. The percent of lysis is plotted against the E:T ratio. **Figure 1** shows CTL activity against HIV-1 envelope protein of a patient followed over one year, PBMC were

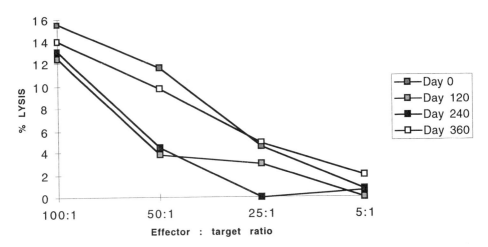

Fig. 1. HIV-1-envelope-specific CTL activity of an HIV-1 infected donor enrolled in a vaccine trial over the course of 1 yr. CTL activity against vaccinia-infected target cells has been subtracted.

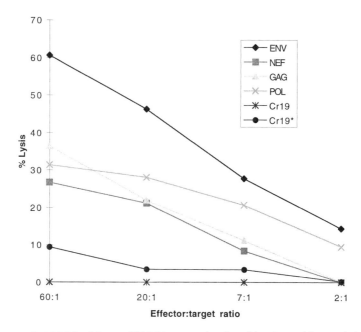

Fig. 2. Fresh PBMC of donor #50546 were stimulated in vitro with vaccinia recombinants expressing env and nef or gag/pol. Post in vitro stimulation, CTL recognition against autologous target cells expressing env, nef, gag, pol, or control vac (Cr19) all with cold targets or control vac alone (Cr19*) were examined at the efferctor:target ratios indicated. Cold target inhibitor cells were added in 40-fold excess.

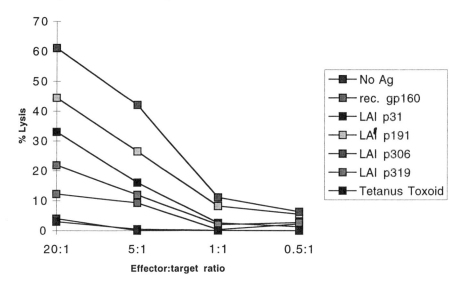

Fig. 3. CD4+ CTL activity against gp160 peptides. A CD4+ gp160-specific line was generated from PMBC of an HIV-1 infected donor by repeated rounds of stimulation with gp160 and IL-2 in vitro. CTL activity against the BLCL target cells pulsed with 5 μg/ML of antigen as indicated. Peptides are from HIV-1-LAI, the LAI numbering includes the signal sequence.

used fresh, i.e., no IVS. The vaccinia-specific lysis was subtracted from the envelope specific lysis. For comparison between different target cells or diferent persons' CTL activity, at least a 10% difference between the lysis of control and test target cells (vaccinia or peptide) over at least two different E:T ratios is generally considered significant. **Figure 2** shows CTL responses after IVS of fresh PBMC with either gp160-IIIB env and nef, or gag and rt-pol vaccinia recombinants. CTL activity was tested against autologous B cells infected with the indicated vaccinia recombinants and cold target inhibitor cells. CTL activity of the control vaccinia alone was <10% and was completely inhibited in the presence of cold targets. MHC-restricted CTL activity can be demonstrated using MHC mismatched target cells. Depletion of either CD4+ or CD8+ populations by magnetic bead separation should indicate class I or II restricted responses. **Figure 3** shows CD4+ CTL activity against HIV-1-gp160 peptide-pulsed target cells.

2. CTL activity can also be expressed as lytic units (LU). An LU is defined as the number of lymphocytes required to yield a particular percent of lysis (e.g. the LU20 is the number of lytic units at 20% lysis for a particular number of effector cells). Plot the percent of specific lysis vs the log of the effector cell number for each E:T ratio. For example, in the standard CTL setup described above, at the 100:1 ratio there are 5×10^5 cells/well, at 50:1 there are 2.5×10^5 effector cells/well, etc. Select a percent of lysis value that encompasses most of the patients' percent of lysis values (e.g., 20%). Determine the LU20 per million effector cells

LU20/10⁶ PBMC, by extrapolating along the axis. The patient values for LU may have to be presented as values greater than or less than the arbitrarily selected LU. The author can be contacted to obtain an easy to use LU program.

3. Precursor frequencies of HIV-1 epitope-specific CTL by limiting dilution analysis. For a semiquantitative assessment of CTL precursors, the number of positive wells are scored by selecting wells showing ⁵¹Cr release CPM of test BLCL (in the presence of effector CTL) greater than the mean ⁵¹Cr release CPM + 3SD of the 24 control target BLCL alone. Alternatively, the number of positive wells in the stimulated cultures is scored by selecting wells showing >10% difference in lysis compared with the mean percent of lysis of non-MHC matched or non-HIV-1 antigen-expressing target cells. A further discussion of quantitation of the HIV-1 specific Cytotoxic T cell response is included in **ref.** *24* and software package information is included in **refs.** *25–26*. To properly quantitate the data, a statistical software package should be used and data presented as CTL precursor frequencies/10⁶ PBMC.

4. Notes

1. To harvest EBV from B95-8 cultures, the culture supernatant is centrifuged at 400*g* for 15 min at 20°C to remove most cells, then filtered twice through a 0.45 m membrane filter to remove all viable cells. The EBV stock can be tested by examining its ability to transform normal human B cells. Filtered EBV stocks are stored in aliquots of 1.0 mL at −70°C, since viral infectivity declines if the preparations are kept above this temperature. Repeated freezing and thawing inactivates the virus.

2. A superb database that is frequently updated of all published MHC restricted CTL peptides is available from B. Korber at the Los Alamos National Laboratory, Los Alamos, NM. The HIV Molecular Immunology Database is also available online at http://hiv-web.lanl.gov/immuno/. If using peptides, it is necessary to MHC type the study subjects. This can be done using PBMC or BLCL by an MHC typing laboratory.

3. The slant tubes allow for close inspection of the cells in the early stages of the transformation process. If the number of cells is limited, this is the best vessel to use. The authors has used as few as 1×10^6 PBMC for transformation; however, it is best to start with at least 5×10^6 PBMC. Alternatively, PBMC can be resuspended at a concentration of 1×10^6/mL, and 5–10 mL of cells are placed in a 25 cm² flask.

4. BLCL show considerable variation in their growth characteristics, some grow very slowly and need to be split only once a week, whereas others grow rapidly and need splitting a couple of times a week. Healthy dividing cultures will turn the culture media yellow within 2–3 d, and large clumps of cells should form. When splitting the cells, these clumps should be disrupted by either vigorously shaking the flask or by resuspending the cells with a pipet. It is possible to maintain some cultures for several months without compromising their viability or ability to present antigen. However for the CTL assay, since good target viability

is critical, it is best to keep a close eye on the cells and thaw new BLCL if the viability is poor. BLCL should be thawed out at least two weeks prior to being used as targets in a CTL assay to allow a few cell divisions to occur. To conserve reagents, BLCL can be passaged in 25 cm^2 flasks in a volume of 10 mL. The week prior to use, the contents of the 25 cm^2 flask should be transferred to a 75 cm^2 flask in a volume of 30–40 mL, so there will be enough target cells for use in the CTL assay.

5. While an input range of 1–20 PFU of vaccinia is generally sufficient to get good expression of the required antigen in the BLCL, it is best to test this in-house. As well as confirming the titer of the virus by standard methods on adherent cells *(19)*, the author also infects BLCL for 6 or 16 h as described and examines their viability and antigen expression. Antigen expression can be examined by standard Western Blot (*see* Chapter 29) or by immunohistochemistry. Using immunohistochemistry, expression of the HIV-specific antigen in 70–100% of the vaccinia virus-infected BLCL is routinely seen. Viability after the 6 h infection period is around 70–90%, but sometimes after the 16 h infection period, the viability can drop as low as 50%. In these cases it is better to lower the input of virus, while still maintaining good antigen expression.

6. In the example of a standard CTL assay for fresh PBMC given above, recommended E:T ratios are 100:1, 50:1, 25:1, and 5:1. If the number of PBMC is limiting the E:T, ratios can be lowered (i.e., to 50:1, 25:1, 5:1, and 1:1) or the number of target cells can be lowered while keeping the same E:T ratio (i.e., 2.5×10^3 targets/well). If fewer than 2.5×10^3 target cells are used, problems are likely to be encountered with detection of low levels of radioactivity. For PBMC that have been restimulated in vitro, a lower E:T ratio can be used (i.e., starting at 50:1 or 25:1). If several assays are performed in one day all with similar E:T ratios, serial dilutions of the effector cells can more easily be performed in the 96-well plate.

7. The authors have also used psoralen (Calbiochem, made up at 1 mg/mL in DMSO) and UV irradiation to fix infected BLCL or other stimulator cells. For psoralin fixation, resuspend at 5×10^5 cells/mL in medium with 10% FCS. Add psoralen at 1 µg/mL to the cell suspension. Dispense 1 mL/well of the cell suspension into wells of a 6-well plate and UV irradiate for 5 min. Wash BLCL thoroughly to remove psoralin, since it is toxic to cells. Ultraviolet (UV) alone and γ irradiation (approx 3000 Rads) can also be used for fixing infected BLCL or other stimulator cells. All these methods seem to work equally well. Before using these fixation procedures, it is advisable to make sure that the BLCL is fixed (i.e., for the UV method, different sources of UV will have different strengths, so the UV exposure time and distance from the UV source may have to be tested). This can be verified quite simply by putting the fixed BLCL in culture and checking for cell growth. Inactivation of vaccinia although important is not as crucial as ablating B cell growth, since vaccinia does not readily infect PBMC at a low PFU input.

8. Since most humans, including HIV-1 infected humans have CTL precursors for EBV *(27)*, there is a strong possibility of obtaining EBV-specific CTL by using

this restimulation technique. Likewise for HIV-1-infected persons who have been immunized with smallpox, there remains the possibility of inducing vaccinia-specific CTL. Both of these drawbacks can be controlled by including either of the following in the CTL assay: BLCL infected with a control vaccinia, containing an irrelevant antigen or no antigen (any killing of this target might be a result of either vaccinia specific CTL- or EBV-specific CTL and can be subtracted from the antigen specific lysis, or cold target inhibition. Add a 20–30-fold excess of unlabeled control vaccinia infected BLCL (cold targets). Any vaccinia or EBV-specific CTL lyse the excess cold targets, and HIV-1-specific CTL can then be detected by lysis of the ^{51}Cr labeled HIV-1-antigen-expressing BLCL. For cold target inhibition, if the CTL assay is being setup with 5×10^3-labeled BLCL targets/well, an additional $1–1.5 \times 10^5$ of unlabeled BLCL would be added/well. Cold targets should also be added to the max and spon wells.

9. Post in vitro culture, there is initially a significant drop in the number of cells recovered. However the cell recovery increases as the CTL expand because of antigen-driven activation. Optimum CTL activity can vary between patients and depends on the in vitro stimulation method. In addition to IL-2 there are some reports showing that IL-7 can significantly enhance class I restricted CTL responses of HIV-1 -infected patients *(28,29)*. The IL-7 appears to increase CTL expansion. CTL cultures can be tested more than once for CTL activity, providing sufficient cells are recovered. It is worthwhile to harvest the culture supernatants, store them, and later test for the presence of lymphokines such as IFN and IL-4 or chemokines.

10. An alternative method of harvesting the supernatant is to carefully remove the plate from the incubator, taking care not to disturb the cell pellets. With a 12-well multichannel pipet, gently remove 50 or 100 μL of the supernatant, and place into small dilution tubes (these do not need to be sterile, but it is useful to have them in a 96-well type of format, so that supernatants can be directly transferred from the 96-well plate). If care is taken, the pellet should not be disturbed by removal of the supernatant. However, to avoid this problem, the plates can be centrifuged so then the pellet is less likely to be disturbed. To inactivate HIV-1 in the supernatant, add an equal volume of formalin or bleach to the tubes before counting. The tube is placed in the gamma counter for detection of ^{51}Cr.

11. Detection of ^{51}Cr in supernatants can also be measured using liquid scintillation counting. Recently, several companies have started marketing 96-well format scintillation counters for detection of gamma emitting isotopes such as ^{51}Cr and ^{125}I. If a standard beta counter is available, a 20 μL aliquot of the supernatant can be spotted onto filter mats laminated with plastic on one side (LKB, Gaithersburgh, MD, 1205-402). The filter mats are then dried by heating for 5 min in a microwave. Filter mats are then processed in the same way as the filter mats used in proliferation assays (*see* Chapter 38, Subheading 3.3.). Alternatively, 35 μL of supernatant can be transferred to special microplates containing a solid scintillator, e.g., LumaPlate (Packard, Meriden, CT). Virus is inactivated by addtion of 10 μL of bleach, the plates are dried and then counted on, e.g., TopCount (Packard).

Nonradioactive methods for detection of cytolytic assays are currently available. However, most of these assays suffer from poor reproducibility and sensitivity. The Europium release assay (LKB Wallac), however, appears to be a suitable alternative *(30,31)*, providing good reproducibility and sensitivity in the author's hands.

12. In cytotoxicity assays, attention should be paid to the spontaneous release of ^{51}Cr from the BLCL. The spontaneous release for vaccinia-infected BLCL should be <20%, ideally <10%. If higher values than 20% are obtained, it suggests that the BLCL are being infected with too many PFU/cell (*see* **Note 5**).

References

1. Rowland-Jones, S. and McMichael, A. (1993) Cytotoxic T lymphocytes in HIV infection. *Semin. Virol.* **4,** 83–94.
2. Lederman, M. M. (1996) Role of cytotoxic T lymphocytes in the control of HIV-1 infection and HIV-1 disease progression. *Cur. Opin. Infect. Dis.* **9,** 14–18.
3. Koup, R. A., Safrit, J. T., Cao, Y., Andrews, C. A., McLeod, G., Borkwosky, W., Farthing, C., and Ho, D. D. (1994) Temporal association of cellular immune responses with the initial viremia in primary human immunodeficiency virus type 1 syndrome. *J. Virol.* **68,** 4650–4655.
4. Borrow, P., Lewicki, H., Hahn, B. H., Shaw, G. M., and Oldstone, M. B. A. (1994) Virus-specific CD8+ cytotoxic T lymphocyte activity associated with control of viremia in primary human immunodeficiency virus type 1 infection. *J. Virol.* **68,** 6103–6110.
5. Harrer, T., Harrer, E., Kalams, S. A., Elbeik, T., Staprans, S. I., Feinberg, M. B., et al. (1996) Strong cytotoxic T cell and weak neutralizing antibody responses in a subset of persons with stable nonprogressing HIV Type 1 infection. *AIDS Res. Hum. Retrovir.* **12,** 585–592.
6. Klein, M. R., van Baalen, C. A., Holwerda, A. M., Kerkhof Garde, S. R., Bende, R. J., Keet, I. P., et al. (1995) Kinetics of Gag-specific cytotoxic T lymphocyte responses during the clinical course of HIV-1 infection: a longitudinal analysis of rapid progressors and long term asymptomatics. *J. Exp. Med.* **181,** 1365–1372.
7. Rowland-Jones, S., Sutton, J., Ariyoshi, K., Dong, T., Gotch, F., McAdam, S., et al. (1995) HIV-specific cytotoxic T-cells in HIV-exposed but uninfected Gambian women. *Nat. Med.* **1,** 59–64.
8. Cheynier, R., Langlade-Demoyen, P., Marescot, M. R., Blanche, S., Blondin, G., Wain-Hobson, S., et al. (1992) Cytotoxic T lymphocyte responses in the peripheral blood of children born to human immunodeficiency virus-1 infected mothers. *Eur. J. Immunol.* **2,** 2211–2217.
9. Rowland-Jones, S., Nixon, D. F., Aldhous, M. C., Gotch, F., Ariyoshi, K., Hallam, N., et al. (1993) HIV-specific cytotoxic T-cell activity in an HIV-exposed but uninfected infant. *Lancet* **341,** 860–861.
10. Walker, B. D., Chakrabarti, S., Moss, B., Paradis, T. J., Flynn, T., Durno, A. G., et al. (1987) HIV-specific cytotoxic T lymphocytes in seropositive individuals. *Nature* **328,** 345–348.
11. Hoffenbach, A., Langlade-Demoyen, P., Dadaglio, G., Vilmer, E., Michel, F., Mayaud, C., et al. (1989) Unusually high frequencies of HIV-specific cytotoxic T lymphocytes in humans. *J. Immunol.* **142,** 452–462.

12. Koenig, S., Earl, P., Powell, B., Pantaleo, G., Merli, S., Moss, B., et al. (1988) Group-specific, major histocompatibility complex class I-restricted cytotoxic responses to human immunodeficiency virus I (HIV-1) envelope proteins by cloned peripheral blood T cells from an HIV-1-infected individual. *Proc. Natl. Acad. Sci. USA* **85,** 8638–8642.

13. Riviere, Y, Tanneau-Salvadori, F., Regnault, A., Lopez, O., Sansonetti, P., Guy, B., et al. (1989) Human immunodeficiency virus-specific cytotoxic responses of seropositive individuals: distinct types of effector cells mediate killing of targets expressing gag and env proteins. *J. Virol.* **63,** 2270–2277.

14. Blazevic, V., Ranki, A., and Krohn, K. J. E. (1995) Helper and cytotoxic T cell responses of HIV Type-1 infected individuals to synthetic peptides of REV. *AIDS Res. and Hum. Retrovir.* **11,** 1335–1342.

15. Nixon, D. F. and McMichael, A. J. (1991) Cytotoxic T-cell recognition of HIV proteins and peptides. *AIDS* **5,** 1049–1059.

16. Hammond, S. A., Bollinger, R. C., Stanhope, P. E., Quinn, T. C., Schwartz, D., Clements, M. L., and Siliciano, R. F. (1992) Comparative clonal analysis of human immunodeficiency virus type-1 (HIV-1)-specific CD4+ and CD8+ cytolytic T lymphocytes isolated from seronegative humans immunized with candidate HIV-1 vaccines. *J. Exp. Med.* **176,** 1531–1542.

17. Curiel, T. J., Wong, J. T., Gorczyca, P. F., Schooley, R. T., Walker, B. D., et al. (1993) CD4+ human immunodeficiency virus type-1 (HIV-1) envelope-specific cytotoxic T lymphocytes derived from the peripheral blood of an HIV-infected individual. *AIDS Res. Hum. Retrovir.* **9,** 61–68.

18. Ratto, S., Sitz, K. V., Scherer, A., Loomis, L. D., Cox, J. H., Redfield, R. R., and Birx, D. L. (1996) CD4+ T-lymphocyte lines developed from HIV-1 seropositive patients recognize difference epitopes within the V3 loop. *J. AIDS* **11,** 128–136.

19. Earl, P. L. and Moss, B. (1992) Expression of proteins in mammalian cells using vaccinia. *Current Protocols In Molecular Biology, vol 2* (Ausubel, F. M., Brent, R., Kingston, R. E., Moore, D. D., Seidman, J. G., Smith, J. A., and Struhl, K., eds.) units 15.1–18.9.

20. van Baalen, C. A., Klein, M. R., Geretti, A. M., Keet, R. I., Miedema, F., van Els, C. A., and Osterhaus, A. D. (1993) Selective in vitro expansion of HLA Class I-restricted HIV-1 gag-specific CD8+ T cells: cytotoxic T-lymphocyte epitopes and precursor rrequencies. *AIDS* **7,** 781–786.

21. Gotch, F., McAdam, S. N., Allsopp, C. E. M., Gallimore, A., Elvin, J., Kieny, M. P., et al. (1993) Cytotoxic T cells in HIV-2 seropositive Gambians. *J. Immunol.* **151,** 3361–3369.

22. McElrath, M., Siliciano, R. F., and Weinhold, K. J. (1997) HIV type 1 vaccine-induced cytotoxic T cell responses in phase I clinical trials: detection, characterization and quantitation. *AIDS Res. Hum. Retrovir.* **13,** 211–216.

23. Ferrari, G., Humphrey, W., McElrath, M.J., Excler, J. L., Duliege, A. M., Clements, M. L., et al. (1997). Clade B-based HIV-1 vaccines elicit cross-clade cytotoxic T lymphocyte reactivities in uninfected volunteers. *P.N.A.S.* **94,** 1396–1401.

24. Carmichael, A., Alp, N., and Borysiewicz, L. (1992) Quantitating the HIV-1 specific cytotoxic T cell response, in *Cytotoxic T Cells in HIV and Other Retroviral*

Infections (Racz, P., Letvin N. L., and Gluckman, J. C., eds.), S. Karger, Basel, pp. 30–39.

25. Fazekas de St Groth, S. (1982) The evaluation of limiting dilution analysis. *J. Immunol. Methods* **49,** R11–R23.

26. Strijbosch, L. W. J., Does, R. J. M. M., and Buurman, W. A. (1988) Computer aided design and evaluation of limiting and serial dilution experiments. *Int. J. Biomed. Comput.* **23,** 279–290.

27. Geretti, A. M., Dings, M. E., van Els, C. A. van Baalen, C. A., Wijnholds, F. J., Borleffs, J. C., and Osterhaus, A. D. (1996) Human immunodeficiency virus Type 1 (HIV-1) - and Epstein-Barr Virus specific cytotoxic T lymphocyte precursors exhibit different kinetics in HIV-1 infected persons. *J. Infect. Dis.* **174,** 34–45.

28. Carini, C. and Essex, M. (1994) Interleukin 2-dependent interleukin 7 activity enhances cytotoxic immune response of HIV-1-infected individuals. *AIDS Res. Hum. Retrovir.* **10,** 121–130.

29. Ferrari, G., King, K., Rathbun, K., Place, C. A., Packard, M. V., Bartlett, J. A., et al. (1995) IL-7 enhancement of antigen-driven activation/expansion of HIV-1-specific cytotoxic T lymphocyte precursors (CTLp*) Clin. Exp. Immunol.* **101,** 239–248.

30. Blomberg, K., Granberg, C., Hemmilä, I., and Lövgren, T. (1986) Europium-labeled target cells in an assay of natural killer cell activity. I. A novel non-radioactive method based on time-resolved fluorescence. *J. Immunol. Methods* **86,** 225–233.

31. Blomberg, K., Hautala, R., Lovgren, J., Mukkala, V. M., Lindqvist, C., and Akerman, K. (1996) Time resolved fluorimetric assay for natural killer activity using target cells labeled with a fluorescence enhancing ligand. *J. Immunol. Methods* **193,** 199–206.

39

HIV-1-Specific Antibody-Dependent Cellular Cytotoxicity (ADCC)

Josephine H. Cox

1. Introduction

Antibodies elicited during the course of HIV-1 infection can act as a bridge between cytolytic cells and HIV-1-infected cells or other cells that have passively absorbed appropriate HIV-1-antigens. These cytolytic cells cause lysis of the HIV-1-infected cells thereby decreasing viral load *(1–5)* . The effector cells for ADCC are natural killer (NK) cells, that mediate lysis in a non-MHC restricted fashion. NK cells expressing CD16$^+$ low affinity Fc-receptors bind to antibody which specifically binds to the antigen expressed on target cells. Two types of ADCC activity can be demonstrated in HIV-1-infected patients. The first type, the classical or indirect ADCC, is assayed using normal donor lymphocytes and HIV-1 patient sera. Lysis of HIV-1 envelope protein-coated or HIV-1-infected target cells is detected in a chromium 51 [^{51}Cr] release assay. Sera from HIV-1-infected individuals appear to mediate indirect ADCC regardless of their disease status. A second type, or direct ADCC, uses NK cells freshly isolated from HIV-1-infected individuals. These NK cells are coated with anti-HIV-1 cytophilic antibodies and can readily lyse envelope-coated or HIV-1-infected target cells. The latter may be a more pertinent measure of ADCC activity since the activity of this type of NK-mediated ADCC declines as HIV-1 disease progresses *(6)*.

The experimental design for indirect ADCC described here takes into account the fact that ADCC activity can be mediated by normal donor NK cells and that specificity of the reaction is determined by the antibody and the target cell. Serum positive for HIV-1 antibodies is used as the antibody bridge between effector and target cells in the ADCC assay. Controls consist of target cells and effector cells without the addition of serum, and of target cells and

From: *Methods in Molecular Medicine, Vol. 17: HIV Protocols*
Edited by: N. L. Michael and J. H. Kim © Humana Press Inc., Totowa, NJ

serum alone. A method for detection of ADCC using the NK resistant cell line CEM.NK^r coated with gp120 protein is described here.

2. Materials
2.1. Effector and Target Cells

1. Effector cells are peripheral blood mononuclear cells (PBMC) isolated by standard Ficoll-Hypaque procedure (Chapter 37, Subheading 3.1.). For one serum tested at 5 different dilutions, 10–15 mL of whole blood are generally required, or 15×10^6 isolated PBMC. For each additional serum, approx 5 mL of blood are required or 5×10^6 isolated PBMC. Since large numbers of PBMC are required for testing multiple sera, it is recommended that donor PBMC that have demonstrable ADCC activity in the presence of serum from an HIV-1 patient are used (*see* **Note 1**).
2. The CEM.NK^r human T-lymphoblastoid target cells can be obtained from the AIDS Research and Reference Reagent Program (Rockville, MD) (Catalog # 458). The cell line can be maintained in continuous culture for multiple passages. The critical requirements are that the CEM.NK^r cells should be in log phase and have a high viability >95% on the day of the assay. 1×10^6 CEM.NK^r cells are sufficient for testing up to six sera. Several other cell lines make good target cells for ADCC (*see* **Note 2**).

2.2. Solutions and Reagent

All solutions should be sterile filtered before use and proper sterile technique used in setting up the assay.

1. Complete medium (CM): The CM will be used for culture of CEM.NK^r target cells, preparation of the effector cells, and all assay procedures. RPMI 1640 media supplemented with 2% L-glutamine, 1% penicillin/streptomycin, 10% heat-inactivated fetal calf serum (FCS), and 2.5% HEPES buffer are used (all reagents can be obtained from Gibco, Gaithersburg, MD). Complete medium should be warmed to 37°C before use in all procedures described below.
2. Sodium chromate, $Na_2{}^{51}CrO_4$ [^{51}Cr], (NEN, Dupont, Boston, MA, or Amersham Life Sciences, Arlington Heights, IL): The concentration should be adjusted to 1 mCi/mL in sterile phosphate-buffered saline (PBS). The half-life of ^{51}Cr is 27.7 d; stocks can be used for up to 6 wk after their calibration date. The isotope should generally be stored at 4°C. Proper training in safety and handling of radio chemicals is required.
3. 10% sodium dodecyl sulfate (SDS): SDS can be made in PBS and sterile filtered or can be purchased ready-made and sterile from Gibco (Gaithersburg, MD). Stock SDS has a long shelf life at room temperature.
4. Recombinant gp-120, (Intracel Corporation, Cambridge, MA): The stock is made up at a concentration of 100 µg/mL and aliquots of about 12 µL stored at –70°C. One microgram of protein is required for 1×10^6 target cells. Several other recombinant proteins from different HIV-1 isolates can be obtained commercially. Since glycosylation of the protein is important, such proteins should be

produced in a eukaryotic system such as a Chinese hamster ovary (CHO) cell system. ADCC reactivity against envelope proteins from HIV-1 isolates other than laboratory isolates may be of interest, thus techniques that isolate and purify envelope protein directly from HIV-1 virions may be employed. Alternatively, vaccinia recombinants that express primary envelope proteins or cell lines that are permissive to primary isolates of HIV-1 may be used providing that the criteria in **Note 2** are followed.

5. Normal human serum: A source of pooled normal donor human serum is required for use as the negative control. The normal donor serum should be heat-inactivated and stored at $-70°C$ in aliquots of 12–15 µL.

6. Human anti-HIV-1 serum: A source of human anti-HIV-1 serum with demonstrable ADCC activity is required for screening normal donor PBMC and for use as a positive control in the ADCC assay. Patient sera may be used or aliquots for screening may be obtained commercially (North American Biologics Inc., Baton Rouge, LA). The serum should be heat inactivated at $56°C$ for 30 min and stored at $-70°C$ in aliquots of 12–15 µL.

7. Patient serum: Approx 10 µL of serum are required for each assay. Plasma may also be used, but generally the ADCC activity is lower. An aliquot of 50 µL of serum or plasma should be heat-inactivated at $56°C$ for 30 min; the serum can then be used immediately or stored in the freezer at $-70°C$ until use.

2.3. Equipment

Measurement of ^{51}Cr released during ADCC assays is usually performed with a gamma-counter or liquid scintillation counter.

3. Methods
3.1. PBMC Preparation

1. If using cryopreserved PBMC, on the day prior to the ADCC assay, gently thaw at least 30×10^6 normal human PBMC/sample to be tested. Resuspend the cells in 10 mL of CM and count the number of viable cells. The PBMC preparation should be at least 90% viable after thawing.

2. Adjust the cell concentration to 2×10^6 cells/mL and place in 75 cm² flasks standing upright and putting no more than 40 mL of cell suspension into a single flask. Incubate at $37°C$ overnight. This step not only allows the PBMC to recover from the thawing process, but also allows the adherence of macrophages and some B cells, partially purifying the cell population. If using freshly isolated cells, the PBMC can also be incubated overnight or for at least 1 h for macrophage depletion. If performing the 1 h incubation for macrophage depletion, it is best to lay the 75 cm² flasks down flat in the incubator to increase the surface area.

3. After macrophage depletion, pool the contents of the flasks, pellet the PBMC, and adjust the concentration with CM to 2.5×10^6 cells/mL. This will give an effector:target (E:T) ratio of 50:1 for the assay. A higher E:T ratio will give greater percent lysis and therefore increased sensitivity.

3.2. CEM.NK' Preparation

1. In order to ensure that the target cells are in log phase, one day prior to the ADCC assay the required number of CEM.NK^r cells (>95% viable) should be removed from the stock flask, pelleted, and placed into a 25 cm^2 flask along with fresh complete media to make a total volume of 10 mL. One million CEM.NK^r cells are sufficient for testing five sera at five different dilutions.

2. On the day of the assay, place the log phase CEM.NK^r cells (prepared above) in a 15-mL centrifuge tube, pellet the cells, decant the supernatant, and resuspend the pellet in 1 mL of CM. Count the cells, remove 1 × 10^6 CEM.NK^r cells per five samples, and place in a fresh 15 mL tube labeled with the cell type and a radiation hazard sticker

3. Pellet the cells, decant the supernatant, and add 100 μCi of ^{51}Cr per 1 × 10^6 CEM.NK^r cells (the volume of ^{51}Cr needs to be adjusted to allow for the decay of the isotope). Add 10% v/v of fetal bovine serum (FBS).

4. Incubate the CEM.NK^r cells for 1 h at 37°C; shake the tube every 15 min to resuspend the cells and ensure uniform labeling.

5. After incubation, add 10 mL CM, centrifuge the tube, decant the supernatant (radioactive liquid must be handled appropriately), and gently break up the pellet by flicking the tube. Resuspend the pellet in 300 μL of CM and add 10 μL (1 μg) of gp120 per 1 × 10^6 cells. Transfer the cell suspension to a sterile 1 mL microcentrifuge tube. Incubate for 1 h at room temperature on a platform rocker.

6. Remove contents of the microcentrifuge tube and place into a 15-mL centrifuge tube. Rinse the microcentrifuge tube with CM and add to remainder of cells. Wash cells three times with 10 mL of CM. After the third wash, decant the supernatant, and resuspend the pellet in 1 mL CM. Count the cells, and adjust the concentration to 1 × 10^5 cells/mL with CM.

3.3. Serum Preparation

1. During the CEM.NK^r target preparation, the serum dilutions for the patient samples can be prepared and plated. Remove serum from freezer, and thaw vial completely at room temperature, then heat-inactivate the serum in a water bath for 30 min at 56°C.

2. For each patient's serum sample, the ADCC positive control serum and normal human serum, dilutions are prepared as follows 1:25, 1:250, 1:2,500, 1:25,000, 1:250,000, in a 96-well plate. A total of 150 μL of each serum dilution is required. Perform the serial dilutions as indicated in **Table 1**.

3.4. Assay Setup

1. Dispense 50 μL of serum dilutions into a 96-well, sterile U-bottomed microtiter plate in triplicate. **Do not** put serum in the maximum release, spontaneous release, or no serum wells.

2. Dispense 50 μL of CEM.NK^r target cells/well, concentration of 1 × 10^5 cells/mL to every well, including maximum release, spontaneous release, and no serum wells in triplicate.

Table 1
Serial Dilutions for ADCC Sera

Formula	Dilution	Final dilution (in assay plate)
10 μL serum sample + 240 μL CM	(1:25)	1:100
20 μL of (1:25) + 180 μL CM	(1:250)	1:1000
20 μL of (1:250) + 180 μL CM	(1:2,500)	1:10,000
20 μL of (1:2,500) + 180 μL CM	(1:25,000)	1:100,000
20 μL of (1:25,000) + 180 μL CM	(1:250,000)	1:1,000,000

3. Incubate target cells and serum for 20 min at room temperature.
4. Dispense 100 μL of PBMC/well. Add to every well **except** maximum release and spontaneous release.
5. Dispense 150 μL of CM to the spontaneous release wells in triplicate, 50 μL of CM to the no serum wells in triplicate, and 150 μL of 10% SDS to the maximum release wells in triplicate.
6. Incubate for 6 h at 37°C

3.5. Harvesting the Assay Plate

1. Remove the plate from the incubator. Supernatant fluid is harvested using the Skatron Harvesting System (the manual supplied with the harvester gives very clear directions) (*see* **Notes 3** and **4**).
2. The level of ADCC activity as denoted by the percent specific lysis of labeled CEM.NK^r target cells is determined by the following formula:

$$\% \text{ lysis} = \frac{\text{mean test cpm} - \text{mean spon CPM}}{\text{mean max cpm} - \text{mean spon CPM}} \times 100$$

CPM = counts per minute (mean CPM is usually average of three replicates), test cpm = cpm released by the target cells in the presence of effector cells, spon = cpm released by the target cells in the absence of any effector cells (*see* **Note 5**), and max = cpm released by the target cells in the presence of SDS.

3.6. Data Analysis

There are several ways in which patient ADCC activities can be compared:

1. **Figure 1** shows ADCC activity of sera from two patients followed over five years, as well as ADCC activity of pooled normal human serum and a known ADCC-active serum. It should be noted that at low serum dilution (up to 1:1000 dilution) there is a significant inhibition of ADCC activity. This phenomenon is commonly seen with CEM.NK^r cells in the presence of saturating amounts of envelope protein, but is less likely to be seen in chronically infected cell lines

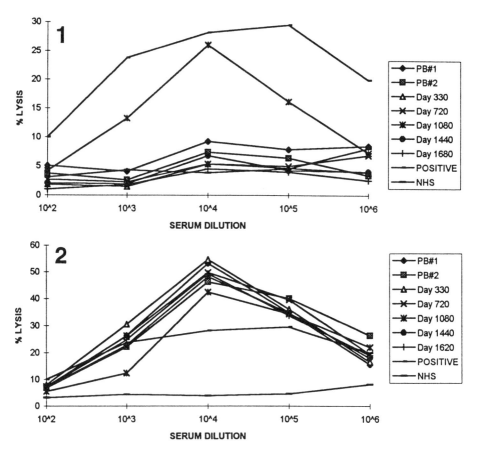

Fig. 1. ADCC activity of two patients enrolled in a vaccine trial followed over 5 yr. ADCC activity was tested against CEM.NKr cells absorbed with HIV-1-gp120-IIIB. Patient #1 has low ADCC activity compared to normal human serum (NHS), while patient #2 has high activity. Positive = serum with known high ADCC activity. PB = prevaccine bleed.

where the surface density of envelope proteins is substantially less than that seen with cell lines incubated with envelope protein. Data can be presented more simply by subtracting the percent lysis of target cells in the presence of NHS from the percent lysis of target cells in the presence of the test serum and then plot the corrected percent lysis vs serum dilution.

The ratio of % lysis in the presence of test serum – percent lysis in the presence of NHS/percent lysis in the presence of NHS, is also useful for comparing ADCC activities of a patient over time. For patient #1 at serum dilution of 1:10,000 the ratio is <1 on all study days except d 1080. For patient #2, the ratio is around 9 for all of the study days.

2. ADCC activity can also be expressed as lytic units (LU) titers. An LU titer is defined as the serum dilution that yields a particular percent lysis (e.g., the LU_{20} is the number of lytic units at 20% lysis for a particular serum dilution). Plot the percent specific lysis versus the serum dilution. Select a percent lysis value that encompasses most of the patients' percent lysis values (e.g., if 20%, then determine the LU_{20} titer by extrapolating along the axis).

4. Notes

1. PBMC from normal donors do not always exhibit good ADCC activity in the presence of a serum with known ADCC activity. Therefore, for testing a large panel of sera, it is best to freeze PBMC from several donors, screen the donors for ADCC activity, and then use donor PBMC exhibiting good ADCC activity for assaying the test sera. The author uses PBMC from leukapheresis donors; by using PBMC from a single donor, day to day variations in ADCC activity can be minimized. It has been found that ADCC activity in fresh and cryopreserved PBMC is comparable. In addition, ADCC activity of sera from nonhuman primates and rabbits can be examined using human PBMC, provided that the correct target cells are used (*see* **Note 2**).

2. Two critical requirements are necessary for target cells used in ADCC assays. First, at least 80% of the target cells should express the specific antigen (usually envelope protein) of interest. For surface expression of the envelope protein, the target cells should be screened by flow cytometric methods (Chapter 30). For the protocol described here, >95% of the cells routinely express surface gp120 as determined by flow cytometry. Second, the chosen target cell should not be lysed by effector cells in the absence of test antibody. For example, many T-cell lines can readily be infected with isolates of HIV-1 or SIV virus and express surface envelope proteins; however, they are lysed by normal donor NK in the absence of any HIV-1 or SIV-specific antibodies. CEM.NK^r infected with HIV-1 (laboratory adapted) isolates make good ADCC target cells. U937 cells and A301 cells can also be chronically infected with HIV-1 and make suitable target for ADCC assays *(7,8)*. It will generally take a couple of weeks to establish a cell line. HIV-1 infection can initially be screened by p24 quantitation in the supernatant. For use in the ADCC assay, the targets should pass the criteria defined above. It has also been found that CEM.NKr cells infected with vaccinia recombinants encoding envelope proteins make good targets for ADCC (*see* Chapter 39). Cells infected with control vaccinia also need to be included in the assay.

3. An alternative method of harvesting the supernatant is to carefully remove the plate from the incubator, taking care not to disturb the cell pellets. With a 12-well multichannel pipet, gently remove 50 or 100μL of the supernatant from the test samples, spon and max wells, and place in small dilution tubes (these do not need to be sterile, but it is useful to have them in a 96-well type of format, so that supernatants can be directly transferred from the 96-well plate). If care is taken, the pellet should not be disturbed by removal of the supernatant. However, to avoid this problem, the plates can be centrifuged and then the pellet is less likely

to be disturbed. To inactivate HIV-1 in the supernatant, add an equal volume of formalin to the tubes before counting. The tube is placed in the gamma-counter for detection of ^{51}Cr.

4. Detection of ^{51}Cr in supernatants can also be measured using liquid scintillation counting. Recently, several companies have started marketing 96-well format beta-counters for detection of gamma-emitting isotopes such as ^{51}Cr and ^{125}I. If a standard beta-counter is available, a 20 μL aliquot of the supernatant can be spotted onto filter mats laminated with plastic on one side (LKB-Wallac, Gaithersburg, MD, 1205-402). The filter mats are then dried by heating for 5 min in a microwave. Filter mats are then processed in the same way as the filter mats used in proliferation assays (see Chapter 38, Subheading 3.3.).

   Nonradioactive methods for detection of cytolytic assays are currently available, but most of these assays suffer from poor reproducibility and sensitivity. However, the Europium release assay (LKB Wallac) appears to be a suitable alternative (9,10) providing good reproducibility and sensitivity in the author's hands.

5. In cytotoxicity assays, attention should be paid to the spontaneous release of ^{51}Cr from the CEM.NK^r cells. The spontaneous release should ideally be less than 10% of the total release. Generally for well-maintained CEM.NK^r, the spontaneous release is <5%. If higher values than 10% are obtained, it suggests that the target cells have either been handled roughly or mycoplasma contamination may is present. If using HIV-1 infected or vaccinia infected target cells, the spontaneous release is likely to be higher (10–20%).

References

1. Tyler, D. S., Lyerly, H. K., and Weinhold, K. J. (1990) Minireview: Anti-HIV-1 ADCC. AIDS Res. Hum. Retrovir. 5, 557–563.
2. Ojo-Amaize, E. A., Nishanian, P., Keith, D. E., et al. (1987) Antibodies to human immunodeficiency virus in human sera induced cell-mediated lysis of human immunodeficiency virus-infected cells. J. Immunol. 139, 2458–2463.
3. Blumberg, R. S., Paradis, T., Hartshorn, K. L., et al. (1987) Antibody-dependent cell mediated cytotoxicity against cells infected with the human immunodeficiency virus. J. Infect. Dis. 156, 878–884.
4. Weinhold, K. J., Lyerly, H. K., Matthews, T. J., et al. (1988) Cellular anti-gp120 cytolytic reactivities in HIV-1 seropositive individual. Lancet 1, 902–905.
5. Tyler, D. S., Stanley, S. D., Nastala, C. A., Austin, A. A., Bartlett, J. A., Stine, K. C., Lyerly, H. K., Bolognesi, D. P., and Weinhold, K. J. (1990) Alterations in Antibody dependent cellular cytotoxicity during the course of HIV-1 infection. J. Immunol. 144, 3375–3384.
6. Ahmad, A. and Menezes, J. (1994) Positive correlation between the natural killer and gp120/41 specific antibody dependent cellular cytotoxic effector functions in HIV-infected individuals. J. AIDS Hum. Retrovir. 10, 115–19.
7. Ljunggren, K., Bötiger, B., Biberfeld, G., Karlsson, A., Fenyö, E. M., and Jondal, M. (1987) Antibody-dependent cellular cytotoxicity-inducing antibodies against human immunodeficiency virus. Presence at different clinical satges. J. Immunol. 139, 2263–2267.

8. Vogel, T., Kurth, R., and Norley, S. (1994) The majority of neutralizing Abs in HIV-1-infected patients recognize linear V3 loop sequences. Studies using HIV-1$_{MN}$ multiple antigenic peptides. *J. Immunol.* **153,** 1895–1904.

9. Blomberg, K., Granberg, C., Hemmilä, I., and Lövgren, T. (1986) Europium-labelled target cells in an assay of natural killer cell activity. I. A novel non-radioactive method based on time-resolved fluorescence. *J. Immunol. Methods* **86,** 225–233.

10. Blomberg, K et al (1996) Time resolved fluorimetric assay for natural killer activity using target cells labelled with a fluorescence enhancing ligand. *J. Immunol. Methods.* **193,** 199–206.

40

Evaluation of Natural Killer Cell Activity

Josephine H. Cox *[handwritten annotation: contains comments equal as Dg6 & T Dg6 3]*

1. Introduction

The immune response to a virus infection involves both nonspecific and specific immune mechanisms. Natural killer (NK) cells are naturally-occurring cytolytic cells capable of lysing various tumor cells and virus-infected cells without previous sensitization or with a requirement for major histocompatibility (MHC) restriction. The molecular mechanisms that explain how NK cells are able to kill virus-infected cells and tumor cells while sparing self-cells have recently been elucidated *(1)*. NK cells may play a role as a first line of defense against virus infection by mediating lysis of virus-infected cells prior to the development of specific humoral and cell-mediated defense mechanisms. Although the percentage of NK cells in HIV-1-infected patients may remain normal, the absolute numbers of some NK subsets are substantially reduced in the blood of HIV-1 patients and NK function decreases as HIV-1 infection proceeds *(2–4)*. The interplay between NK cells and other cells of the innate and specific immune system is mediated, in part, through the release of cytokines, in particular interleukin-2 (IL-2) and γ-interferon (γ-IFN). Thus, it seems plausible that the generalized immunosuppression seen in HIV-1-infected patients may contribute to the impairment of NK activity. A dynamic balance between NK cells and cytotoxic T lymphocytes (CTL) is likely to occur *(5)*. Therefore, any alterations in NK or CTL activity are likely to impair anti-HIV-1 cytolytic function.

NK cell activity can be detected in freshly isolated human peripheral blood mononuclear cells (PBMC) and does not require prior in vitro sensitization. Preparations of PBMC are examined for NK activity immediately following isolation from heparinized blood samples in a classic chromium 51 (^{51}Cr) release assay. The cell line K-562, derived from a patient with chronic myelogenous leukemia in blast crisis, is the standard target cell for measuring NK activity.

From: *Methods in Molecular Medicine, Vol. 17: HIV Protocols*
Edited by: N. L. Michael and J. H. Kim © Humana Press Inc., Totowa, NJ

2. Materials

2.1. Effector and Target Cells

1. Effector cells are PBMC isolated by standard Ficoll-Hypaque procedure (Chapter 38, Subheading 3.1.). For one NK assay, 5–10 mL of whole blood are generally required or 5×10^6 isolated PBMC.
2. The K562 target cells obtained from ATCC (Rockville, MD) (human chronic myelogenous leukemia, ATCC #CCL-243) can be maintained in continuous culture for up to six passages. The critical requirements are that the K562 cells should be in log phase and have a high viability (>95%).

2.2. Solutions and Reagents

All solutions should be sterile filtered before use and proper sterile technique used in setting up the assay.

1. Complete medium (CM): Used for culture of K562 target cells, preparation of the effector cells and all assay procedures, RPMI 1640 media supplemented with 2% L-glutamine, 1% penicillin/streptomycin, 10% heat inactivated fetal calf serum (FCS), and 2.5% HEPES buffer is used (all reagents can be obtained from Gibco, Gaithersburg, MD). Complete medium should be warmed to 37°C before use in all procedures described below.
2. Sodium chromate, $Na_2{}^{51}CrO_4$ (^{51}Cr), (NEN, Boston, MA, Dupont or Amersham Life Sciences, Arlington Heights, IL): The concentration should be adjusted to 1 mCi/mL in sterile phosphate-buffered saline (PBS). The half-life of ^{51}Cr is 27.7 d; stocks can be used for up to 6 wk after their calibration date. Generally, the isotope should be stored at 4°C. Proper training in safety and handling of radio chemicals is required.
3. 10% sodium dodeycl sulfate (SDS): SDS can be made in PBS and sterile filtered or can be purchased ready-made and sterile from Gibco (Gaithersburg, MD). Stock SDS has a long shelf life at room temperature.

2.3. Equipment

Measurement of ^{51}Cr released during an NK assay is usually performed with a gamma-counter or liquid scintillation counter.

3. Methods

3.1. Preparation and Labeling of K562 Target Cells

1. In order to ensure that the target cells are in log phase, one day prior to the NK assay, the required number of K562 cells (>95% viable) should be removed from the stock flask, centrifuged, and placed into a 25 cm² flask along with fresh complete media to make a total volume of 10 mL. One million K562 cells are sufficient for setting up 3–4 NK assays. Therefore, on the day prior to the assay, 1–3 million K562 cells should be placed into a flask with fresh CM (*see* **Note 1**).

2. On the day of the assay, place the log phase K562 cells (prepared above) in a 15-mL centrifuge tube. Pellet the cells, decant the supernatant, and resuspend the pellet in 1 mL of CM. Count the cells, remove 1×10^6 K562 cells/three samples, and place in a fresh 15-mL tube labeled with the cell type and a radiation hazard sticker (e.g., if 6 patient NK assays are to be performed, 2×10^6 K562 cells should be prepared).

3. Pellet the cells, decant the supernatant, and add 100 μCi of ^{51}Cr per 1×10^6 K562 cells (the volume of ^{51}Cr needs to be adjusted to allow for the decay of the isotope). Add 10% v/v of fetal bovine serum (FBS).

4. Incubate the K562 cells for 1 h at 37°C; shake the tube every 15 min to resuspend the cells and ensure uniform labeling.

5. After incubation, add 10 mL CM, pellet the cells, decant the supernatant (radioactive liquid must be handled appropriately), and gently resuspend the pellet by flicking the tube. Repeat this step two more times to wash the cells free of excess ^{51}Cr.

6. After the final wash, resuspend the cells in 1 mL of CM, count cells using a hemacytometer, and adjust the concentration to 5×10^5 viable K562 cells/mL. Adjust the 5×10^5 cells/mL to 5×10^4 cells/mL by making a 1:10 dilution with CM. This is the stock required for plating the target cells.

3.2. Effector Preparation

1. Separate PBMC from whole blood using Ficoll-Hypaque (Chapter 37, Subheading 3.1.), and resuspend 5×10^6 cells in 5 mL of CM. In order to partially purify the PBMC population, adherent macrophages can be removed by placing the PBMC suspension in a 25 cm^2 tissue culture flask and incubating the cells at least 1 h at 37°C. The flask should be laid down flat in the incubator.

2. After incubation, collect the PBMC, and dispense into a 15-mL centrifuge tube. Gently rinse the flask with an additional 3 mL CM, and avoid disturbing the adherent macrophages, and add to remaining cells. Pellet the cells, decant supernatant, and resuspend the pellet in 500 μL of CM.

3. Count the PBMC, and adjust the concentration to 5×10^6 cells/mL; this concentration is for the effector:target (E:T) ratio of 100:1, assuming that 5×10^3 target cells are used/well. If 5×10^6 PBMC were provided for the assay, there should be plenty of cells to perform all of the required dilutions to give E:T ratios of 100:1, 50:1, 25:1, and 5:1. Stepwise dilutions of the PBMC are performed in CM medium to generate aliquots of cells at 2.5, 1.25, and 0.25×10^6, respectively, for the required E:T ratios. The dilutions are usually performed in dilution tubes, using CM. Each E:T incubation is performed in triplicate, therefore a minimum of 300 μL of each concentration of PBMC is required (*see* **Notes 2** and **3**).

3.3. Plating of Effectors and Targets

1. In a 96-well U-bottomed microtiter plate, dispense 100 μL of each effector cell concentration in triplicate. For example, place 100 μL of effectors for the 100:1 ratio for patient #1 into wells C1–3, for the 50:1 ratio into D1–3, and so on. For

patient #2, place 100 μL of effectors for the 100:1 ratio into wells C4–6, for the 50:1 ratio into D4–6, and so on.

2. Dispense 100 μL of K562 target cells, adjusted to 5×10^4 cells/mL to every well containing effector cells. Dispense 100 μL of K562 target cells in wells A1–3 and H1–3 for patient #1, A4–6 and H4–6 for patient #2, and so forth. To row A add 100 μL of sterile 10% SDS. Addition of 10% SDS lyses the target cells and releases all the ^{51}Cr from the target cells; the ^{51}Cr released from the SDS-treated cells is used to calculate the maximum release (max). To row H, add 100 μL of CM; the ^{51}Cr released from these wells is used to calculate the spontaneous release (spon).

3. Incubate microtiter plate (with lid on) for 4 h at $37°C$.

3.4. Harvesting the Assay Plate

1. Remove the plate from the incubator. Supernatant fluid is harvested using the Skatron Harvesting System (the manual supplied with the harvester gives very clear directions). The principal of this system is that supernatant from individual wells is absorbed onto a cartridge with a filter disk on the end closest to the cells, the latter prevents transfer of cells to the cartridge. The cartridge is then removed from the plate leaving the filter disk in the plate. The cartridge is then placed in a macrowell tube and the tube is placed in the gamma counter for detection of ^{51}Cr (*see* **Notes 4** and **5**).

2. The level of NK activity as denoted by the percent specific lysis (% lysis) of labeled targets is determined by the following formula.

$$\% \text{ lysis} = \frac{\text{mean test cpm} - \text{mean spon CPM}}{\text{mean max cpm} - \text{mean spon CPM}} \times 100$$

CPM = counts/min (mean CPM is usually average of three replicates), test cpm = cpm released by the target cells in the presence of effector cells, spon = cpm released by the target cells in the absence of any effector cells (*see* **Note 6**) and max = cpm released by the target cells in the presence of SDS.

3.5. Data Analysis

1. Most gamma-counters can be programed to calculate the percent specific lysis (percent lysis). This value alone can suffice as a measure of NK activity or nonparametric tests, such as Kruskall-Wallis or Wilcoxon tests can be used to determine significant statistical differences between slopes of response curves at different E:T ratios and different groups of patients and controls (**Fig. 1**).

2. NK cytotoxic activity can also be expressed as lytic units (LU). An LU is defined as the number of lymphocytes required to yield a particular percent lysis, (e.g., the LU_{20} is the number of lytic U at 20% lysis for a particular number of effector cells). Plot the percent specific lysis vs the log of the effector cell number for each E:T ratio (i.e., in the standard NK set up described above, at the 100:1 ratio there are 5×10^5 cells/well, at 50:1 there are 2.5×10^5 effector cells/well, etc).

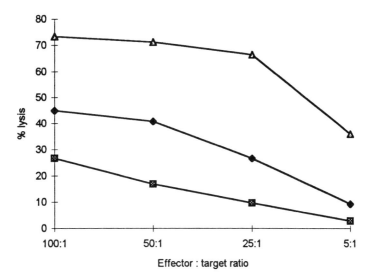

Fig. 1. NK lysis of K562 target cells by two HIV-1-infected seropositives (■ and ◆) and a seronegative (▲). LU_{20} are 4, 12, and 48, respectively, per 10^6 PBMC.

Select a percent lysis value that encompasses most of the patients' percent lysis values (e.g., 20%). Then determine the LU_{20} per million effector cells $LU_{20}/10^6$ PBMC, by extrapolating along the axis. The patient values for LU may have to be presented as values greater than or less than the arbitrarily selected LU. The author can be contacted to obtain an easy to use LU program.

4. Notes

1. Providing that K562 target cells are available, several NK assays can be performed in a single working day. Patient blood drawn early in the morning can be processed within 2–3 h. The target cells can be labeled while the macrophages are being depleted and the assay can be set up within 2 h of receipt of blood. After allowing for the 4 h incubation of effector and target cells, the whole setup should take 8–10 h. Ficolled PBMC incubated overnight in CM can also be used successfully in NK assays.

2. In the example of a standard NK assay given above, recommended E:T ratios are 100:1, 50:1, 25:1, and 5:1. If the number of PBMC is limiting the E:T, ratios can be lowered (e.g., 50:1, 25:1, 5:1, and 1:1) or the number of target cells can be lowered while keeping the same E:T ratio (e.g., 2.5×10^3 targets/well). If fewer than 2.5×10^3 target cells are used, problems are likely to be encountered with detection of low levels of radioactivity.

   If several assays are performed in one day, all with similar E:T ratios, the dilutions of the effector cells can be performed in the plate. Also, instead of having several spontaneous and maximum release wells, one set of spontaneous and maximum release wells can suffice for all assays set up on one day. It is recommended that if the assay is performed in this way, then five or six replicate wells should be set up instead of the usual triplicate set of wells.

3. For NK assays, normal PBMC can provide a positive control for the ability of the labeled K562 cells used in the assay to be killed and to determine the range of variation of the normal donor population in this assay. Because NK cell activity is highly variable among individuals, direct comparison of patient values and normal donor values will not necessarily yield statistically significant differences in levels of NK activity at varying effector:target ratios. Under ideal circumstances, each NK assay performed on an HIV-1-infected patient sample should be accompanied by a similar assay performed on a normal patient sample. Repeat bleeding of an individual allows for detection of changing NK activity levels associated with various modalities of treatment or with changing clinical status. Although NK activity is readily detectable in freshly isolated human PBMC, very low or borderline NK responses can be detected in thawed preparations of PBMC. The NK activity can be augmented in serial samples or thawed backup PBMC by a preincubation overnight with 10 U/mL IL-2. To a certain extent, the defect in NK function of PBMC from HIV-1-infected patients can also be restored by incubation overnight with 10 U/mL of recombinant IL-2. In assays employing addition of IL-2, it is important to compare IL-2-treated patient samples with other IL-2-treated patient samples.

4. An alternative method of harvesting the supernatant is to carefully remove the plate from the incubator, taking care not to disturb the cell pellets. With a 12-well multichannel pipet, gently remove 50 or 100 μL of the supernatant from the test samples, spon and max wells, and place in small dilution tubes (these do not need to be sterile, but it is useful to have them in a 96-well type of format, so that supernatants can be directly transferred from the 96-well plate). With care, the pellet should not be disturbed by removal of the supernatant. However, to avoid this problem, the plates can be centrifuged so the pellet is less likely to be disturbed. To inactivate HIV-1 in the supernatant, add an equal volume of formalin to the tubes before counting. The tube is placed in the gamma counter for detection of ^{51}Cr.

5. Detection of ^{51}Cr in supernatants can also be measured using liquid scintillation counting. Recently, several companies have started marketing 96-well format beta-counters for detection of gamma emitting isotopes such as ^{51}Cr and ^{125}I. If a standard beta-counter is available, a 20-μL aliquot of the supernatant can be spotted on filter mats laminated with plastic on one side (LKB, 1205-402). The filter mats are then dried by heating for 5 min in a microwave. Filter mats are then processed in the same way as the filter mats used in proliferation assays (see Chapter 38, Subheading 3.3.).

   Nonradioactive methods for detection of cytolytic assays are currently available; however, most of these assays suffer from poor reproducibility and sensitivity. However, the Europium release assay (LKB Wallac, Gaithersburg, MD) appears to be a suitable alternative (6,7), providing good reproducibility and sensitivity in the author's hands.

6. In cytotoxicity assays, attention should be paid to the spontaneous release of ^{51}Cr from the K562 cells. The spontaneous release should ideally be <10% of the total

release. Generally for well-maintained K562 cells, the spontaneous release should be <5%. If higher values than 10% are obtained, it suggests that the target cells have either been handled roughly or mycoplasma contamination may be present.

References

1. Moretta, A., Bottino, C., Vitale, M., Pende, D., Biassoni, R., Mingari, M. C., and Moretta, L. (1996) Receptors for HLA class-I molecules in human natural killer cells. *Ann. Rev. Immunol.* **14,** 619–648.
2. Cai, Q., Huang, X.-L. Rappocciolo, G., and Rinaldo, C. R. (1990) Natural killer cell response in homosexual men with early HIV infection. *J. Acq. Immune Defic. Syndr.* **3,** 669–676.
3. Ullum, H., Gotzsche, P. C., Victor, J., Dickmeiss, E., Skinhoj, P., and Pederson, B. K. (1995) Defective natural immunity: an early manifestation of human immunodeficiency virus infection. *J. Exp. Med.* **182,** 789–799.
4. Hu, P-F., Hultin, L. E., Hultin, P. Hausner, M. A., Hirji, K., Jewett, A., et al (1995) Natural killer cell immunodeficiency in HIV disease is manifest by profoundly decreased numbers of $CD16^{+}CD56^{+}$ cells and expansion of a population of $CD16^{dim}CD56^{-}$ cells with low lytic activity. *J. Acq. Imm. Def. Synd.* **10,** 331–340.
5. Kos, F. J. and Engleman, E. G. (1996) Immune regulation: a critical link between NK and CTLs. *Immunol. Today* **17,** 174–176.
6. Blomberg, K., Granberg, C., Hemmilä, I., and Lövgren, T. (1986) Europium-labeled target cells in an assay of natural killer cell activity. I. A novel non-radioactive method based on time-resolved fluorescence. *J. Immunol. Methods* **86,** 225–233.
7. Blomberg, K., Hautala, R., Lovgren, J., Mukkala, V. M., Lindqvist, C., and Akerman, K. (1996) Time resolved fluorimetric assay for natural killer activity using target cells labeled with a fluorescence enhancing ligand. *J. Immunol. Methods* **193,** 199–206.

41

Generation and Expansion
of HIV-1 CD4+ Antigen-Specific T Cell Lines

Silvia Ratto-Kim

1. Introduction

T-helper (Th) lymphocytes play a pivotal role in the immune response to viral pathogens. Understanding of the mechanisms governing the Th response to human immunodeficiency virus type 1 (HIV-1) is key to unveiling the pathogenesis of HIV-1 disease given the primary role the CD4+ T-cell plays as both a viral target and host effector cell. Determining the fine specificity of these T-cells can be correlated with patient outcome and used as a tool for specific immune reconstitution. The classic approach that has been used to study the interaction between the virus and its target cells has been the use of transformed CD4+ T-cell lines. Although easy to grow and maintain in culture, these transformed T-cell lines do not reflect the exact behavior of primary CD4+ lymphocytes *(1,2)*. Therefore, nontransformed CD4+ antigen-specific T-cell lines should be considered the definitive model for the cellular study of HIV infection and pathogenesis in vivo.

Another usage of these antigen-specific T-cell lines is immune reconstitution. These T-cell lines either unmodified or after genetic modification would be re-infused into patients to serve as effector cells. For example, HIV-1 specific helper cells transduced with cytokine genes could induce beneficial local effects while maximizing the toxicity associated with systemic cytokine delivery. The antigen-specificity of such reagents would also serve to reduce unwanted collateral responses.

The following protocol will focus primarily on the generation and expansion of antigen-specific T-cell lines and will give some helpful hints on their subsequent use.

From: *Methods in Molecular Medicine, Vol. 17: HIV Protocols*
Edited by: N. L. Michael and J. H. Kim © Humana Press Inc., Totowa, NJ

2. Materials

2.1. Solution and Medium for Mononuclear Cells Isolation

1. Ficoll-Hypaque solution (density 1.077g/L).
2. Phosphate-buffered saline (PBS): 1.15 g anhydrous Na_2HPO_4, 0.23 g anhydrous NaH_2PO_4, 9.00 g NaCl, 950 mL distilled water, pH adjusted to between 7.2 and 7.4 with either 1 M HCl or 1 M NaOH. Adjust final volume to 1000 mL with distilled H_2O; autoclave sterilized. This solution is available commercially from several sources.
3. Heparinized phlebotomy tubes.
4. Beckman GPR-5 centrifuge (or equivalent).
5. Microscope.
6. Hemocytometer.
7. 0.4% Trypan blue.

2.2. Culture Medium

RPMI 1640 (Gibco, Grand Island, NY) supplemented with 4 mM L-glutamine, 5×10^{-5} M 2-mercaptoethanol, 100 U/mL penicillin , 100 µg/mL streptomycin, and 5% heat-inactivated normal human AB serum (ABI, Columbia, MD).

2.3. Antigens

Virtually any soluble protein kept in physiologic buffer can be used as an antigen. Typical antigens used in developing HIV-1 specific CD4+ T-cell lines have been the envelope glycoprotein gp160 or gp120 *(3,4)*. It is important that titration is performed for any given antigen to choose the optimum concentration for the assay (*see* Chapter 1). A typical antigen concentration range is 5–50 µg/mL.

2.4. Freezing Solution

1. Ninety percent fetal calf serum, 10% dimethylsulfoxide (*see* **Note 1**).

2.5. Special Equipment

1. Gamma irradiator (^{60}Co or ^{137}Cs source).

3. Methods

Peripheral blood mononuclear cells (PBMC) are a mixture of CD4+ and CD8+ T lymphocytes, monocytes, and B cells. The goal of this technique is to select and then enrich for the CD4+ antigen-specific T-cells population. CD4+ T lymphocytes respond and grow in response to antigens processed and presented on the surface of antigen presenting cells (APC) in the context of MHC class II antigens. Adding a soluble antigenic protein to PBMC in culture will prime a proliferative response by CD4+ T-lymphocytes specifically recognizing the antigen, resulting in a CD4+ antigen-specific T-cell line.

The technique reported below is divided into four sections:

1. Start an antigen-specific mononuclear T-cell line;
2. Cell expansion;
3. Cyclic stimulations in order to enrich for antigen-specific CD4+ T-cells; and
4. Specificity determination.

3.1. Starting an Antigen-Specific Mononuclear T-Cell Line

The easiest source for CD4+ T lymphocytes is whole blood. Lymphoid cells are purified using Ficoll-Hypaque gradient centrifugation which takes advantage of the density difference between mononuclear cells and other blood components.

1. Perform venipuncture into heparinized blood tubes (or ACD tubes).
2. Dilute heparinized blood 1:1 with PBS.
3. Slowly layer an equal volume of Ficoll-Hypaque solution underneath the blood/PBS mixture by placing the tip of the pipet at the bottom of the sample tube.
4. Centrifuge 20 min. at $900g$ (brake off).
5. Using a sterile pipet, remove the aqueous layer that contains the platelet-rich plasma. Collect the white ring of peripheral blood mononuclear cells (PBMC) right above the Ficoll-Hypaque solution in a separate 50-mL conical sterile tube and approximate its volume.
6. Wash the cells in ≥ 3 vol of PBS.
7. Centrifuge 10 min at $400g$.
8. Resuspend mononuclear cells in 2–5 mL of PBS. Count the cells and determine viability by Trypan blue exclusion.
9. Add 40 mL of PBS and centrifuge 10 min at $400g$.
10. Resuspend the cells at a density of 1×10^7 cells/mL in culture medium.
11. Pulse PBMC at 1×10^7 cells/mL with antigen (5–50 µg/mL) for 4 h at 37°C.
12. Dilute the cells in culture medium to 2×10^6 cells/mL
13. Plate at 2×10^6 cells/mL in 24-well plates (Costar, Cambridge, MA), and incubate for 4 d at 37°C, 5% CO_2.

3.2. Cell Expansion in Culture

1. After 4 d, feed the cells with 10 U/mL recombinant interleukin-2 (rIL-2) (Boehringer-Mannheim, Germany).
2. After 1 wk of culture, and every 2–3 d thereafter, replace half of the medium with fresh medium containing 10 U/mL of rIL-2.
3. Split the culture 1:2 as needed (*see* **Notes 2–9**).

3.3. Cyclic Stimulations to Enrich for Antigen-Specific CD4+ T-Cells

1. After 15–20 d of culture, harvest T cells, wash, and resuspend at a final concentration of 5×10^5/mL.
2. Pulse 1×10^7 autologous PBMC with antigen (5–50 µg/mL) for 4 h at 37°C.

3. Irradiate PBMC with 30 Gy from a ^{60}Co or ^{137}Cs source.
4. Dilute the antigen-pulsed PBMC to 1×10^6 cells/mL.
5. Add 1×10^6 antigen presenting cells (APC) to 5×10^5 of the harvested T-cells in a 24-well plate. (It is possible to use ratios as low as 1:1 APC:T-cells though these low ratios may lower success.)
6. After 2 d, add rIL-2, and expand the culture by splitting after 5 d and every 2 d thereafter.
7. Perform the third stimulation after 15 d of culture as described in **steps 1–6**.

3.4. Determination of Antigen Specificity

The technique used to assess the specificity of the CD4+ T-cells is similar to the lymphoproliferative assay described in Chapter 1. The proliferative response of the T-cell lines is measured by incubating the growing T-cells with autologous antigen pulsed or nonpulsed, irradiated PBMC.

1. Incubate 3×10^4 T cells in a 96-well flat bottom plate (Costar, Cambridge, MA) with either 1×10^5 autologous antigen pulsed or nonpulsed, irradiated PBMC. The assay should be done in triplicate or duplicate wells.
2. After 2 d of incubation, pulse the cells with 1.67 μCi/well of ^{3}H thymidine.
3. After 16–18 h, harvest the plate using the Skatron harvesting system (Skatron Instruments, Sterling, VA) and count in a β-counter (BetaPlate, Model 1205, Wallac, Uppsala, Sweden).
4. The data can be expressed as an LSI [Lymphocyte Stimulation Index = (T cell + antigen pulsed PBMC cpm)/(T cell + unpulsed PBMC cpm)] to define antigen specificity. Lines can be designated as antigen-specific if their LSI is ≥3.

4. Notes

1. Caution: All solutions, material, and equipment coming in contact with cultured cells must be sterile, and proper sterile techniques must be adhered to strictly.
2. The key to the success of this technique is to evaluate the cell growth every 2 d under the microscope to determine the amount of IL-2 needed. After the first 7 d in culture, some clumps of cells should appear. Usually they are positioned around the plate edge. The medium should start turning yellow in 7–10 days. The cells should be split 1:2 adding half of fresh medium. When the cells start dividing, it is usually necessary to split the culture every 2 d. When the medium no longer turns yellow and the cells start to be reduced in size, it is time for the next restimulation. If the cells fail to grow after 7–10 d, change half of the medium and keep adding IL-2 for another week. If the cells fail to grow after 15 d, harvest the cells anyway and proceed with the restimulation. Sometimes the antigen-specific precursor cell frequency is so low that cell growth is not apparent.
3. To obtain maximum expansion, the cell concentration in the well has to be maintained optimally. If the split occurs too early, the cells will stop growing. On the other hand, if the well is overgrown the cells will die because of lack of nutrients. Evaluating the cell growth under the microscope helps to determine all these parameters.

4. It is usually better after 15 d of cell culture to harvest the cells off of the plate and plate them into a new tissue culture plate. This passage will clean the cells from debris and old monocytes that stick to the old plate. It is useful also to keep the cells resting for 1 d before restimulation and proliferation assay assess specificity (always at the same time as restimulation). The day before restimulation T-cells should be harvested, counted and plated at 1×10^6 cells/mL without IL-2. The next day cells are diluted to 5×10^5 and plated with the antigen pulsed-irradiated PBMC.

5. Instead of using autologous-antigen-pulsed PBMC as feeder cells it is possible to use an autologous or HLA class II matched B-lymphoblastoid cell line (B-LCL) (*see* Chapter 39). It is important that these cells present antigen and support proliferation. This will solve the problem of continuously phlebotomizing patients. Once the lines are established, it is also possible to freeze the cells and thaw them when the patient is available again. Freeze $1–2 \times 10^6$ cells/aliquot.

7. It is useful to check what markers the cells have on their surface. It is essential to check the percentage of CD4+ and CD8+. It is common to have an enrichment in nonspecific CD8+ cells that can overcome the growth of CD4+ cells.

8. Once the antigen-specific T-cell line has been established, it may be used to map the epitopes recognized by that particular patient. T-cell lines should be rested as described in **Note 4** at the end of the restimulation cycle and challenged with a panel of peptides spanning the entire antigen (or some part of it) in a proliferation assay as described in **Subheading 3.4.** Peptides should be used 1–5 μg/mL. Assays should be run in duplicate.

9. It has been demonstrated that CD4+ T-cell lines may possess cytotoxic activity. Cytotoxic activity was mainly attributed in the past to CD8+ T-cells but it is now clear that CD4+ T-cells can kill target cells *(3,4)*. The killing has been demonstrated to be class II restricted so the preparation of the target cells differs from the classic vaccinia infected target cells (*see* Chapter 39). CD4+ T cell lines should be tested for specific cytotoxicity after 7–10 d from the stimulation. 2×10^6 cells/mL of target cells (B-LCL) should be pulsed with the antigen/peptide for 10–16 h and then washed and loaded with [^{51}Cr]. The standard protocol for CTL assay should be followed thereafter.

References

1. Sawyer, L. S., Wrin, M. T., Crawford, M. L., Potts, B., Wu, Y., Weber, P. A., et al. (1994) Neutralization sensitivity of human immunodeficiency virus type 1 is determined in part by the cell in which the virus is propagated. *J. Virol.* **68,** 1342–1349.
2. Wrin, T., Loh, T. P., Vennari, J. C., Schiutemaker, H., and Nunberg, J. H. (1995) Adaptation to persistent growth in the H9 cell line renders a primary isolate of human immunodeficiency virus type 1 sensitive to neutralization by vaccine sera. *J. Virol.* **69,** 39–48.
3. Siliciano, R. F., Bollinger, R. C., Callahan, K. M., Hammond, S. A., Liu, A. Y., Miskovsky, E. P., et al. (1992) Clonal analysis of T-cell responses to the HIV-1 envelope proteins in AIDS vaccine recipients. *AIDS Res. Hum. Retroviruses* **8,** 1349–1352.
4. Ratto, S., Sitz, K. V., Scherer, A. M., Manca, F., Loomis, L. D., Cox, J. H., et al. (1995) Establishment and characterization of human immunodeficency virus type 1 (HIV-1) envelope-specific CD4+ T-lymphocyte lines from HIV-1 seropositive patients. *J. Infect. Dis.* **171,** 1420–1430.

42

Immunophenotyping and Assessment of Cell Function by Three-Color Flow Cytometry of Peripheral Blood Lymphocytes

Stephen P. Perfetto and Gilbert McCrary

1. Introduction

Infection by the human immunodeficiency virus type 1 (HIV-1) is known to cause a number of changes in the immunophenotypic profile of patients even in the early asymptomatic stages of disease. Such "surrogate markers" are known to correlate with the stage of HIV disease and often are predictive of outcomes. The best known of these is the absolute count of T helper lymphocytes, or CD4 cells, which undergoes a gradual decline as the virus infects greater and greater numbers of these cells *(1)*. A number of other markers have been found, some of which also are predictive of outcome in many cases. These include prevalence and intensity of the CD38 marker on CD8 T cells, percentage of CD4 cells exhibiting loss of the CD26 and CD28 markers, and percentage of CD4 cells with the CD95 marker *(2)*. The CD38 intensity of CD3/CD8 cells has, in fact, been more closely correlated with future disease progression in patients than the CD4 count *(3)*. The following method is a comprehensive immunophenotyping panel that incorporates all of these markers and provides several parameters by which to monitor disease progression and advise clinicians on treatment options.

2. Materials

2.1. Sample Collection

Whole blood specimens are collected from both HIV-positive and normal healthy control donors into blood collection tubes that contain tripotassium EDTA or sodium heparin.

From: *Methods in Molecular Medicine, Vol. 17: HIV Protocols*
Edited by: N. L. Michael and J. H. Kim © Humana Press Inc., Totowa, NJ

Table 1
Monoclonal Anitbody Core Panel

IgG1 FITC	CD26 PE
IgG1 PE	CD28 FITC
CD3 FITC	CD29 FITC
CD3 PerCP	CD38 PE
CD4 FITC	CD45 FITC
CD4 PE	CD14 PE
CD4 PerCP	CD45RA FITC
CD8 PE	CD56 PE
CD8 PerCP	CD62L PE
CD20 FITC	CD95 PE

2.2. Sample Preparation

1. Specimen buffer: Dulbecco's phosphate-buffered saline (PBS) (without Ca, Mg, or phenol red), with 0.1% (w/v) bovine serum albumin (BSA) (Fraction V from Sigma, St. Louis, MO) and 0.5% (v/v) sodium azide stock solution (*see* **step 2**). Reagent is stable for 1 mo, kept at 4°C.
2. Sodium azide stock solution: 20% (w/v) sodium azide in Dulbecco's PBS, stable for 1 yr at room temperature. Note: sodium azide is highly toxic, and can form explosive compounds; consult MSDS (*see* **Note 1**).
3. Formaldehyde, 1%: prepared from a stock of 20% buffered formaldehyde (Tousimis) and stable for 1 mo at 4°C. Stock is stable for one year at 4°C.
4. Monoclonal antibody core panel (*see* **Table 1**).

2.3. Sample Analysis

Samples are analyzed on a flow cytometer using (Elite-ESP, Coulter-Beckman Corp.) 88-nm argon laser illumination and equipped with Elite software version 4.0.

3. Method

3.1. Sample Collection

Whole blood samples are taken from both healthy control donors and HIV-positive individuals, drawn into sodium EDTA or heparin collection tubes. Samples are always drawn at the same time of day to cancel the effects of diurnal variation. The samples, once drawn, must be kept at room temperature (18–22°C) and transported to the laboratory as soon as possible. Samples must be less than 24 h old to be analyzed. Samples should be refused under certain conditions (*see* **Note 2**) *(4–6)*.

Table 2
Monoclonal Antibody-Fluorescent Conjugate Combination

Tube	FITC	PE	PerCP
1	(Unstained control)		
2	CD45	CD14	CD3
3	IgG1	IgG1	
4	CD3	CD4	
5	CD3	CD8	
6	CD3	CD38	CD3
7	CD28	CD95	CD4
8	CD29	CD26	CD4
9	CD45RA	CD62L	CD4
10	CD45RA	CD62L	CD8
11	CD20	CD56	CD3

3.2. Sample Preparation

1. Label 12 × 75-mm polystyrene centrifuge tubes for each monclonal antibody (MAb) combination for each sample. The panel is provided in **Table 2**.
2. Add the amount of MAb and specimen buffer (diluent) recommended by the manufacturer to stain 1×10^6 cells to the appropriate tubes. Note that the first tube is an unstained control and will receive only buffer.
3. Add 100 μL of whole blood from the samples to each appropriate assay tube.
4. Incubate the tubes at 4°C for 20 min.
5. Add 3 mL of buffer to each tube.
6. Centrifuge 400g for 5 min at 4°C.
7. Decant or aspirate off supernatant, vortex.
8. Repeat **steps 5–7** a second time.
9. Prepare a working solution of Coulter Immunolyse: Dilute stock 1:25 in specimen buffer, preparing 1 mL for each tube to be lysed. Chill at 4°C. Reagent may be used up to 2 h after dilution if kept cold.
10. Add lysing solution to each tube, vortex, wait 1–2 min.
11. Add 250 μL Coulter fixative. Vortex.
12. Repeat **steps 5–7** three times.
13. Add 125 μL of 1% formaldehyde (approx 1:1). Store at 4°C at least 30 min before analysis.

3.3. Sample Analysis

Collect data on the flow cytometer. Prior to collecting data, the FCM is aligned and standardized with the appropriate beads.

1. Run the unstained control. Use this sample to optimize flow rate, instrument alignment, etc. Look for distinguishable populations of lymphocytes, monocytes,

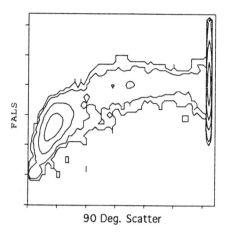

Fig. 1. 90 Deg. vs FALS.

and PMNs on the FALS vs 90LS histogram (*see* **Fig. 1**). Set a gate around the lymphocyte population that appears on this histogram. Confirm that RBC lysis was complete and that >99% of the lymphocytes are negative for all measured fluorescent parameters. This data does not have to be saved *(6, 7)*.

2. Run the CD45/14/3 control tube. This combination allows the purity of the population within the lymphocyte gate to be determined. Debris, dead cells, etc., are usually CD45 negative, whereas all normal leukocytes are CD45 positive. The CD14 marker enables detection of monocytes which, due to sample aging or other factors, may fall into the lymphocyte gate. To determine the purity of the gated lymphocyte population, set a scatter gate (as above) and look at the percentage of CD45+/CD14- cells. A rough three-part differential of lymphocytes, monocytes, and granulocytes can also be obtained by gating on CD45+ events and plotting them on a YFL vs 90LS histogram (*see* **Fig. 2**). Save this and all subsequent tubes on this patient as listmode files, and print the histograms after analysis *(6, 7)*.

3. Run the isotypic control tube (IgG1-FITC and IgG1-PE). This is a control for nonspecific staining of lymphocytes by fluorescent MAbs. Ideally, >99% of events in the lymphocyte gate should be negative for both FITC and PE. If <95% of events are negative for both, then the percent positive events for each parameter should be subtracted from the total in subsequent tubes.

4. Run the CD3/CD4 and CD3/CD8 tubes to determine the percentages of CD4-positive and CD8-positive T cells, respectively. Note that monocytes are dimly positive for CD4 but not for CD3, and that a subpopulation of natural killer (NK) cells is positive for CD8 but not CD3 (*see* **Figs. 3** and **4**).

5. Run the CD3/38/8 tube. The percent of CD8 T-cells positive for CD38 increases significantly in HIV infection, as does the intensity of the CD38 signal on positive cells. Gate on CD3 vs 90LS, then on CD8, to obtain the CD38 data. There is a marked correlation between the intensity of CD38-PE on CD8+ T cells and disease progression in HIV patients (*see* **Figs. 5** and **6**).

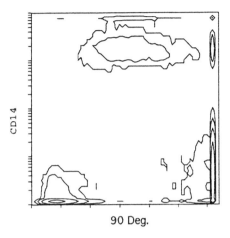

Fig. 2. 90 Deg vs CD14.

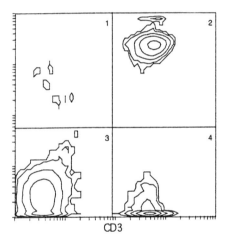

Fig. 3. CD3 vs CD4.

6. Run the CD28/95/4 tube. Gate on CD4 vs 90LS to obtain a bivariate histogram of CD28 vs CD95. CD28 is progressively lost on CD4 cells during HIV infection (*see* **Figs. 7** and **8**).
7. Run the CD29/26/4 tube, again gating on CD4 vs 90LS to obtain a bivariate histogram of CD29 vs CD26. Loss of CD26 and gain of CD29 on CD4+ T cells are both correlated with disease progression (*see* **Figs. 7** and **9**).
8. Run the CD45RA/62L/4 and CD45RA/62L/8 tubes, gating first on CD4 or CD8 vs 90LS and counting the cells positive for both 45RA and 62L. These markers of naive T cells are both expected to decline with progression of HIV disease (*see* **Figs. 7** and **10**).

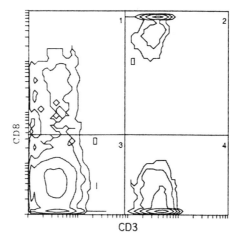

Fig. 4. CD3 vs CD8.

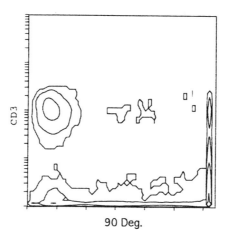

Fig. 5. 90 Deg vs CD3

9. Run the CD20/56/3 tube, gating on FALS vs 90LS to obtain a count of the lineage markers of the lymphocyte population: CD20 for B lymphocytes, CD56 for NK cells, and CD3 for T lymphocytes.

4. Notes

1. After the azide is completely dissolved in the PBS, filter the solution through a 0.2 or 0.45-μm apparatus. This removes compounds that can oxidize hemoglobin. If buffer made with this solution does oxidize hemoglobin (causing a whole blood sample to darken to black after several minutes' exposure to the buffer), discard the buffer, filter the azide solution again, and make fresh buffer.

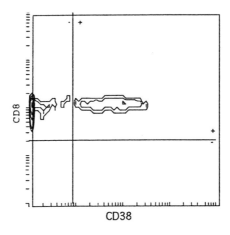

Fig. 6. CD38 vs CD8.

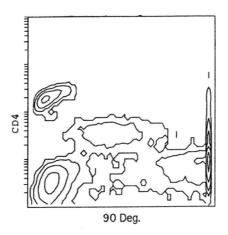

Fig. 7. 90 Deg vs CD4.

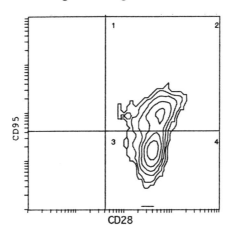

Fig. 8. CD9 vs CD28.

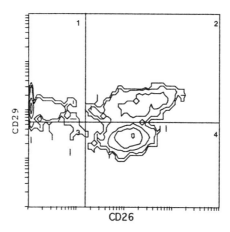

Fig. 9. CD29 vs CD26.

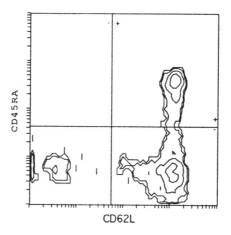

Fig. 10. CD62L vs CD45RA.

2. Criteria for sample refusal include:
   a. Hemolyzed specimens.
   b. Insufficient amount of peripheral blood.
   c. Specimen is clotted.
   d. Wrong anticoagulant (heparin, ACD, and EDTA are acceptable).
   e. Specimens over 24 h old in heparin with viability of >85%.
   f. Specimens over 6 h old in EDTA with viability <85%.
   g. Specimens that have been refrigerated or frozen (<15°C) or exposed to very warm temperatures (>30°C) with viability >85%.
   h. Specimens held in water, alcohol, formalin, etc.
   I. Specimens that are not clearly labeled and cannot be identified.

References

1. Redfield, R. R. and Burke, D.S. (1987) Shadow on the land: the epidemiology of HIV infection. *Vir. Immunol.* **1,** 69–81.
2. Perfetto, S., Hickey, T., Blair, P., Maino, V., Wagner, K., Zhou, S., et al. (1997) Measurement of CD69 induction in the assessment of immune function in asymptomatic HIV-infected individuals. *Cytometry* **30,** 1–9.
3. Liu, Z., Hultin, L. E., Cumberland, W. G., Hultin, P., Schmid, I., Matud, J., et al. (1996) Elevated relative fluorescence intensity of CD38 antigen expression in CD8+ T cells is a marker of poor prognosis in HIV infection: results of 6 years of follow-up. *Cytometry* **26,** 1–7.
4. Malone, J. L., Simms, T. E., Gray, G. C., Wagner, K. F., Burge, J. R., and Burke, D. S. (1990) Sources of variability in repeated T-helper lymphocyte counts from human immunodeficiency virus type 1-infected patients: total lymphocyte count fluctuations and diurnal cycle are important. *J. Acquir. Immune Defic. Synd.* **2,** 144–151.
5. Center for Disease Control (1994) 1994 revised guidelines for the performance of CD4+ T-cell determinations in persons with human immunodeficiency virus (HIV) infections—United States. *Morb. Mortal. Wkly. Rep.* **43,** 1–21.
6. Center for Disease Control (1997) 1997 Revised guidelines for the performance of CD4+ T-cell determinations in persons with human immunodeficiency virus (HIV). *Morb. Mortal. Wkly. Rep.* **46,** 1–29.
7. National Institutes of Health (1993) *NIAID Division of AIDS Guidelines for Flow Cytometric Immunophenotyping.* NIH, Bethesda, MD.

43

Detection of Apoptosis
in HIV-Infected Cell Populations using TUNEL

Patrick J. Blair and Stephen P. Perfetto

1. Introduction

Cells within an organism undergo two common forms of cell death. Sudden injury resulting from physical or chemical insult leads to a form of cell death called necrosis. A more subtle programmed form of cell death is termed apoptosis. Apoptosis describes a genetically encoded pathway that plays an important role in regulating the immune response *(1,2)*. Apoptotic cell death is characterized by distinct biochemical and morphologic changes and the fragmentation of DNA into nucleosomal-sized multimers *(3)*. Apoptosis plays a crucial role in viral infections and in the host response to viral insult *(4)*.

Direct HIV-mediated cytopathicity is one mechanism that has been proposed to account for the depletion of CD4[+] T cells in HIV-infected individuals based on the rapid turnover of virus *(5,6)*. Apoptosis may also contribute to the depletion of CD4[+] cells and the functional defects that follow HIV-infection. The role of apoptosis in HIV disease is supported by reports of increased apoptotic T cell death in vivo within the lymph nodes *(7)* and by observations of increased levels of activation-induced cell death (AICD) in vitro in CD4[+] and CD8[+] T-cells from HIV-infected individuals *(8–13)*. Recent observations suggest that apoptosis is an indirect effect of HIV infection as apoptosis occurs predominantly in bystander cells, rather than in cells productively infected with HIV *(14–15)*, perhaps because of interactions with HIV-specific proteins *(16–18)*.

Although many methods have been developed for the analysis of apoptosis, methods that utilize flow cytometry offer the advantage of analyzing large number or cells as well as the identification and quantitation of subpopulations of cells. Outlined here is a simple, highly sensitive protocol that utilizes flow

From: *Methods in Molecular Medicine, Vol. 17: HIV Protocols*
Edited by: N. L. Michael and J. H. Kim © Humana Press Inc., Totowa, NJ

cytometric analysis to measure terminal deoxylnucleotidyl transferase-mediated d-UTP-biotin nick end-labeling (TUNEL) of apoptotic cells that exhibit DNA fragmentation *(19–20)*. TUNEL can be performed following cell-surface immunophenotyping to quantitatively measure cell death in specific populations of cells.

2. Materials

2.1. Cell Preparation

Freshly-isolated peripheral blood mononuclear cells (PBMC) were obtained from the buffy-coat of blood that had been diluted 1:1 with sterile Hank's balances saline soultion (HBSS) (BioWhittaker, Walkersville, MD) and centrifuged over Ficoll-Hypaque. Viability of samples was generally >95%. Unless otherwise indicated, PBMC were cultured for 48 h at 1×10^6 cells/mL in RPMI 1640 supplemented with 10% fetal calf serum (FCS) in 24-well plates. In order to induce high amounts of apoptosis in PBMC from HIV-infected patients *(13)*, some samples were stimulated in the presence of poke weed mitogen (PWM) (Sigma Chemical Company, St. Louis, MO) at 10 µg/mL.

2.1. Solutions and Reagents for TUNEL Assay

1. Phosphate-buffered saline (PBS): 137 mM NaCl, 2.7 mM KCL, 14.1 mM Na$_2$HPO$_4$, and 2.9 mM KH$_2$PO$_4$ (*see* **Note 1**).
2. Paraformaldehyde fixative: Dissolve 1% (w/v) paraformaldehyde in PBS with 0.01% Tween-20 at 68°C, pH to 7.4.
3. 95% ethanol, stored at –20°C.
4. Terminal deoxynucleotidyl transferase (TdT) reaction mixture: 0.1 M cacodylic acid, 1 mM CoCl$_2$, 0.1 mM dithiothreitol, and 50 µg/mL bovine serum albumin (BSA).
5. TdT/biotin-dUTP solution: In the TdT reaction buffer dilute dUTP (Boehringer Mannheim) to a final concentration of 0.5 to 1 µM, and add 8 µL of TdT (25 U/µL, Boehringer Mannheim) per mL.
6. Staining solution: 4X SSC (0.015 M Na$_3$C$_6$H$_5$O$_7$ x 2H$_2$0, 0.15 M NaCl), 0.1% Triton X-100, and 5 % nonfat dry milk.
7. Streptavidin-fluorescein isothiocyanate solution: Make a 1:10 dilution of streptavidin-fluorescein isothiocyanate (Gibco-BRL, Gaithersburg, MD) with staining solution.
8. 12 × 75-mm round-bottom centrifuge tubes.
9. 0.1% Triton X-100 solution: Dissolve 100 µL of Triton X-100 (Sigma) in 100 mL PBS. Place on a stir plate for 30 min to insure that the Triton is in solution. Store at 4°C.
10. Trypan blue solution: Dissolve 0.4 g of trypan blue into 100 mL PBS.

3. Methods

3.1. Preparation of TUNEL-Stained Cells

1. While observing appropriate biosafety protocols for HIV-infected cells, harvest cultures and assess cell viability by trypan blue exclusion (*see* **Note 2**).

2. Place an aliquot of 0.5–1 × 10⁶ cells into centifugation tubes. Perform immunof-luorescence staining if subset analysis is desired. Add 2 mL of PBS and centri-fuge at 400*g*, decanting supernatant before TUNEL staining (*see* **Note 3**).

3. Flick tube to resuspend in residual PBS. Slowly add 1 mL of 1% paraformalde-hyde solution dropwise while vortexing gently (*see* **Note 4**). Incubate for 15 min on ice.

4. Add 2 mL of PBS, then centrifuge cells 5 min at 600*g* at 4°C. Decant the super-natant. A higher centrifugation speed is necessary to pellet the cells once they are fixed.

5. Flick tube to resuspend cells in 250 μL PBS. Slowly add 750 μL ice-cold 95% ethanol dropwise while gently vortexing tube. Store samples at –20°C for 2 h to 3 d.

6. Centrifuge the cells 5 min at 600*g* at 4°C. Decant the supernatant. Flick pellet, and resuspend in 50 μL of a TdT reaction mixture (*see* **Note 5**) containing 0.5 n*M* biotin 16-dUTP and 10 U of TdT (Boehringer) for 45 min at 37°C (*see* **Note 6**).

7. After a wash in PBS as in **step 6**, decant supernatant, and add 100 μL of staining solution containing 2.5 μg/mL FITC-avidin (*see* **Note 7**). Incubate samples 30 min at room temperature.

8. Add 2 mL of 0.1% Triton X-100 solution to each sample, and then centifuge at 600*g*. Decant supernatant, flick pellet, and resuspend in 500 μL of PBS. Samples can be stored at 4°C in the dark for up to 24 h before FACS analysis.

3.2. Flow Cytometric Analysis of TUNEL-Stained Samples (see Notes 8 and 9).

1. Dual or single-color analyses can be performed depending on whether surface-staining of other markers is carried out before TUNEL staining. When staining by TUNEL alone, use the bivariant histogram FITC and 90° light scatter to detect fluorescent shifts (*see* **Fig. 1**).

2. Enumerate five to ten thousand cells within the total cell gate using the param-eters of 90° scatter vs log-FITC intensity.

3. Apoptotic cells are generally defined as FITC-positive cells with a low forward angle and low 90° scatter on the light scatter gate. However, the collection gate is set large to capture all cells both apoptotic and non-apoptotic (*see* **Fig. 2**).

4. The cursor and data in **Fig. 2** show the gating strategy used in the TUNEL assay. The cursor divides the positive (cells above the cursor) and negative (cells below the cursor) apoptotic cell populations. The position of this cursor is determined by the negative control.

4. Notes

1. All solutions should be sterilized by sterile filtration before use.

2. In order to accurately determine the cell count and viability, cells were stained with trypan blue (1% in PBS) and enumerated in a hemocytometer.

3. The importance of preparing both negative and positive staining controls to determine the efficiency of the reagents used in the TUNEL procedure cannot be understated. Samples lacking TdT can serve as appropriate negative controls.

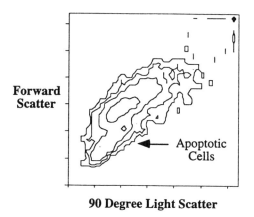

Fig. 1.

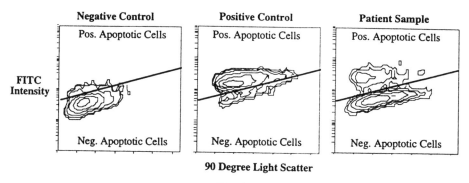

Fig. 2.

There are many protocols that describe the induction of apoptosis *(21)*. However, the best positive control in our hands has been the utilization of Fas-mediated cell death *(22–24)* in Jurkat cells (ATCC TIB-152). Treatment of Jurkat cells cultured in RPMI with 10% FCS at 1×10^6 cells/mL for 18 h with 0.5 µg/mL human anti-Fas antibody (Upstate Biotechnology, Inc.) results in approx 70–95% apoptosis (*see* **Fig. 2**).

4. Fixation of the cells can result in cell clumping. Therefore, paraformaldehyde and ethanol should be added slowly while the samples are gently vortexed. Ethanol fixation also results in cell-shrinkage, necessitating higher centrifugation spins in order to pellet cells.

5. The reagents used to label DNA fragments, namely the dUTP and TdT, should be aliquoted and stored at –20°C. The TdT/biotin-dUTP solution should be made up just prior to use. Unused portions should be thrown away rather than frozen and stored for later use.

6. Samples containing the TdT/biotin-dUTP solution should be wrapped in parafilm and placed in a 37°C water bath (rather than an incubator set at 37°C) to insure that samples are kept at constant temperature.

7. Optimal staining for apoptotic populations by TUNEL utilizes FITC-conjugated streptavidin. Other fluorochromes such as PerCP and PE are of higher molecular weight and do not penetrate fixed cells as efficiently resulting in weaker signals.

8. An advantage of using the TUNEL technique is that it serves as the most direct method to analyze DNA fragmentation within the cell itself. TUNEL can be performed in conjunction with cell-surface staining, thereby providing information about subset analysis. Also, because DNA fragmentation is an early event within the programmed cell death pathway, TUNEL provides analysis of events occurring very early in the process.

9. A potential disadvantage of the TUNEL method is that DNA fragmentation does not occur in all cell types undergoing apoptosis. Additionally, the reagents used in the TUNEL reaction, dUTP, and TdT are expensive, making this method a costly means by which to detect apoptotic cells. These reagents can be titrated to determine the appropriate concentrations for use in the assay.

References

1. Kroemer, G., Petit, P., Zamzami, N., Vayssiere, J. L., and Mignotte B. (1995) The biochemistry of programmed cell death. *FASEB J.* **9**, 1277-1287.

2. Cohen, J. J. (1994) Apoptosis. *Immunol. Today* **14**, 126–130.

3. Wyllie, A. H., Kerr, J. F. R., and Currie, A. R. (1980) Cell death: the significance of apoptosis. *Int. Rev. Cytol.* **68**, 251–306.

4. Razvi, E. S. and Welsh, R. M. (1995) Apoptosis in viral infections. *Adv. Virus Res.* **45**, 1–60.

5. Ho, D. D., Neumann, A. U., Perelson, A. S., Chen, W., Leonard, J. M., and Markowitz M. (1995) Rapid turnover of plasma virions and CD4 lymphocytes in HIV-1 infection. *Nature* **373**, 123–126.

6. Wei, X., Ghosh, S. K., Taylor, M. E., Johnson, V. A., Emini, E. A., et al. (1995) Viral dynamics in human immunodeficiency virus type 1 infection. *Nature* **373**, 117–122.

7. Muro-Cacho, C., Pantaleo, G., and Fauci, A. S. (1995) Analysis of apoptosis in lymph nodes of HIV-infected persons. Intensity of apoptosis correlates with the general state of activation of the lymphoid tissue and not with stage of disease or viral burden. *J. Immunol.* **154**, 5555–5566.

8. Oyaizu, N., McCloskey, T. W., Coronesi, M., Chirmule, N., Kalyanaraman, V. S., and Pahwa S. (1995) Accelerated apoptosis in peripheral blood mononuclear cells (PBMCs) from human immunodeficiency virus type-1 infected patients and in CD4 cross-linked PBMCs from normal individuals. *Blood* **82**, 3392–3400.

9. Ucker, D. S., Ashwell, J. D., and Nickas G. (1989) Activation-driven T cell death. I. Requirements for de novo transcription and translation and association with genome fragmentation. *J. Immunol.* **143**, 3461–3469.

10. Jaleco, A. C., Covas, M. J., and Victorino, R. (1994) Analysis of lymphocyte cell death and apoptosis in HIV-2-infected patients. *Clin. Exp. Immunol.* **98**, 185–189.

11. Gougeon, M. L., Laurent, C. A., Hovanessian, A. G., and Montagnier, L. (1993) Direct and indirect mechanisms mediating apoptosis during HIV infection: contribution to in vivo CD4 T cell depletion. *Semin. Immunol.* **5,** 187–194.

12. Gougeon, M. L., Garcia, S., Heeney, J., Tschopp, R., Lecoeur, H., Guetard, D., et al. (1993) Programmed cell death in AIDS-related HIV and SIV infections. *AIDS Res. Hum. Retrovir.* **9,** 553–563.

13. Groux, H., Torpier, G., Monte, D., Mouton, Y., Capron, A., and Ameisen, J. C. (1992) Activation-induced death by apoptosis in CD4+ T cells from human immunodeficiency virus-infected asymptomatic individuals. *J. Exp. Med.* **175,** 331–340.

14. Finkel, T. H., Tudor, W. G., Banda, N. K., Cotton, M. F., Curiel, T., Monks, C., et al. (1995) Apoptosis occurs predominantly in bystander cells and not in productively infected cells of HIV- and SIV-infected lymph nodes. *Nat. Med.* **1,** 129–134.

15. Su, L., Kaneshima, H., Bonyhadi, M., Salimi, S., Kraft, D., Rabin, L., and McCune, J. M. (1995) HIV-1-induced thymocyte depletion is associated with indirect cytopathogenicity and infection of progenitor cells in vivo. *Immunity* **2,** 25–36.

16. Li, C. J., Friedman, D. J., Wang, C., Metelev, V., and Pardee, A. (1995) Induction of apoptosis in uninfected lymphocytes by HIV-1 Tat protein. *Science* **268,** 429–431.

17. Westendorp, M. O., Frank, R., Ochsenbauer, C., Stricker, K., Dhein, J., Walczak, H., et al. (1995) Sensitization of T cells to CD95-mediated apoptosis by HIV-1 Tat and gp120. *Nature* **375,** 497–500.

18. Nardelli, B., Gonzalez, C. J., Schechter, M., and Valentine, F. T. (1995) CD4+ blood lymphocytes are rapidly killed in vitro by contact with autologous human immunodeficiency virus-infected cells. *Proc. Natl. Acad. Sci. USA* **92,** 7312–7316.

19. Gorczcan, W., Gong, J., and Darzynkiewicz, Z. (1993) Detection of DNA strand breaks in individual apoptotic cells by the in situ terminal deoxynucleotidyl transferase and nick translational assay. *Cancer Res.* **53,** 1945–1948.

20. Gavrieli, Y., Sherman, Y., and Ben-Sasson, S. A. (1992) Identification of programmed cell death in situ via specific labeling of nuclear DNA fragments. *J. Cell Biol.* **119,** 493–501.

21. Peter, M. A., Heufelder, A. E., and Hengortner, M. O. (1997) Advances in apoptosis research. *Proc. Natl. Acad. Sci. USA* **94,** 12,736–12,757.

22. Dhein, J., Walczak, H., Baumler, C., Debatin, K. M., and Krammer, P. H. (1995) Autocrine T-cell suicide mediated by APO-1/(Fas/CD95). *Nature* **373,** 438–441.

23. Brunner, T., Mogil, R. J., La, F. D., Yoo, N. J., Mahboubi, A., Echeverri, F., et al. (1995) Cell-autonomous Fas (CD95)/Fas-ligand interaction mediates activation-induced apoptosis in T-cell hybridomas. *Nature* **373,** 441–444.

24. Ju, S. T., Panka, D. J., Cui, H., Ettinger, R., El-Khatib, M., Sherr, D. H., et al. (1995) Fas (CD95)/FasL interactions required for programmed cell death after T-cell activation. *Nature* **373,** 444–448.

Index